Essentials of
Ophthalmic Oncology

Edited by

Arun D. Singh, MD

Director, Department of Ophthalmic Oncology, Cole Eye Institute, Cleveland Clinic Foundation
Cleveland, OH

Bertil E. Damato, MD, PhD, FRCOphth

Professor of Ophthalmology, Ocular Oncology Service, The Royal Liverpool University Hospital
Liverpool, United Kingdom

Jacob Pe'er, MD

Professor of Ophthalmology, Department of Ophthalmology, Kiryat Hadassah
Jerusalem, Israel

A. Linn Murphree, MD

Director, The Retinoblastoma Center, Childrens Hospital Los Angeles
Los Angeles, CA

Julian D. Perry, MD

Section Head, Orbital and Oculoplastic Surgery, Cole Eye Institute, Cleveland Clinic Foundation
Cleveland, OH

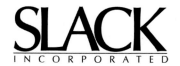
SLACK
INCORPORATED

ISBN: 978-1-55642-917-0

Copyright © 2009 by SLACK Incorporated

Published by: SLACK Incorporated
                  6900 Grove Road
                  Thorofare, NJ 08086 USA
                  Telephone: 856-848-1000
                  Fax: 856-848-6091
                  www.slackbooks.com

Contact SLACK Incorporated for more information about other books in this field or about the availability of our books from distributors outside the United States.

Library of Congress Cataloging-in-Publication Data
Essentials of ophthalmic oncology / edited by Arun D. Singh ... [et al.].
    p. ; cm.
Includes bibliographical references and index.
ISBN 978-1-55642-917-0 (alk. paper)
1. Eye--Cancer. I. Singh, Arun D.
[DNLM: 1. Eye Neoplasms. WW 149 E78 2009]
RC280.E9E77 2009
616.99'484--dc22
                        2009005737

Printed in the United States of America.

Last digit is print number: 10   9   8   7   6   5   4   3   2   1

CONTENTS

Acknowledgments .... *ix*

Contributing Authors .... *xi*

Introduction .... *xvii*

SECTION 1   Basic Principles

Chapter 1   Principles of Clinical Epidemiology 1
          Annette C. Moll, Michiel R. de Boer, and Lex M. Bouter

Chapter 2   Cancer Etiology 3
          Evelyn X. Fu and Arun D. Singh

Chapter 3A   Cancer Pathology 4
          Stefan Seregard and Charlotta All-Ericsson

Chapter 3B   Cancer Angiogenesis 6
          Werner Wackernagel, Lynn Schoenfield, and Arun D. Singh

Chapter 4   Cancer Immunology 9
          Martine J. Jager, Jihan Dennaoui, and Willem Maat

Chapter 5   Cancer Genetics 11
          J. William Harbour and Michael D. Onken

Chapter 6   Principles of Cryotherapy 13
          Dan S. Gombos

Chapter 7   Principles of Laser Therapy 15
          Stefan Sacu and Ursula Schmidt-Erfurth

Chapter 8   Principles of Radiation Therapy 18
          Carryn Anderson, Peter Fleming, Allan Wilkinson, and Arun D. Singh

Chapter 9   Ocular Complications of Radiotherapy 21
          Mehran Taban, Mehryar Taban, James P. Bolling, and Arun D. Singh

Chapter 10   Principles of Chemotherapy 25
          Michael Levien, Jennifer Gravette, and Joanne Hilden

Chapter 11   Counseling Patients With Cancer 28
          Sharon Cook and Bertil E. Damato

SECTION 2   Eyelid Tumors

Chapter 12   Examination Techniques 29
          Julian D. Perry

Chapter 13   Classification and Differential Diagnosis of Eyelid Tumors 30
          Jacob Pe'er

Chapter 14   Benign Epidermal Tumors 31
          Edoardo Midena, Valentina de Belvis, Lynn Schoenfield, and Arun D. Singh

Chapter 15   Basal Cell Carcinoma 33
          Mordechai Rosner

Chapter 16   Squamous Cell Carcinoma 35
          Mordechai Rosner

Chapter 17   Sebaceous Gland Carcinoma 37
          Mordechai Rosner

Chapter 18   Melanoma of the Eyelid 39
          Jacob Pe'er and Robert Folberg

Chapter 19   Eyelid Adnexal Tumors 41
          Karin U. Loeffler

Chapter 20   Eyelid Stromal Tumors 43
          Geeta K. Vemuganti and Santosh G. Honavar

Chapter 21   Surgical Techniques...46
Jennifer I. Hui and David T. Tse

Chapter 22   Systemic Associations of Eyelid Tumors...49
Arun D. Singh and Elias I. Traboulsi

SECTION 3   Conjunctival and Corneal Tumors

Chapter 23   Examination Techniques, Classification, and Differential Diagnosis of Conjunctival and Corneal Tumors 51
Jacob Pe'er

Chapter 24   Benign Conjunctival Tumors...53
Jacob Pe'er

Chapter 25   Ocular Surface Squamous Neoplasia 55
Jacob Pe'er and Joseph Frucht-Pery

Chapter 26   Primary Acquired Melanosis 57
Jacob Pe'er and Robert Folberg

Chapter 27   Conjunctival Melanoma...59
Jacob Pe'er and Robert Folberg

Chapter 28   Conjunctival Stromal Tumors...61
Jacob Pe'er

Chapter 29   Surgical Techniques 63
Anat Galor, Bennie H. Jeng, and Arun D. Singh

Chapter 30   Systemic Associations of Conjunctival and Corneal Tumors...65
Arun D. Singh and Elias I. Traboulsi

SECTION 4   Uveal Tumors

Chapter 31   Examination Techniques...67
Nikolaos Trichopoulos and Bertil E. Damato

Chapter 32   Diagnostic Techniques 69
Sophie Bakri, LuAnne Sculley, and Arun D. Singh

Chapter 33   Classification of Uveal Tumors 72
Bertil E. Damato, Sarah E. Coupland, and Paul Hiscott

Chapter 34   Tumors of the Uvea: Benign Melanocytic Tumors...73
Arun D. Singh

Chapter 35   Uveal Malignant Melanoma: Epidemiologic Aspects..78
Arun D. Singh, Louise Bergman, and Stefan Seregard

Chapter 36   Uveal Malignant Melanoma: Clinical Features..81
Leonidas Zografos

Chapter 37   Uveal Malignant Melanoma: Differential Diagnosis 85
Devron H. Char

Chapter 38   Uveal Malignant Melanoma: Histopathologic Features..89
Tero Kivelä

Chapter 39   Management of Patients With Uveal Melanoma 92
Bertil E. Damato

Chapter 40   Uveal Malignant Melanoma: Management Options—Thermotherapy..94
Hanneke J. G. Journée-de Korver, Nicoline E. Schalij-Delfos, and Saskia M. Imhof

Chapter 41   Uveal Malignant Melanoma: Management Options—Brachytherapy..98
Stefan Seregard, Bertil E. Damato, and Peter Fleming

Chapter 42   Uveal Malignant Melanoma: Management Options—Proton Beam Radiotherapy 102
Anne Marie Lane and Evangelos S. Gragoudas

Chapter 43   Uveal Malignant Melanoma: Management Options—Stereotactic Radiotherapy...............................104
Karin Dieckmann, Gerald Langmann, Roy Ma, Mona Schmutzer, Richard Poetter, Werner Wackernagel, and Martin Zehetmayer

Chapter 44   Uveal Malignant Melanoma: Management Options—Resection Techniques 106
Bertil E. Damato and Carl Groenewald

Chapter 45   Uveal Malignant Melanoma: COMS Results..109
Arun D. Singh and Tero Kivelä

Chapter 46   Uveal Malignant Melanoma: Prognostic Factors..113
Robert Folberg and Jacob Pe'er

Chapter 47   Uveal Malignant Melanoma: Mortality..116
Bertil E. Damato and Azzam Taktak

Chapter 48   Uveal Malignant Melanoma: Metastasis 119
             Arun D. Singh, Julie Bray, and Ernest C. Borden

Chapter 49   Uveal Vascular Tumors 121
             Arun D. Singh and Peter K. Kaiser

Chapter 50   Uveal Neural Tumors 125
             Arun D. Singh and Jonathan E. Sears

Chapter 51   Uveal Osseous Tumors 127
             Arun D. Singh

Chapter 52   Uveal Myogenic, Fibrous, and Histiocytic Tumors 131
             Paul Rundle, Hardeep Singh Mudhar, M. Andrew Parsons, and Ian G. Rennie

Chapter 53   Uveal Lymphoproliferative Tumors 133
             Sarah E. Coupland

Chapter 54   Uveal Metastatic Tumors 136
             Norbert Bornfeld

Chapter 55   Intraocular Manifestations of Proliferative Hematopoietic Disorders 140
             Hayyam Kiratli

Chapter 56   Intraocular Biopsy 142
             Devron H. Char

SECTION 5   Tumors of the Retina and Retinal Pigment Epithelium

Chapter 57   Retinal Vascular Tumors 144
             Arun D. Singh, Paul Rundle, and Ian G. Rennie

Chapter 58   Coats' Disease 147
             Thomas M. Aaberg, Jr

Chapter 59   Retinal Astrocytic Tumors 149
             Mehryar Taban, Mehran Taban, and Arun D. Singh

Chapter 60   Tumors of the Retinal Pigment Epithelium 151
             Elias I. Traboulsi, Martin Heur, and Arun D. Singh

Chapter 61   Tumors of the Ciliary Pigment Epithelium 154
             Javier Elizalde, María de la Paz, and Rafael I. Barraquer

Chapter 62   Lymphoma of the Retina and Central Nervous System 156
             Arun D. Singh, Hilel Lewis, Andrew P. Schachat, and David Peereboom

Chapter 63   Ocular Paraneoplastic Diseases 159
             Rishi P. Singh and Arun D. Singh

Chapter 64   Neuro-Oculocutaneous Syndromes (Phakomatoses) 162
             Arun D. Singh, Elias I. Traboulsi, and Lynn Schoenfield

SECTION 6   Retinoblastoma

Chapter 65   Retinoblastoma and Cancer Genetics 168
             Alfred G. Knudson, Jr

Chapter 66   Genetic and Cellular Events in Retinoblastoma 170
             Michael A. Dyer and J. William Harbour

Chapter 67   Geographic and Environmental Factors 172
             Greta R. Bunin and Manuela Orjuela

Chapter 68   Retinoblastoma: An International Perspective 174
             Guillermo L. Chantada and Carlos Leal-Leal

Chapter 69   Staging and Grouping of Retinoblastoma 176
             A. Linn Murphree and Guillermo L. Chantada

Chapter 70   Heritable Retinoblastoma: The RB1 Cancer Predisposition Syndrome 179
             A. Linn Murphree and Arun D. Singh

Chapter 71   Non-Ocular Tumors 181
             Cari E. Lyle, Carlos Rodriguez-Galindo, and Matthew W. Wilson

Chapter 72   Trilateral Retinoblastoma 183
             Cari E. Lyle, Carlos Rodriguez-Galindo, and Matthew W. Wilson

Chapter 73A Genetic Testing and Counseling 184
             Robin D. Clark and Nancy C. Mansfield

Chapter 73B Family Counseling 186
             Nancy C. Mansfield and Robin D. Clark

viii   Contents

Chapter 74   Chemotherapy for Retinoblastoma: An Overview 187
              Rima F. Jubran, Judith G. Villablanca, and Anna T. Meadows

Chapter 75   Local Therapy, Brachytherapy, and Enucleation.. 189
              A. Linn Murphree

Chapter 76   Teletherapy: Indications, Risks, and New Delivery Options................................. 193
              Thomas E. Merchant

Chapter 77   Histopathologic Features and Prognostic Factors 195
              Patricia Chévez-Barrios, Ralph C. Eagle, Jr, and Eduardo F. Marback

Chapter 78   Orbital Retinoblastoma 198
              Santosh G. Honavar

Chapter 79   Metastatic Retinoblastoma.. 200
              Ira J. Dunkel and Guillermo L. Chantada

Chapter 80   Retinocytoma or Retinoma... 202
              Arun D. Singh, Aubin Balmer, and Francis Munier

Chapter 81   Children's Oncology Group Trials for Retinoblastoma 204
              *Anna T. Meadows, Murali Chintagumpala, Ira J. Dunkel, Debra Friedman, Julie A. Stoner,
              and Judith G. Villablanca*

Chapter 82   Retinoblastoma: At-Risk Pregnancies 206
              Lisa Paquette and David A. Miller

Chapter 83   Future Directions 207
              A. Linn Murphree

SECTION 7   Orbital Tumors

Chapter 84   Examination Techniques... 208
              Mehryar Taban and Julian D. Perry

Chapter 85   Imaging Techniques 209
              Patrick De Potter

Chapter 86   Classification of Orbital Tumors 214
              Mehran Taban and Julian D. Perry

Chapter 87   Evaluation of a Child With Orbital Tumor 215
              Paul L. Proffer, Jill A. Foster, and Julian D. Perry

Chapter 88   Evaluation of an Adult With Orbital Tumor 216
              Benson Chen, Julian D. Perry, and Jill A. Foster

Chapter 89   Non-Specific Orbital Inflammation 218
              Roberta E. Gausas, Kimberly Cockerham, and Madhura Tamhankar

Chapter 90   Vascular Orbital Tumors.. 221
              Benson Chen and Julian D. Perry

Chapter 91   Benign Tumors of the Orbit 224
              Bhupendra Patel

Chapter 92   Tumors of the Optic Nerve... 227
              Jonathan Dutton

Chapter 93   Tumors of the Lacrimal Gland 230
              Omar M. Durrani and Geoffrey E. Rose

Chapter 94   Tumors of the Lacrimal Sac 232
              Jacob Pe'er

Chapter 95   Orbital and Adnexal Lymphoma 234
              David S. Bardenstein

Chapter 96   Malignant Tumors of the Orbit... 237
              Bhupendra Patel

Chapter 97   Rhabdomyosarcoma.. 240
              Benson Chen and Julian D. Perry

Chapter 98   Enucleation and Orbital Implants... 243
              David R. Jordan and Stephen R. Klapper

Chapter 99   Principles of Orbital Surgery.. 246
              José Perez-Moreiras, Javier Coloma, and Consuelo Prada

Index *253*

ACKNOWLEDGMENTS

To my parents, who educated me beyond their means; my wife, Annapurna; and my children, Nakul and Rahul, who make all my efforts worthwhile.
—*ADS*

To my family, Frankanne, Erika, and Stephen.
—*BED*

To my wife, Edith, and my children, Liron, Neta, and Doron, for years of support and patience.
—*JP*

To my family, Rogel, Nancy, Gary, Gayle, and Maxine.
—*ALM*

To Clifford, Agnes, Jim, and Bud for my foundation; to Bob, Norm, and Neil for my education; to Wendy, Julian, Liam, and Remy for my inspiration.
—*JDP*

Thanks to Elsevier, publishers of our book *Clinical Ophthalmic Oncology*, from which this book, *Essentials of Ophthalmic Oncology,* is derived.
—*ADS, BED, JP, ALM, JDP*

Essentials of Ophthalmic Oncology was derived from material in our book *Clinical Ophthalmic Oncology*, which was published by Elsevier in 2007.

—ADS, BED, JP, ALM, JDP

CONTRIBUTING AUTHORS

Thomas M. Aaberg, Jr, MD
Associated Retinal Consultants
Grand Rapids, MI

Charlotta All-Ericsson, MD, PhD
Senior Staff Ophthalmic Surgeon
Ocular Oncology Service
Department of Vitreoretinal Diseases
St. Erik Eye Hospital
Stockholm, Sweden

Carryn Anderson, MD
Radiation Oncology Resident
Department of Radiation and
Ophthalmic Oncology
Cole Eye Institute
Cleveland Clinic Foundation
Cleveland, OH

Sophie Bakri, MD
Retina Fellow
Cole Eye Institute
Cleveland Clinic Foundation
Cleveland, OH

Aubin Balmer, MD
Lecturer
Deparment of Ophthalmology
Jules Gonin Eye Hospital
Lausanne, Switzerland

David S. Bardenstein
Director of Ocular Oncology and
Ocular Pathology
Departments of Ophthalmology and
Pathology
Case Western Reserve University
School of Medicine
University Hospitals of Cleveland
Cleveland, OH

Rafael I. Barraquer, MD, PhD
Assistant Director, Centro de
Oftalmologia Barraquer
Director, Ocular Oncology Service
Barcelona, Spain

Valentina de Belvis, MD
Lecturer
Department of Ophthalmology
University of Padova
Padova, Italy

Louise Bergman
Senior Vitreoretinal Surgeon
Department of Vitreoretinal Diseases
Karolinska Institute
St. Erik Eye Hospital
Stockholm, Sweden

Michiel R. de Boer, PhD
Senior Lecturer in Epidemiology and
Applied Biostatistics
Faculty of Earth and Life Sciences
Institute of Health Sciences
VU University
Amsterdam, Netherlands

James P. Bolling, MD
Associate Professor and Chair
Department of Ophthalmology
Mayo Clinic
Jacksonville, FL

Ernest C. Borden, PhD
Staff Hematologist Oncologist
Department of Oncology
Cleveland Clinic Foundation
Cleveland, OH

Norbert Bornfeld, MD
Professor of Ophthalmology
Zentrum für Augenheilkunde
Universitätsklinikum Essen
Essen, Germany

Lex M. Bouter, PhD
Professor of Epidemiology
Scientific Director
Institute for Research in Extramural
Medicine
VU University Medical Center
Amsterdam, Netherlands

Julie Bray
Nurse Practitioner
Taussig Cancer Center
Cleveland Clinic Foundation
Cleveland, OH

Greta R. Bunin, PhD
Research Associate Professor of
Pediatrics
Children's Hospital of Philadelphia
Division of Oncology
Philadelphia, PA

Guillermo L. Chantada, MD
Principal Physician
Hemato-Oncology Department
Hospital J. P. Garrahan
Buenos Aires, Argentina

Devron H. Char, MD
President
The Tumori Foundation
Clinical Professor
Stanford University
San Francisco, CA

Benson Chen, MD
Research Fellow
Cole Eye Institute
Cleveland Clinic Foundation
Cleveland, OH

Patricia Chévez-Barrios, MD
Associate Professor of Pathology
Department of Pathology
Weill Medical College of
Cornell University
The Methodist Hospital
Houston, TX

Murali Chintagumpala, MD
Associate Professor of Pediatrics
Texas Children's Cancer Center at
Baylor College
Houston, TX

Robin D. Clark, MD
Associate Clinical Professor of
Medical Genetics
Departments of Pediatrics and
Ophthalmology
Keck School of Medicine
Riverside, CA

Kimberly Cockerham, MD
Associate Professor
Department of Ophthalmology
University of California
San Francisco, CA

Javier Coloma, MD
Ophthalmologist
Centro Oftalmologico Moreiras
Orbital-Ophthalmoplastic and
Reconstructive Surgery
A Coruna, Spain

Sharon Cook, MD
Health Psychologist
Ocular Oncology Service
University of Liverpool
Liverpool, United Kingdom

Sarah E. Coupland, MBBS, PhD
Senior Lecturer in Ophthalmic Pathology
Department of Cellular and
Molecular Pathology
University of Liverpool
Liverpool, United Kingdom

Bertil E. Damato, MD, PhD, FRCOphth
Professor of Ophthalmology
Ocular Oncology Service
The Royal Liverpool University Hospital
Liverpool, United Kingdom

Jihan Dennaoui
Research Student
Department of Ophthalmology
Leiden University Medical Center
Leiden, Netherlands

Karin Dieckmann, MD
Staff
Department of Radiation Oncology
Medical University of Vienna
General Hospital Vienna
Vienna, Austria

Ira J. Dunkel, MD
Associate Attending Pediatrician
Department of Pediatrics
Memorial Sloan-Kettering Cancer Center
New York, NY

Omar M. Durrani, MD, FRCS
Oculoplastic and Orbit Surgeon
Birmingham and Midland Eye Centre
City Hospital
Birmingham, United Kingdom

Jonathan Dutton, MD
Professor and Vice Chair
Department of Ophthalmology
University of North Carolina
Chapel Hill, NC

Michael A. Dyer, PhD
Associate Member
Department of
Developmental Neurobiology
St. Jude Children's Research Hospital
Memphis, TN

Ralph C. Eagle, Jr, MD
Director
Department of Pathology
Wills Eye Hospital
Thomas Jefferson University
Philadelphia, PA

Javier Elizalde, MD
Ophthalmologist
Vitreous Retina Service
Ocular Oncology Service
Centro de Oftalmologia Barraquer
Barcelona, Spain

Peter Fleming, MD
Staff Radiation Oncologist
Department of Radiation and
Ophthalmic Oncology
Cole Eye Institute
Cleveland Clinic Foundation
Cleveland, OH

Robert Folberg, MD
Frances B. Geever Professor and Head
Department of Pathology
University of Illinois College of
Medicine
Chicago, IL

Jill A. Foster, MD
Assistant Clinical Professor
The Ohio State University
The William H. Havener Eye Institute
Columbus, OH

Debra Friedman, MD
Associate Professor of Pediatrics
Fred Hutchinson Cancer Research Center
Seattle, WA

Joseph Frucht-Pery, MD
Associate Professor of Ophthalmology
Head of the Cornea and
Refractive Surgery Unit
Department of Ophthalmology
Hadassah-Hebrew University
Medical Center
Jerusalem, Israel

Evelyn X. Fu, MD
Resident Physician
Department of Ophthalmic Oncology
Cole Eye Institute
Cleveland Clinic Foundation
Cleveland, OH

Anat Galor
Chief Resident
Cole Eye Institute
Cleveland Clinic Foundation
Cleveland, OH

Roberta E. Gausas, MD
Associate Professor of Ophthalmology
Scheie Eye Institute
University of Pennsylvania
Medical School
Philadelphia, PA

Dan S. Gombos, MD, FACS
Assistant Professor of Ophthalmology
Department of Head and Neck Surgery
The University of Texas
MD Anderson Cancer Center
Houston, TX

Evangelos S. Gragoudas, MD
Director, Retina Service
Professor of Ophthalmology
Harvard Medical School
Massachusetts Eye and Ear Infirmary
Boston, MA

Jennifer Gravette, RN, BS, CPON
Nurse
Department of Pediatric
Hematology/Oncology
Cleveland Clinic Foundation
Cleveland, OH

Carl Groenewald, MD
Consultant Vitreoretinal Surgeon
St. Paul's Eye Unit
Royal Liverpool University Hospital
Liverpool, United Kingdom

J. William Harbour, MD
Paul A. Cibis Distinguished Professor of
Ophthalmology, Cell Biology, and
Molecular Oncology
Director, Ocular Oncology Service
Department of Ophthalmology
Washington University
School of Medicine
St. Louis, MO

Martin Heur, MD
Resident
Cole Eye Institute
Cleveland Clinic Foundation
Cleveland, OH

Joanne Hilden, MD
Chair, Pediatric Hematology/Oncology
Medical Director, Pediatric
Palliative Care
Cleveland Clinic Foundation
Cleveland, OH

Paul Hiscott, MD
Professor of Ophthalmology
Unit of Ophthalmology
School of Clinical Science
University of Liverpool
Liverpool, United Kingdom

Santosh G. Honavar, MD
Director
Ocular Oncology Service
LV Prasad Eye Institute
Hyderabad, India

Jennifer I. Hui, MD
Lecturer
Bascom Palmer Eye Institute
University of Miami
Miller School of Medicine
Miami, FL

Saskia M. Imhof, MD, PhD
Doctor
VU University Medical Center
Amsterdam, Netherlands

Martine J. Jager, MD, PhD
Head, Laboratory of Ophthalmology
Department of Ophthalmology
Leiden University Medical Center
Leiden, Netherlands

Bennie H. Jeng, MD
Associate Staff
Cornea and External Disease
Cole Eye Institute
Cleveland Clinic Foundation
Cleveland, OH

David R. Jordan, MD, FACS, FRCS(C)
Professor of Ophthalmology
University of Ottawa
Ottawa, Ontario, Canada

Hanneke J. G. Journée-de Korver, PhD
Senior Scientist
Scientific Research
Department of Ophthalmology
Leiden University Medical Center
Leiden, Netherlands

Rima F. Jubran
Pediatric Oncologist
Childrens Hospital Los Angeles
Los Angeles, CA

Peter K. Kaiser, MD
Director of Clinical Research
Cole Eye Institute
Cleveland Clinic Foundation
Cleveland, OH

Hayyam Kiratli, MD
Professor of Ophthalmology
Department of Ophthalmology
Hacettepe University School of Medicine
Sihhiye, Ankara, Turkey

Tero Kivelä, MD, FEBO
Professor of Ophthalmology
Department of Ophthalmology
Helsinki University Central Hospital
Helsinki, Finland

Stephen R. Klapper, MD, FACS
Ophthalmologist
Klapper Eyelid and Facial Plastic Surgery
Carmel, IN

Alfred G. Knudson, Jr, MD, PhD
Senior Member
Division of Population Science
Fox Chase Cancer Center
Philadelphia, PA

Anne Marie Lane, MPH
Manager
Retina Research Unit
Massachusetts Eye and Ear Infirmary
Boston, MA

Gerald Langmann
Ophthalmologist
Department of Ophthalmology
Universitaets-Augenklinik Graz
Graz, Austria

Carlos Leal-Leal, MD
Pediatric Oncologist
Instituto Nacional de Pediatra
Mexican Retinoblastoma Group
Mexico

Michael Levien, MD
Staff Pediatric Oncologist
Department of Pediatric Oncology
Cleveland Clinic Foundation
Cleveland, OH

Hilel Lewis, MD
Director of Cole Eye Institute
Professor and Chairman
Division of Ophthalmology
Cleveland Clinic Foundation
Cleveland, OH

Karin U. Loeffler, MD
Professor of Ophthalmology
Department of Ophthalmology
University of Bonn
Bonn, Germany

Cari E. Lyle, MD
Instructor
Department of Ophthalmology
University of Tennessee Health
Sciences Center
Memphis, TN

Roy Ma, MD
Staff
Department of Radiation Oncology
Medical University of Vancouver
BC Cancer Agency
Vancouver, Canada

Willem Maat, MD
Resident in Ophthalmology
Department of Ophthalmology
Leiden University Medical Center
Leiden, Netherlands

Nancy C. Mansfield, PhD
Assistant Clinical Professor of
Ophthalmology
Keck School of Medicine
Institute for Families
Los Angeles, CA

Eduardo F. Marback, MD
Consultant Ophthalmologist
Ophthalmology Clinic
Federal University of Bahia
Salvador, Brazil

Anna T. Meadows, MD
Professor of Pediatrics
University of Pennsylvania
Children's Hospital of Philadelphia
Philadelphia, PA

Thomas E. Merchant, DO, PhD
Chief of Radiation Oncology
St. Jude Children's Research Hospital
Memphis, TN

Edoardo Midena, MD
Professor of Ophthalmology and
Visual Sciences
Department of Ophthalmology
University of Padova
Padova, Italy

David A. Miller, MD
Associate Professor
Clinical Obstetrics, Gynecology, and
Pediatrics
Keck School of Medicine
Los Angeles, CA

Annette C. Moll, MD, PhD, FEBOphth
Associate Professor of Ophthalmology
Department of Ophthalmology
VU University Medical Center
Amsterdam, Netherlands

Hardeep Singh Mudhar, BSc, PhD,
MBBChir, MRCPath
Consultant Ophthalmic Histopathologist
Department of Histopathology
Royal Hallamshire Hospital
Sheffield, United Kingdom

Francis Munier, MD
Associate Professor
Hôpital Ophtalmique Jules Gonin
Lausanne, Switzerland

A. Linn Murphree, MD
Director
The Retinoblastoma Center
Childrens Hospital Los Angeles
Los Angeles, CA

Michael D. Onken, PhD
Post-Doctoral Fellow
Department of Ophthalmology and
Visual Sciences
Washington University
School of Medicine
St. Louis, MO

Manuela Orjuela
Assistant Professor of Clinical Pediatrics
(Oncology)
Department of Environmental Health
Sciences
Mailman School of Public Health
Columbia University
New York, NY

Lisa Paquette, MD
Assistant Professor of Pediatrics
Division of Neonatal Medicine
University of Southern California
Keck School of Medicine
Childrens Hospital Los Angeles
Los Angeles, CA

M. Andrew Parsons, MB, ChB, FRCPath
Senior Lecturer and Honorary Consultant
in Ophthalmic Pathology
Department of Ophthalmology and
Orthoptics
University of Sheffield
Royal Hallamshire Hospital
Sheffield, United Kingdom

Bhupendra Patel
Professor of Ophthalmology and Chief
Division of Ocuplastic and Orbital
Service
John A. Moran Eye Center
Salt Lake City, UT

María de la Paz, MD
Ophthalmologist
Centro de Oftalmologia Barraquer
Barcelona, Spain

Jacob Pe'er, MD
Professor of Ophthalmology
Department of Ophthalmology
Kiryat Hadassah
Jerusalem, Israel

David Peereboom, MD
Staff Physician
Brain Tumor Institute
Solid Tumor Oncology
Cleveland Clinic Foundation
Cleveland, OH

José Perez-Moreiras, MD, PhD
Ophthalmologist
Calle Eduardo Pondal
A Coruna, Spain

Julian D. Perry, MD
Section Head
Orbital and Oculoplastic Surgery
Cole Eye Institute
Cleveland Clinic Foundation
Cleveland, OH

Richard Poetter, MD
Chair
Department of Radiation Oncology
Medical University of Vienna
General Hospital Vienna
Vienna, Austria

Patrick De Potter
Professor of Ophthalmology
Ophthalmology Department
Cliniques Universitaires St Luc
Brussels, Belgium

Consuelo Prada, MD
Ophthalmologist
Calle Eduardo Pondal
A Coruna, Spain

Paul L. Proffer, MD, FACS
Assistant Clinical Professor
Ohio State University
Columbus, OH

Ian G. Rennie, MB, ChB, FRCS(Ed),
FRCOphth, FEBO
Professor of Ophthalmology
Academic Unit of Ophthalmology and
Orthoptics
Royal Hallamshire Hospital
Sheffield, United Kingdom

Carlos Rodriguez-Galindo, MD
Associate Member
Department of Hematology/Oncology
Division of Solid Tumors
St. Jude's Children's Research Hospital
Memphis, TN

Geoffrey E. Rose, BSc, MBBS, MS, DSc,
MRCP, FRCS, FRCOphth
Consultant Ophthalmic Surgeon
Moorfields Eye Hospital
London, United Kingdom

Mordechai Rosner, MD
Associate Clinical Professor and
Vice-Chairman
Goldschleger Eye Institute
Sheba Medical Center
Sackler School of Medicine
Tel-Aviv University
Israel

Paul Rundle, MBBS, FRCOphth
Consultant Ophthalmologist
Ocular Oncology Clinic
Royal Hallamshire Hospital
Sheffield, United Kingdom

Stefan Sacu, MD
Ophthalmologist
Department of Ophthalmology and
Optometry
Medical University of Vienna
Vienna, Austria

Andrew P. Schachat, MD
Vice Chairman for Clinical Affairs
Cole Eye Institute
Cleveland Clinic Foundation
Cleveland, OH

Nicoline E. Schalij-Delfos, MD, PhD
Doctor
Leiden University Medical Center
Leiden, Netherlands

Ursula Schmidt-Erfurth
Professor and Chair
Department of Ophthalmology and
Optometry
Medical University of Vienna
Vienna, Austria

Mona Schmutzer, MD
Ophthalmology Resident
Department of Ophthalmology
Medical University Graz
Graz, Austria

Lynn Schoenfield, MD
Staff Pathologist
Department of Anatomic Pathology
Cleveland Clinic Foundation
Cleveland, OH

LuAnne Sculley
Ultrasonographer
Cole Eye Institute
Cleveland Clinic Foundation
Cleveland, OH

Jonathan E. Sears, MD
Vitreoretinal Fellow
Cleveland Clinic Foundation
Cleveland, OH

Stefan Seregard, MD, PhD
Professor and Chairman
St. Erik Eye Hospital
Stockholm, Sweden

Arun D. Singh, MD
Director
Department of Ophthalmic Oncology
Cole Eye Institute
Cleveland Clinic Foundation
Cleveland, OH

Rishi P. Singh, MD
Retina Fellow
Department of Ophthalmic Oncology
Cole Eye Institute
Cleveland Clinic Foundation
Cleveland, OH

Julie A. Stoner, PhD
Associate Professor of Biostatistics
University of Nebraska Medical Center
Omaha, NE

Mehran Taban, MD
Ophthalmology Resident
Cole Eye Institute
Cleveland Clinic Foundation
Cleveland, OH

Mehryar Taban, MD
Ophthalmology Resident
Cole Eye Institute
Cleveland Clinic Foundation
Cleveland, OH

Azzam Taktak, MD
Clinical Scientist
Ocular Oncology Service
Department of Clinical Engineering
Royal Liverpool University Hospital
Liverpool, United Kingdom

Madhura Tamhankar, MD
Associate Professor
Department of Ophthalmology
University of Pennsylvania
Medical School
Philadelphia, PA

Elias I. Traboulsi, MD
Head, Department of
Pediatric Ophthalmology
Director, The Center for
Genetic Eye Diseases
Cole Eye Institute
Cleveland Clinic Foundation
Cleveland, OH

Nikolaos Trichopoulos, MD
Ocular Oncology Fellow
Ocular Oncology Service
Royal Liverpool University Hospital
Liverpool, United Kingdom

David T. Tse, MD, FACS
Professor of Ophthalmology
Department of Ophthalmology
Bascom Palmer Eye Institute
Miami, FL

Geeta K. Vemuganti, MD, DNB
Director, Ophthalmic Pathology Service
Head, Stem Cell Laboratory
Ophthalmic Pathology Service
L.V. Prasad Eye Institute
Hyderabad, India

Judith G. Villablanca, MD
Associate Professor of Clinical Pediatrics
Hematology/Oncology
Childrens Hospital of Los Angeles
Los Angeles, CA

Werner Wackernagel, MD
International Fellow
Cole Eye Institute
Cleveland Clinic Foundation
Cleveland, OH

Allan Wilkinson, PhD
Vice-Chief of Medical Physics
Department of Radiation Oncology and
the Department of Ophthalmic Oncology
Cole Eye Institute
Cleveland Clinic Foundation
Cleveland, OH

Matthew W. Wilson, MD, FACS
Associate Professor of Ophthalmology
University of Tennessee
Health Science Center
Memphis, TN

Martin Zehetmayer, MD
Staff
Department of Ophthalmology-Oncology
Service
Medical University of Vienna
General Hospital Vienna
Vienna, Austria

Leonidas Zografos, MD
Professor of Ophthalmology
Jules Gonin Eye Hospital
Lausanne, Switzerland

INTRODUCTION

The management of patients with ophthalmic tumors presents particular challenges. Ophthalmic tumors are rare and diverse so that their diagnosis can be quite complex. Treatment usually requires special expertise and equipment and in many instances is controversial. The field is advancing rapidly, because of accelerating progress in tumor biology, pharmacology, and instrumentation. Increasingly, the care of patients with an ocular or adnexal tumor is provided by a multidisciplinary team, comprising ocular oncologists, general oncologists, radiotherapists, pathologists, psychologists, and other specialists. Such expertise may only be available far from the patient's home, in which case the local ophthalmologist will continue to be involved in the patient's care. For all these reasons, we felt that there was scope for a textbook of ophthalmic oncology, which would amalgamate knowledge from several different disciplines, thereby helping the various specialists to understand each other better and to cooperate more efficiently.

Essentials of Ophthalmic Oncology was derived from our book *Clinical Ophthalmic Oncology,* a large textbook specifically for oncologists and published by Elsevier. Sensing a need for an oncology book geared more toward general ophthalmologists, we compiled the pertinent material into this book—*Essentials of Ophthalmic Oncology.*

The purpose of *Essentials of Ophthalmic Oncology* is to provide up-to-date information of the whole spectrum of eyelid, conjunctival, intraocular, and orbital tumors. The first section is devoted to basic principles of chemotherapy, radiation therapy, cancer epidemiology, angiogenesis, and cancer genetics. We have also included a chapter on counseling patients with ophthalmic cancer.

Special attention has been paid to make the text easily readable. Each chapter has a similar layout; features include boxes that highlight the key features, tables that provide comparison, and flow diagrams that outline therapeutic approaches. Several chapters authored by radiation oncologists, medical physicists, pediatric oncologists, hematologist-oncologists, and medical geneticists have been included to provide a broader perspective.

All 128 authors from 18 countries were gracious to accept editorial changes so as to present a balanced view of clinical practice. As evidence-based data are sparse in the field of ophthalmic oncology, it is anticipated that *Essentials of Ophthalmic Oncology* will act as a stimulus for further thought and investigation.

Principles of Clinical Epidemiology

Annette C. Moll, Michiel R. de Boer, and Lex M. Bouter

INTRODUCTION

During the past decade, evidence-based medicine (EBM) has become a dominant approach in many medical fields, including ophthalmology.[1] Clinical epidemiological studies provide evidence that can aid the decision-making processes.

OUTCOME MEASURES

Prevalence

Prevalence refers to the proportion of the population with the condition of interest. Usually, prevalence is given for a specific moment in time (point prevalence), but sometimes it is estimated for a period of time (eg, 1 year or lifetime prevalences).

Incidence

Whereas prevalence relates to existing cases, incidence relates to the proportion of new cases in a certain population. There are two different measures of incidence: cumulative incidence (CI) and incidence density (ID). CI is the proportion of new cases in a population at risk over a specified period of time.

Mortality

Mortality refers to the incidence of death. The mortality rates can be all-cause, indicating all deaths, or disease-specific, for instance mortality caused by melanoma or retinoblastoma. Case fatality rate refers to the proportion of patients with a given disease who will die from that disease and thus reflects the seriousness of the condition.

Quality of Life

With the increasing survival rate and severe side effects of some treatment modalities, quality-of-life measures such as the measure of outcome in ocular disease (MOOD) have become increasingly important in ophthalmic oncology.[2]

MEASURES OF ASSOCIATION

Relative Risk

The ratio of cumulative incidence between a group of exposed and unexposed individuals or treated and untreated patients is the relative risk (RR).

Hazard Ratio

The ratio of incidence density between a group of unexposed and exposed patients is the hazard ratio (HR), which has a similar interpretation as the RR. This measure is often used in relation to mortality because we are generally not only interested in the proportion of patients who die, but also in the time from baseline (diagnosis or start treatment) until death. A special application of the HR is the ratio of the observed to the expected number of cases (O/E ratio).

Odds Ratio

Odds ratio (OR) is the ratio of the odds of outcome of interest between the exposed and the unexposed.

Differences in Risk

The risk difference is easy to interpret and can be used to calculate the number of patients needed to treat (NNT) to prevent one extra event (eg, death) compared to the standard treatment or placebo. The NNT can be calculated as the inverse of RD (1/RD).

Differences in Mean Score

For scores on interval scales, such as quality of life, differences in mean score between exposed and unexposed participants are the only measure of interest.

BIAS

An estimate can be very precise but still not be accurate because of bias. Three main sources of bias exist: confounding, selection, and information bias.

Confounding occurs when the association between exposure and outcome is influenced by a third variable that is both related to the exposure and the outcome.

Selection bias may occur when the chance of being included in the study population is not random for all members of the source population. For example, patients with an advanced tumor stage are more likely to be referred to a special cancer center than patients with a less advanced tumor stage. This form of selection bias is called referral bias. Selection bias could also be introduced in a study by choosing the wrong control group, especially if controls are selected from hospital patients.

Table 1-1. The Relation Between Outcome, Measures of Association, Study Design, and Statistical Methods

Outcome	Measure of Association	Computation	Study Design	Statistical Method
Prevalence	Prevalence rate	P_1/P_2	Cross-sectional	χ^2 test Logistic regression analysis
	Prevalence difference	$P_1 - P_2$	Cross-sectional	χ^2 test
Odds of exposure	Odds ratio	Odds of exposure group 1/odds of exposure group 2	Case control study (cohort study, RCT)	χ^2 test Logistic regression
Cumulative incidence (CI)	Relative risk	CI_1/CI_2	Cohort study/RCT	χ^2 test
	Risk difference	$CI_1 - CI_2$	RCT	
Incidence density (ID)	Hazard ratio	ID_1/ID_2	Cohort study/RCT	Kaplan-Meier Cox regression
	Risk difference	$ID_1 - ID_2$	RCT	Kaplan-Meier
	O/E ratio	Observed ID/expected ID in general population	Cohort study/registry study	
Quality of life	Difference in mean score	$\chi_1 - \chi_2$	Cohort study/RCT	Independent t-test Linear regression analyses

P_1, prevalence group 1; P_2, prevalence group 2; CI, cumulative incidence; CI_1, CI group 1; CI_2, CI group 2; ID, incidence density; ID_1, ID group 1; ID_2, ID group 2; O/E ratio, observed to expected ratio; RCT, randomized controlled trial; χ_1, mean score group 1; χ_2, mean score group 2.

Information bias occurs when outcome or exposure variables are not accurately assessed. A well-known type of information bias is recall bias. This refers to the phenomenon that patients tend to remember more details about exposures that are possibly related to their disease than controls.

STUDY DESIGNS

There are several research designs, such as case series, cross-sectional, cohort, randomized control trial, and case control study that can be adopted in order to address the research questions (Table 1-1).

Case Series

In case series, the authors present the clinical data regarding a group of patients. The disadvantage is that this kind of study is not randomized, does not have a comparative design, and does not permit an answer to a question such as, "there is a good response, but compared to what?"

Cross-Sectional Study

In a cross-sectional study, the outcome (and exposure) are assessed at one point in time. The cross-sectional study design has the advantages that it is relatively easy to plan, only one measurement is needed, it is inexpensive, and it is quick to perform. As both exposure and outcome are measured at the same time, we cannot be sure that the exposure preceded the outcome (the most important criterion for causality).

Cohort Study

Some of the problems listed above can be overcome by conducting a cohort study. At baseline, one starts with a cohort of people free from disease and the exposure(s).

During or at the end of follow-up, incident cases in both the unexposed and the exposed group are identified, and RRs or HRs can be calculated. The cohort studies are often expensive because they need large sample sizes and long follow-up for meaningful analyses.

Randomized Controlled Trial

A randomized controlled trial is a specific type of cohort study. Participants are randomly assigned to the intervention group (treatment under investigation) or a control group (no treatment, placebo, or standard treatment). The randomization, if successful, ensures that confounding factors are evenly distributed between the intervention and control groups.

Case-Control Study

In contrast to cohort studies, the starting point in case-control is not to assess the exposure status, but the disease status. People with the disease of interest are selected, and a control group of people without the disease is subsequently recruited.

A pilot study is often performed before the start of a large study. Its aim is to improve the methodological quality and to evaluate the feasibility.

Systematic Review

In a systematic review, all available evidence (literature) on a certain topic is reviewed in a systematic, transparent, and reproducible manner. When the studies in a systematic review are reasonably homogenous, their results can be pooled in a meta-analysis.

REFERENCES

1. Sackett DL. Clinical epidemiology. What, who, and whither? *J Clin Epidemiol.* 2002;55:1161-1166.
2. Foss AJ, Lamping DL, Schroter S, et al. Development and validation of a patient based measure of outcome in ocular melanoma. *Br J Ophthalmol.* 2000;84:347-351.

Cancer Etiology

Evelyn X. Fu and Arun D. Singh

INTRODUCTION

Cancer is an abnormal mass of tissue resulting from the clonal expansion of a single precursor cell that has incurred genetic damage.

CARCINOGENIC AGENTS

Carcinogenic agents may be classified as chemical, radiation, and microbial (Table 2-1).

GENETIC SUSCEPTIBILITY

Retinoblastoma, being the most striking example, shows an autosomal dominant inheritance pattern. Xeroderma pigmentosum has an autosomal recessive inheritance (Chapter 16).

IATROGENIC CANCERS

Immunosuppression

Patients with immunosuppression have increased risks for lymphomas and carcinomas.[1]

Chemotherapy

Second primary cancers have been estimated to occur in 5% to 10% of patients who have received chemotherapy.[2]

Radiation Therapy

Follow-up of survivors of atomic bombs and nuclear power plant accidents show marked increase in the incidences of leukemia and solid tumors involving breast, colon, thyroid, and lung.[3]

REFERENCES

1. Opelz G, Dohler B. Lymphomas after solid organ transplantation: a collaborative transplant study report. *Am J Transplant.* 2004;4:222-230.
2. Kaldor JM, Day NE, Clarke EA, et al. Leukemia following Hodgkin's disease. *N Engl J Med.* 1990;322:7-13.
3. Williams D. Cancer after nuclear fallout: lessons from Chernobyl accident. *Nat Rev Cancer.* 2002;2:543-549.

Table 2-1. Various Types of Carcinogen				
Chemicals	Radiation	Infectious	Dietary	Iatrogenic
Occupational	UV light	Virus	Fat	Radiation
Arsenic	X-ray	HPV	Calorie	Immunosuppression
Asbestos	g-ray	EBV	Low fiber	Chemotherapy
Coal tars	Nuclear radiation	KSHV		
Soot		HTLV-1		
Benzene		HEP B/C		
Vinyl chloride				
Behavioral		Bacteria		
Tobacco		*H. pylori*		
Alcohol		*C. psittaci*		
		Fungus		
		A. flavus		
		Parasite		
		Schistosoma		
		Clonorchis		

Cancer Pathology

Stefan Seregard and Charlotta All-Ericsson

INTRODUCTION

Neoplasia (Greek for new growth) indicates cell growth that may be distinct (a lump or tumor) or diffuse (eg, leukemia). Originally used to denote a lump of any origin (neoplastic or inflammatory), tumor as a concept is now often perceived as identical to neoplasia.

CLASSIFICATION OF NEOPLASIA

Tumors may be either benign or malignant. Moreover, benign tumors may be precursors to malignant tumors. Characteristic differences between benign and malignant tumors are summarized in Table 3A-1.

Benign Tumors

Benign tumors are usually labeled by the suffix –oma. For example, adenoma of the lacrimal gland is a benign tumor composed of cells originating from the glandular epithelium of the lacrimal gland.

- Hamartoma: a benign tumor composed of histologically normal cells normally occurring at the affected site.
- Choristoma: a benign tumor composed of cells not normally occurring at the affected site, but otherwise histologically normal.
- Teratoma: composed of pluripotent cells forming different types of tissue originating from one or more of the three germ cell layers. Teratoma may be benign or malignant.

Malignant Tumors

- Carcinoma: a malignant neoplasm of epithelial origin.
- Sarcoma: a malignant neoplasm derived from mesenchymal tissue.
- Blastoma: a malignant tumor of embryonic origin and is identified by the suffix –blastoma.
- Leukemia: a malignancy of blood cells that arises from the bone marrow precursor cells and is present in the peripheral blood.
- Lymphoma: a malignancy derived from lymph nodes, but occasionally may be present in other organs like the lacrimal gland or in peripheral blood.
- Melanoma: a malignant tumor that originates from melanocytes.

Box 3A-1. Microscopic Features of Neoplasia

- Cellular proliferation
- Cellular pleomorphism
- Cellular dedifferentiation
- Nuclear cytoplasmic ratio
- Invasion of surrounding tissues

Table 3A-1. Characteristic Differences Between Benign and Malignant Tumors

Feature	Benign	Malignant
Cellular pleomorphism	None or mild	Mild to severe
Cellular dedifferentiation	None or mild	Mild to severe
Necrosis	Rare	Occasionally
Basement membrane invasion	Never	Frequent
Metastatic spread	Never	Occasionally

MICROSCOPIC FEATURES OF NEOPLASIA

Certain histopathologic features differentiate benign and malignant tumors from surrounding normal tissues (Box 3A-1). In general, the extent of such changes from the normal tissue is more marked in malignant tumors than in benign tumors.

METASTATIC PROCESS

The most significant difference between benign and malignant tumors is the metastatic potential of malignant tumors. Carcinoma tend to have lymphatic spread, whereas sarcoma preferentially undergo hematogenous spread. Cancer dissemination is a complex multifactorial process (Box 3A-2).

TISSUE SAMPLING AND PROCESSING

With cytological sampling, the diagnosis is usually made on the morphological appearance of individual cells because the relationship to surrounding cells is lost.

Exfoliative cytology is sampling of spontaneously exfoliated and dispersed cells.

Aspiration cytology may be applied to palpable lesions or guided by ultrasound or computerized tomography imaging (Chapter 56).

HISTOPATHOLOGIC SAMPLING

Typically, tissue is obtained by incisional (or excisional) biopsy of the lesion. Assessment of the surgical margins is paramount in any excisional tumor biopsy.[1,2]

DIAGNOSTIC TECHNIQUES

Light microscopy samples are usually fixed in formaldehyde and then embedded in paraffin. This allows for the cutting of 3 to 4 microns thin sections. Embedding in epoxy resin (Epon) allows for even thinner (micron) sections, which may be stained with toluidine blue. Paraffin sections are usually routinely stained with hematoxylin and eosin.

Immunohistochemistry has rapidly evolved from a research tool to a diagnostic technique.

Electron microscopy (EM) provides excellent spatial resolution and allows for the visualization of individual cell organelles. While transmission EM (TEM) provides high-resolution tissue cross-sectioning, scanning EM (SEM) is used for tissue surface imaging.

RESEARCH TECHNIQUES

Recent advances in molecular pathology have generated numerous techniques for the study of DNA, RNA, and proteins. Some of these techniques have become a routinely used part of the diagnostic arsenal (flow cytometry in lymphoma and tissue

---

Box 3A-2. Steps in the Metastatic Process

- Tumor invasion of the vasculature or lymph vessels
- Tumor cell survival in the circulation
- Cellular extravasation
- Establish a metastasis at a distant site
- Acquiring an intrinsic vasculature

---

imprints for gene rearrangement studies in rhabdomyosarcoma). In situ hybridization is used to detect messenger RNA transcripts but non-specific background staining or hybridization to homologous transcripts limits the use in diagnostic pathology. The PCR technique, in particular when used as competitive or "real time" PCR, allows for sensitive assays of gene expression at the RNA level. Gene profiling using the microarray technique is still a research tool, but is soon expected to become more readily available. Proteomics holds a similar promise and generates vast amounts of data on protein expression.[3]

REFERENCES

1. Zuidervaart W, van der Velden PA, Hurks MH, et al. Gene expression profiling identifies tumour markers potentially playing a role in uveal melanoma development. *Br J Cancer.* 2003;89:1914-1919.
2. Onken MD, Worley LA, Ehlers JP, Harbour JW. Gene expression profiling in uveal melanoma reveals two molecular classes and predicts metastatic death. *Cancer Res.* 2004;64:7205-7209.
3. Missotten GS, Beijnen JH, Keunen JE, Bonfrer JM. Proteomics in uveal melanoma. *Melanoma Res.* 2003;13:627-629.

Cancer Angiogenesis

Werner Wackernagel, Lynn Schoenfield, and Arun D. Singh

INTRODUCTION

Interest in the role of angiogenesis for the development and treatment of cancer began in the early 1970s, when it was postulated that the formation of new and large vessels in tumors is essential for tumor growth and metastasis.[1] Since then, our growing understanding of the regulation of angiogenesis has revealed an important role in other diseases, such as proliferative diabetic retinopathy and age-related macular degeneration, rheumatoid arthritis, and psoriasis.[2]

TUMOR ANGIOGENESIS

Small tumors can get their nutrients and oxygen by diffusion alone. However, with increasing distance from a capillary vessel, oxygen supply is insufficient for the proliferation of tumor cells.[3] Tumorigenesis is a multistep process, caused by mutations over time.[4] Only those cells that know how to build their own vessels grow to a visible size if experimentally implanted into another location. The others remain microscopic in size without any sign of growth, a phenomenon called "no take."

COOPTION

At an early stage, some tumors and metastases can invade healthy vascularized tissue forming microcylinders up to 200 microns in diameter around pre-existing capillaries, a mechanism called *cooption*.[5]

ANGIOGENIC SWITCH

Ultimately, all tumors rely on the formation of new blood vessels to grow to a clinically detectable size. Tumor cells implanted in rabbit cornea show a low growth rate as long as the cornea remains avascular. With the onset of revascularization, the tumor cells switch to a higher proliferation rate, and the tumor grows rapidly.[6] The same is observed for tumors in the anterior chamber of a rabbit eye. Though revascularization of the iris develops soon, the tumors do not grow to a large size until they are in touch with the iris and the newly formed vessels.[7] The ability of a tumor to induce growth of its own vessels is called angiogenic switch and usually occurs after malignant transformation.[8] However, cervical dysplasia demonstrates an angiogenic phenotype even before definite signs of malignancy are present.[9]

STEPS IN ANGIOGENESIS

Angiogenesis begins with vasodilation and an increase in vascular permeability because of dissolution of adherens junctions with consequent vascular leakage leading to extravasation of plasma.[10] Matrix metalloproteinases degrade the basement membrane and the surrounding extracellular matrix, amplifying the angiogenic stimulus by releasing basic fibroblast growth factor (bFGF) and vascular endothelial growth factor (VEGF). Proliferating endothelial cells now migrate away from the vessel. The new sprout appears to be a solid column, but a lumen is formed either by intracellular vacuolar fusion or by arrangement of cells around a central lumen.[11]

TUMOR VESSELS

The vascular density of a tumor can be many times the density of normal tissue.[12] However, the vessels are disorganized, torturous, and show a chaotic blood flow.[13] Often, they leak fluid or bleed. In some tumors, including uveal melanoma, fluid-conducting structures similar to vessels can be found that do not have endothelial cell lining (vascular mimicry).[14]

METASTATIC CASCADE

The different steps a tumor has to take to successfully metastasize are called the metastatic cascade (Chapter 3A).

PROMOTERS OF ANGIOGENESIS

Angiogenesis can be induced by different factors and different conditions. Inflammation, hypoxia, and mechanical factors can induce the production or the release of proangiogenic factors and cytokines.

VASCULAR ENDOTHELIAL GROWTH FACTOR

Vascular endothelial growth factor (VEGF) was discovered in 1989 for its ability to increase vascular permeability and was named vascular permeability factor (VPF).[15] VEGF promotes endothelial cell motility and the growth of new blood and lymphatic vessels.[16] The VEGF-induced vasculature consists of primitive vascular plexuses that are highly fragile and hemorrhagic. In

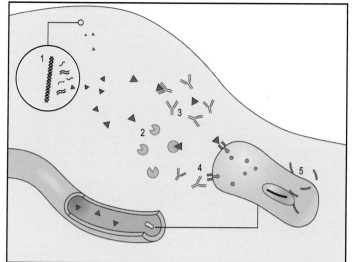

Figure 3B-1. Direct and indirect ways of inhibiting angiogenesis. Antiangiogenic therapy can interfere with pro-angiogenic stimuli on different levels. (1) Antisense oligonucleotides bind to mRNA of pro-angiogenic factors, thus inhibiting translation by the ribosome and inducing degradation. (2) Small molecules, oligonucleotides, and (3) antibodies against diffusible circulating angiogenic factors bind and inactivate those factors before they reach the endothelial cell. (4) Antibodies can also bind to the cell surface/transmembrane receptor and prevent stimulation by angiogenic factors. (5) Direct inhibitors bind to the cell surface or become internalized, exerting an inhibiting function on their target cells.

vivo, it is physiologically expressed in areas of wound healing, bone growth, and the female reproductive organs. VEGF plays a role in the pathogenesis of retinopathy of prematurity (ROP), choroidal neovascularization in age-related macula degeneration, and neovascularization of the iris.

SUBTYPES

VEGF family of growth factors consists of at least six members binding to different VEGF receptors (VEGFR) on the cell surface. In general terms, when VEGF is mentioned, it is the VEGFA that are being referred to. The gene for VEGF is located on the short arm of chromosome 6 (6p21),[17] and alternative splicing results in the different isoforms of protein that are named after the number of their amino acids. VEGF 121, 145, 165, 189, and 206 differ in their affinities to the VEGF receptors and to structures of the extracellular matrix.

VEGF RECEPTORS

The function of VEGF is mediated by different cell surface receptors, a family of transmembrane receptor tyrosine kinases.

REGULATION OF VEGF

Hypoxia induces the expression of two hypoxia-inducible factors (HIF-1 and HIF-2).[18] This induces the expression of VGEF and more than 60 other genes. However, under normoxic conditions, this rarely happens because HIF undergoes rapid degradation. If the VHL protein is missing, mutated, or not functional, HIF is not inactivated properly, and normoxic tissue behaves as if under hypoxic conditions.

Epidermal growth factor, transforming growth factor-beta, keratinocytic growth factor, insulin-like growth factor, fibroblast growth factor, and angiopoietin can all induce VEGF in vitro or in vivo.

INHIBITORS OF ANGIOGENESIS
ENDOGENOUS

Thrombospondin was the first naturally occurring inhibitor.

Angiostatin is a fragment of plasminogen that is generated from plasminogen among others by urokinase plasminogen activator (uPA) and matrix-metallo proteinases (MMP).[19] It has been successfully used in animal models.

Endostatin also plays a critical role in the development of the retinal vessels. In Knobloch syndrome, characterized by a deficiency of endostatin, the hyaloid artery of the vitreous fails to regress.[20] The endostatin levels are elevated in eyes with proliferative diabetic retinopathy.

EXOGENOUS

There are direct and indirect ways to inhibit VEGF (Figure 3B-1). Some of the clinically used agents include Bevacizumab, Ranibizumab, Pegabtanib, Sugen (Semaxanib SU5416), Herceptin, and interferon-alpha 2a.

REFERENCES

1. Folkman J. Tumor angiogenesis: therapeutic implications. *N Engl J Med.* 1971;285:1182-1186.
2. Folkman J. Angiogenesis in cancer, vascular, rheumatoid and other disease. *Nat Med.* 1995;1:27-31.
3. Tannock IF. Population kinetics of carcinoma cells, capillary endothelial cells, and fibroblasts in a transplanted mouse mammary tumor. *Cancer Res.* 1970;30:2470-2476.
4. Achilles EG, Fernandez A, Allred EN, et al. Heterogeneity of angiogenic activity in a human liposarcoma: a proposed mechanism for "no take" of human tumors in mice. *J Natl Cancer Inst.* 2001;93:1075-1081.
5. Holash J, Maisonpierre PC, Compton D, et al. Vessel cooption, regression, and growth in tumors mediated by angiopoietins and VEGF. *Science.* 1999;284:1994-1998.
6. Gimbrone MA, Jr., Cotran RS, Leapman SB, Folkman J. Tumor growth and neovascularization: an experimental model using the rabbit cornea. *J Natl Cancer Inst.* 1974;52:413-427.
7. Gimbrone MA, Jr., Leapman SB, Cotran RS, Folkman J. Tumor dormancy in vivo by prevention of neovascularization. *J Exp Med.* 1972;136:261-276.
8. Hanahan D, Christofori G, Naik P, Arbeit J. Transgenic mouse models of tumour angiogenesis: the angiogenic switch, its molecular controls, and prospects for preclinical therapeutic models. *Eur J Cancer.* 1996;32A:2386-2393.
9. Smith-McCune KK, Weidner N. Demonstration and characterization of the angiogenic properties of cervical dysplasia. *Cancer Res.* 1994;54:800-804.
10. Pepper MS. Role of the matrix metalloproteinase and plasminogen activator-plasmin systems in angiogenesis. *Arterioscler Thromb Vasc Biol.* 2001;21:1104-1117.
11. Milkiewicz M, Ispanovic E, Doyle JL, Haas TL. Regulators of angiogenesis and strategies for their therapeutic manipulation. *Int J Biochem Cell Biol.* 2006;38:333-357.
12. Thompson WD, Shiach KJ, Fraser RA, McIntosh LC, Simpson JG. Tumours acquire their vasculature by vessel incorporation, not vessel ingrowth. *J Pathol.* 1987;151:323-332.

13. Jain RK. Molecular regulation of vessel maturation. *Nat Med.* 2003;9:685-693.

14. Folberg R, Maniotis AJ. Vasculogenic mimicry. *Apmis.* 2004;112:508-525.

15. Dvorak HF. Tumors: wounds that do not heal. Similarities between tumor stroma generation and wound healing. *N Engl J Med.* 1986;315:1650-1659.

16. Ferrara N, Houck K, Jakeman L, Leung DW. Molecular and biological properties of the vascular endothelial growth factor family of proteins. *Endocr Rev.* 1992;13:18-32.

17. Vincenti V, Cassano C, Rocchi M, Persico G. Assignment of the vascular endothelial growth factor gene to human chromosome 6p21.3. *Circulation.* 1996;93:1493-1495.

18. Zagzag D, Zhong H, Scalzitti JM, Laughner E, Simons JW, Semenza GL. Expression of hypoxia-inducible factor 1alpha in brain tumors: association with angiogenesis, invasion, and progression. *Cancer.* 2000;88:2606-2618.

19. O'Reilly MS, Holmgren L, Chen C, Folkman J. Angiostatin induces and sustains dormancy of human primary tumors in mice. *Nat Med.* 1996;2:689-692.

20. Sertie AL, Sossi V, Camargo AA, Zatz M, Brahe C, Passos-Bueno MR. Collagen XVIII, containing an endogenous inhibitor of angiogenesis and tumor growth, plays a critical role in the maintenance of retinal structure and in neural tube closure (Knobloch syndrome). *Hum Mol Genet.* 2000;9:2051-2058.

Cancer Immunology

Martine J. Jager, Jihan Dennaoui, and Willem Maat

INNATE AND SPECIFIC IMMUNE RESPONSES

The most primitive and direct defenses against either microbes, trauma, or abnormal cells is the innate immune response. As soon as "danger" is encountered, granulocytes and macrophages are alerted and will try to inactivate the danger. If this response is inadequate, antigen-presenting cells will pick up parts of the microbes or abnormal cells and take them to the regional lymph node, where specific immune responses will then develop. There are different kinds of T cells: such as T cells that can kill (cytotoxic T cells; CTLs) and that can cause local inflammation (delayed type hypersensitivity T cells), and regulatory T cells, which are able to suppress other T cells. Furthermore, T cells are necessary to stimulate B cells to start production of specific antibodies.

IMMUNOLOGICAL ESCAPE

It appears that the immune responses that do exist are limited in their effectiveness inside the eye, which is known to be an immunologically privileged site. The presence of regulatory T cells may suppress an effective immune response. This is observed when antigens are injected into the anterior chamber of the eye of a mouse, which leads to the induction of an unusual immune response, known as anterior chamber-associated immune deviation (ACAID).[1] ACAID is characterized by the presence of regulatory splenic T cells that prevent the development of delayed-type hypersensitivity and prevent the maturation and differentiation of precursor CTLs.[2] In experimental animal models, it has been shown that tumor cells that are rejected when placed in the skin enjoy the pleasure of an immune-privileged ocular environment when placed inside the eye.

IMMUNOLOGICAL ASPECTS OF UVEAL MELANOMA

The uveal melanoma cells are antigenic, and patients can develop specific anti-tumor antibodies or T cells, as the tumors express a wide range of antigens. However, in spite of these anti-tumor immune responses, the tumor manages to escape immunological destruction and expands inside the eye while especially larger tumors give rise to metastases.

Tumor Antigen Expression in Uveal Melanoma

The first potential tumor antigens were identified by monoclonal antibodies developed against cutaneous melanoma. Van der Pol observed both a differential expression as well as heterogeneity for antigens such as Antigen gp100. The subsequent use of T cells as tools to identify specific tumor antigens led to the recognition of many more antigens considered to be good targets for immunotherapy.[3]

HLA Expression in Uveal Melanoma

Tumors are known to lack specific HLA antigens, and this would block the effectiveness of specific CTL responses. One would expect that tumor cells that can thus escape CTL-mediated lysis would give rise to metastases, but in uveal melanoma the opposite occurs.[4,5] We hypothesized that during the hematogeneous spreading, uveal melanoma micrometastases with a low expression of HLA class I are removed from the blood by circulating NK cells before they can reach the liver.[6] This hypothesis is supported by earlier experimental studies by Ma and Niederkorn in mice; when uveal melanoma cells with a low HLA class I expression were injected into the bloodstream of mice, they did not induce metastases, while cells with a high HLA class I expression did.[7]

Infiltrating Immune Cells in Uveal Melanoma

Uveal melanomas contain varying amounts of lymphocytes and macrophages (Figure 4-1) with inverse relationship to survival.[8,9]

Anti-Uveal Melanoma T Cell Responses

Using leukocyte migration assays and formalinized melanoma cells, Cochran and colleagues demonstrated that the majority of uveal melanoma, conjunctival melanoma, and cutaneous melanoma patients had anti-tumor T cell reactivity.[10]

Antibodies Against Uveal Melanoma

Sera from patients with uveal melanoma often test positively for antibodies against cytoplasmic or cell surface antigens of uveal melanoma and tumor-specific antibodies.[11]

IMPLICATIONS

While uveal melanomas express many different antigens, and as the presence of a wide range of immune responses can be demonstrated, they do not seem to contribute to survival but are more proof of spreading of tumor cells beyond the eye. New techniques have to be used to better stimulate anti-tumor immune responses if immunotherapy is going to help patients clinically.

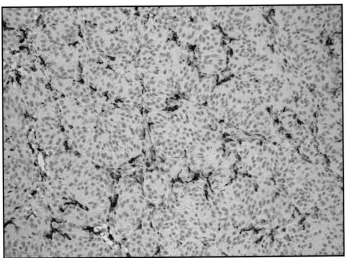

Figure 4-1. Positive staining for macrophages in a uveal melanoma.

REFERENCES

1. Streilein JW. Ocular immune privilege: therapeutic opportunities from an experiment of nature. *Nat Rev Immunol.* 2003;3:879-889.

2. Ksander BR, Rubsamen PE, Olsen KR, Cousins SW, Streilein JW. Studies of tumor-infiltrating lymphocytes from a human choroidal melanoma. *Invest Ophthalmol Vis Sci.* 1991;32:3198-208.

3. van der Pol JP, Jager MJ, de Wolff-Rouendaal D, Ringens PJ, Vennegoor C, Ruiter DJ. Heterogeneous expression of melanoma-associated antigens in uveal melanomas. *Curr Eye Res.* 1987;6:757-765.

4. Blom DJ, Luyten GP, Mooy C, Kerkvliet S, Zwinderman AH, Jager MJ. Human leukocyte antigen class I expression. Marker of poor prognosis in uveal melanoma. *Invest Ophthalmol Vis Sci.* 1997;38:1865-1872.

5. Ericsson C, Seregard S, Bartolazzi A, et al. Association of HLA class I and class II antigen expression and mortality in uveal melanoma. *Invest Ophthalmol Vis Sci.* 2001;42:2153-2156.

6. Jager MJ, Hurks HM, Levitskaya J, Kiessling R. HLA expression in uveal melanoma: there is no rule without some exception. *Hum Immunol.* 2002;63:444-451.

7. Ma D, Luyten GP, Luider TM, Niederkorn JY. Relationship between natural killer cell susceptibility and metastasis of human uveal melanoma cells in a murine model. *Invest Ophthalmol Vis Sci.* 1995;36:435-441.

8. Davidorf FH, Lang JR. Lymphocytic infiltration in choroidal melanoma and its prognostic significance. *Trans Ophthalmol Soc U K.* 1977;97:394-401.

9. Makitie T, Summanen P, Tarkkanen A, Kivela T. Tumor-infiltrating macrophages (CD68(+) cells) and prognosis in malignant uveal melanoma. *Invest Ophthalmol Vis Sci.* 2001;42:1414-1421.

10. Cochran AJ, Foulds WS, Damato BE, Trope GE, Morrison L, Lee WR. Assessment of immunological techniques in the diagnosis and prognosis of ocular malignant melanoma. *Br J Ophthalmol.* 1985;69:171-176.

11. Kan-Mitchell J, Liggett PE, Harel W, et al. Lymphocytes cytotoxic to uveal and skin melanoma cells from peripheral blood of ocular melanoma patients. *Cancer Immunol Immunother.* 1991;33:333-340.

Cancer Genetics

J. William Harbour and Michael D. Onken

INTRODUCTION

A fundamental characteristic of cancer cells is that they proliferate and survive outside of their normal physiologic context. This ability is acquired through genetic mutations and epigenetic alterations in genes responsible for sensing, interpreting, and responding to tissue-specific homeostatic signals. These genes are often referred to as oncogenes and tumor suppressor genes, depending on whether cancer-causing mutations result in gain or loss of function, respectively.

PROLIFERATION AND THE CELL CYCLE

Growth Factor Signaling Pathways

Normal cells are limited in their proliferative capacity by the availability of mitogenic (growth-stimulating) signals (Figure 5-1). Cancer cells often overcome this limitation and become mitogen-independent by mutations in growth factor receptors, which were some of the first oncogenes identified. Gain-of-function mutations in genes encoding proteins such as the epithelial growth factor receptor and the c-Kit receptor circumvent the requirement for growth factors and can lead to constitutive growth signaling and autocrine stimulation.[1] Alternatively, growth factor signaling can be disrupted by mutations downstream of the receptor.

Rb-p16Ink4a-Cyclin D Pathway

The ultimate downstream target of most growth signaling pathways is the core cell cycle machinery, which is regulated by the retinoblastoma protein (Rb) pathway.[2] While the Rb gene itself is mutated in only a subset of cancers, including its namesake, mutations elsewhere in the Rb pathway that functionally inactivate Rb are more common.[3]

Myc

The c-Myc gene is located at chromosome 8q24 within the region that is frequently amplified in uveal melanoma.[4] Moreover, most uveal melanomas overexpress the c-Myc protein.[5]

Apoptosis and Senescence

Normal cells undergo apoptosis (programmed cell death) or senescence (permanent cell cycle withdrawal) if they stray from their normal environmental restraints.[6] The success of cancer cells depends on their ability not only to proliferate, but also to avoid apoptosis and senescence as they deviate further from their normal physiologic milieu.

p53 and HDM2

The p53 tumor suppressor can activate senescence and apoptotic programs in response to abnormalities associated with neoplastic transformation, such as excessive proliferation and DNA damage.[7] More than half of all cancers contain loss-of-function mutations in the p53 gene, and most other cancers functionally inhibit p53. In uveal melanoma, p53 is rarely mutated, but the p53 pathway is functionally impaired by overexpression of the p53 inhibitor HDM2.[8]

Bcl-2 is an anti-apoptotic factor and the namesake of a family of pro- and anti-apoptotic proteins that interact in a complex manner to regulate apoptosis by the intrinsic mitochondrial pathway.[9] The vast majority of uveal melanomas express high levels of Bcl-2.[10]

Telomerase

Cell cycling is normally accompanied by shortening of the telomeres until they are reduced to a critical length that triggers a DNA damage response and p53-mediated senescence or apoptosis.[11] Consequently, cancer cells often commandeer this enzyme by up-regulating its catalytic subunit, TERT, to maintain telomere length.[12]

REFERENCES

1. Bafico A, Aaronson SA. Growth factors and signal transduction in cancer. In: Kufe DW, Pollock R, Weichselbaumet RR, et al, eds. *Cancer Medicine*. 6th ed. Hamilton, Ontario: BC Decker Inc; 2003.
2. Harbour JW, Dean DC. The Rb/E2F pathway: expanding roles and emerging paradigms. *Genes Dev*. 2000;14:2393-2409.
3. Brantley MA Jr, Harbour JW. Inactivation of retinoblastoma protein in uveal melanoma by phosphorylation of sites in the COOH-terminal region. *Cancer Res*. 2000;60:4320-4323.
4. Parrella P, Caballero OL, Sidransky D, Merbs SL. Detection of c-myc amplification in uveal melanoma by fluorescent in situ hybridization. *Invest Ophthalmol Vis Sci*. 2001;42:1679-1684.
5. Royds JA, Sharrard RM, Parsons MA, et al. C-myc oncogene expression in ocular melanomas. *Graefes Arch Clin Exp Ophthalmol*. 1992;230:366-371.
6. Dragovich T, Rudin CM, Thompson CB. Signal transduction pathways that regulate cell survival and cell death. *Oncogene*. 1998;17:3207-3213.

7. Prives C, Hall PA. The p53 pathway. *J Pathol.* 1999;187:112-126.

8. Brantley MA, Jr., Harbour JW. Deregulation of the Rb and p53 pathways in uveal melanoma. *Am J Pathol.* 2000;157:1795-1801.

9. Gross A, McDonnell JM, Korsmeyer SJ. BCL-2 family members and the mitochondria in apoptosis. *Genes Dev.* 1999;13:1899-1911.

10. Harbour JW, Worley L, Ma D, Cohen M. Transducible peptide therapy for uveal melanoma and retinoblastoma. *Arch Ophthalmol.* 2002;120:1341-1346.

11. Blasco MA. Telomeres and human disease: ageing, cancer and beyond. *Nat Rev Genet.* 2005;6:611-622.

12. Heine B, Coupland SE, Kneiff S, et al. Telomerase expression in uveal melanoma. *Br J Ophthalmol.* 2000;84:217-223.

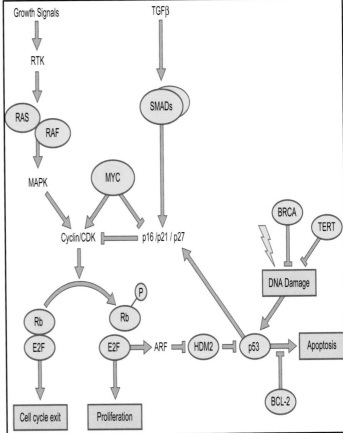

Figure 5-1. Major components of proliferative and apoptotic pathways are linked through a complex, interdependent network of interactions and pose a formidable obstacle to neoplastic transformation and cancer progression. Rb and p53 pathways are interconnected and form a cornerstone for the cellular strategy against neoplastic transformation. When Rb is hypophosphorylated and able to bind E2F transcription factors, it inhibits proliferation and promotes cell cycle exit (differentiation or senescence). Cancer cells overcome these tumor suppressor mechanisms by many different strategies that aim to disrupt the Rb-p53 network.

Principles of Cryotherapy

Dan S. Gombos

INTRODUCTION

Cryotherapy (or cryosurgery) is the technique of precise freezing and thawing of undesirable tissue, resulting in cell death and regression. The commercial availability of liquid nitrogen and the introduction of the cryoprobe by Cooper and Lee in the 1960s heralded significant advancements in the field.[1,2] For the ophthalmologist, modification of the cryoprobe led to significant surgical advances in cataract extraction, glaucoma management, and repair of retinal tears. Subsequent pioneering work by Lincoff,[3] Fraunfelder,[4] and Jakobiec[5] led to application of cryotherapy in the management of various intra- and periocular tumors.

In the mid 19th century, Arnott[1] described the use of crushed ice and salt (NaCl) to freeze advanced breast and uterine malignancies. By the beginning of the 20th century, solid CO_2 was being used to treat various skin and gynecologic cancers.[1]

MECHANISM OF TISSUE INJURY

Initially, the cryoprobe begins cooling the tissues by removing heat (Figure 6-1). Over time, tissue in contact with the probe freezes. Subsequently, the freezing interface progresses in an outward direction, resulting in a temperature distribution that is coldest at the point of contact with the probe. Once freezing is complete, thawing is facilitated by heat from the adjacent tissues.[1,6]

Direct Effects

Microscopically, the initial decline in temperature in the extracellular space forms crystals, leading to a hyperosmotic environment, extracting water from the cells and causing them to shrink. As the temperature lowers, intracellular crystals form, leading to disruption of organelles and cell membranes. This affects the ability of membrane proteins to control intracellular ionic content. During the thawing phase, as the frozen water crystals dissolve, the extracellular space becomes hypotonic. Limited only by a defective cell membrane, extracellular water enters the cell and disrupts it.[7] In addition, the cold temperature physically disrupts the cellular cytoskeleton and denatures proteins.[1,6]

Indirect Effects

Freezing temperatures are also associated with vascular stasis and cellular anoxia. Initially, the cold temperatures lead to vaso-constriction, followed by vasodilation, increased vascular permeability, and edema during the thawing process. Endothelial damage leads to stagnation of blood and the formation of thrombus. The resultant hypoxia promotes tissue necrosis. Some experiments suggest that this mechanism is more important in the death of tumor cells than direct injury from freezing.

TECHNICAL ASPECTS

Certain technical factors, such as tissue temperature, cooling rate, the freeze–thaw cycle, and the number of repetitions influence the efficacy of cryotherapy.[8,9]

Cooling Rate

A rapid cooling rate is more effective in causing cell death.

Freeze-Thaw Cycle

This is the most important factor, with cell death occurring at temperatures between −20°C and −50°C.[10] Studies indicate that a slow thaw is among the most important variables contributing to cell death.

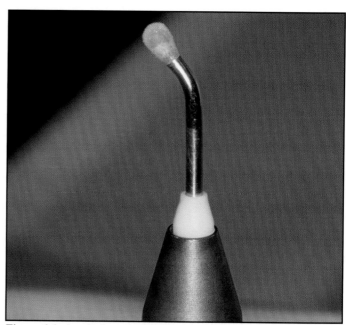

Figure 6-1. A retinal cryoprobe. Note the ice ball on the tip.

SECTION 1 Basic Principles

Number of Repetitions

Multiple freeze-thaw cycles further increase cell damage and death.[11]

INDICATIONS

Eyelid and Conjunctival Tumors

Basal cell carcinoma, particularly lesions less than 1 cm in diameter, can be cured with this approach. Select cases of squamous cell and meibomian gland carcinoma of the lid and conjunctiva have also been treated with cryotherapy as an alternative to surgery and/or radiotherapy.[12,13]

Intraocular Tumors

Certain intraocular tumors (particularly those anterior to the equator) are amenable to cryotherapy as the treatment of choice. Small peripheral retinal capillary hemangiomas,[14] Coats' disease, and retinoblastoma foci (those less than 2-mm thick) respond well to cryotherapy.[15]

Orbital Tumors

The cryoprobe can be used intraoperatively to assist in the excision of orbital lesions such as cavernous hemangioma and dermoid cysts.

COMPLICATIONS

Although cryotherapy is generally safe and effective, there are numerous complications that must be considered. In most instances, transient edema and injection occur at the site of treatment. Lesions on the eyelid and close to the lash margin can develop ptosis, trichiasis, and ectropion. Hypertrophic scarring can occur, as can skin depigmentation in darker patients. The conjunctiva generally tolerates freezing well. However, repeated application can lead to limbal stem cell failure, dry eye, and symblepharon formation. Periocular edema and pain due to uveitis are not uncommon following cryotherapy of intraocular lesions. Cryotherapy can increase the risk of exudative and rhegmatogenous retinal detachment, as well as vitreous hemorrhage.

REFERENCES

1. Rubinsky B. Cryosurgery. *Annu Rev Biomed Eng.* 2000;21:157-187.
2. Cooper I, Lee A. Cryostatic congelation: a system for producing a limited controlled region of cooling or freezing of biological tissue. *J Nerv Ment Dis.* 1961;1961:259-263.
3. Lincoff H, McLean J, Long R. The cryosurgical treatment of intraocular tumors. *Am J Ophthalmol.* 1967;63:389-399.
4. Fraunfelder FT, Wallis TR, Farris HE, et al. The role of cryosurgery in external ocular and periocular disease. *Trans Am Acad Ophthalmol Otolaryngol.* 1977;83:713-724.
5. Jakobiec FA, Rini FJ, Fraunfelder FT, et al. Cryotherapy for conjunctival primary acquired melanosis and malignant melanoma. Experience with 62 cases. *Ophthalmology.* 1988;95:1058-1070.
6. Gage AA, Baust J. Mechanisms of tissue injury in cryosurgery. *Cryobiology.* 1998;37:171-186.
7. Muldrew K, McGann LE. The osmotic rupture hypothesis of intracellular freezing injury. *Biophys J.* 1994;66:532-541.
8. Gage AA, Baust JG. Cryosurgery for tumors—a clinical overview. *Technol Cancer Res Treat.* 2004;3:187-199.
9. Baust JG, Gage AA. Progress towards optimization of cryosurgery. *Technol Cancer Res Treat.* 2004;3:95-101.
10. Gage AA. What temperature is lethal for cells? *J Dermatol Surg Oncol.* 1979;5:459-460.
11. Gill W, Fraser J, Carter D. Repeated freeze-thaw cycles in cryosurgery. *Nature.* 1968;219:410-413.
12. Fraunfelder FT, Zacarian SA, Wingfield DL, et al. Results of cryotherapy for eyelid malignancies. *Am J Ophthalmol.* 1984;97:184-188.
13. Shields JA, Shields CL, De Potter P. Surgical approach to conjunctival tumors. The 1994 Lynn B. McMahan Lecture. *Arch Ophthalmol.* 1997;115:808-815.
14. Singh AD, Nouri M, Shields CL, et al. Treatment of retinal capillary hemangioma. *Ophthalmology.* 2002;109:1799-1806.
15. Shields JA, Parsons H, Shields CL, et al. The role of cryotherapy in the management of retinoblastoma. *Am J Ophthalmol.* 1989;108:260-264.

Principles of Laser Therapy

Stefan Sacu and Ursula Schmidt-Erfurth

INTRODUCTION

In 1949, Meyer-Schwickerath created chorioretinal burns around retinal holes using the sun as the light source. A variety of different light sources were investigated in the prototype instruments before Carl Zeiss developed the first commercial model using a Xenon lamp in 1956.[1] Maiman and Gould (1960) invented the ruby laser, considered to be the first successful laser. The ruby laser was followed by the argon and krypton lasers.

BASIC CONSIDERATIONS

Laser Properties

LASER is an acronym for Light Amplification by the Stimulated Emission of Radiation. A laser beam is a monochromatic (single wavelength), coherent, and parallel beam of light, usually of high energy. The range of laser radiation extends from the ultraviolet through the visible to the infrared regions of the optical spectrum (Figure 7-1).[2]

Laser Output

Laser output can be continuous-wave or pulsed. Retinal photocoagulation is usually performed with a continuous-wave laser.

The output for retinal photocoagulation is usually delivered over a time interval of 0.1 to 1.0 sec.

Tissue Effects

There are two forms of interaction between light and ocular tissue: absorption and ionization. Ionization is primarily used to incise tissues of the eye (YAG capsulotomy). Absorption interaction is used in laser photocoagulation, thermotherapy, and photodynamic therapy.

Treatment Variables

Optical clarity of ocular tissues, the degree of absorption by ocular pigments, specific wavelengths used, spot size, power applied, and the exposure time are some of the important variables that influence the treatment effects.

Clarity of the Media

It is important to take opacities of the media into consideration as scattering and absorption of energy may occur while the laser travels toward the target tissue.[3] Longer wavelengths have less scattering and are more efficient in delivering energy.

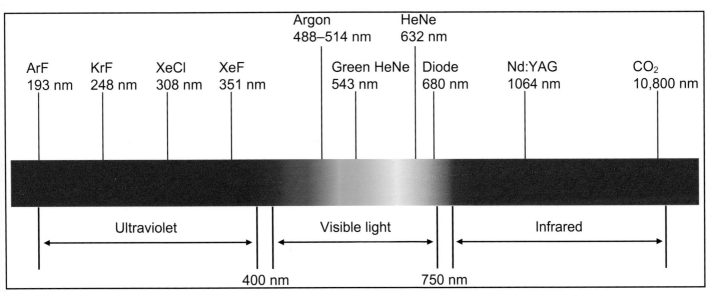

Figure 7-1. Electromagnetic spectrum of lasers used in ophthalmology.

Tissue Absorption

Tissue absorption spectrum of the three ocular pigments (melanin, hemoglobin, and xanthophyll) varies and can be used to achieve tissue selectivity of laser effects. Melanin has a maximum absorption between 400 and 600 nm (blue, green, yellow, and red) with greater absorption for shorter than longer wavelengths (Figure 7-2).[4]

Spot Size

The laser burn is round and proportional to the square of the radius. Decreasing a spot size requires a decrease in power level, while increasing a spot size requires a power increase.

Magnification Factor

The actual spot size on the retina and, therefore, laser irradiance is influenced by the magnification induced by the type of contact lens used.[3,5] With area centralis of the three-mirror Goldmann lens, the spot size setting on the slit lamp is about the same size as the actual burn on the retina.

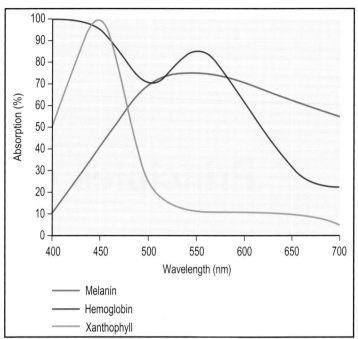

Figure 7-2. Absorption of visible wavelengths by three ocular pigments (melanin, hemoglobin, and xanthophyll). (This data was published in *Surv Ophthalmol,* 28, Peyman GA, Raichand M, Zeimer RC, Ocular effects of various laser wavelengths, 391-404, © Elsevier 1984.)

TYPES OF LASERS

Ruby Laser

A solid-state laser based on a pulsed ruby laser was the first commercially available ophthalmic laser photocoagulator and operated at a constant coagulation or exposure time of about 500 μs.

Argon Laser

This was the first laser system to enjoy broad acceptance. It is a continuous wave laser and emits two wavelengths: 514 nm (green) and 488 nm (blue). It is ideally suited for retinal use because there is excellent absorption at the level of the retinal pigment epithelium and the hemoglobin. Blue light-induced photochemical damage to the macula (due to xanthophyll) can be reduced by incorporating a green filter.

Krypton Laser

Krypton laser sources emitting 647 nm as a continuous wave overcome the absorption difficulties of the argon laser. Krypton is poorly absorbed by hemoglobin because it is a red source, so accidental coagulation of blood vessels can be avoided. The disadvantage of the argon laser and krypton laser is a low efficiency of laser production.[6]

Dye Laser

The dye laser has the same disadvantage as the argon or krypton laser. Additionally, the dye (rhodamine) is carcinogenic and requires special handling. Therefore, dye lasers are infrequently used today.[7]

Diode Laser

The diode laser is compact and portable. Despite their low input power, diode lasers may represent a significant hazard to vision, especially when the output is collimated, invisible, and of higher power (>3 to 5 mW).[8,9]

Holmium Laser

This laser has a CO_2 laser-like action. The holmium laser crystal is similar to the Nd:YAG laser in that the holmium atoms are distributed throughout a YAG host.

Excimer Laser

The excimer laser is a gas laser that generates a powerful ultraviolet beam. This technique can be used to ablate cornea to any depth.

TECHNIQUES OF LASER THERAPY

Laser Photocoagulation

This is the thermal denaturation of tissues using a high-intensity laser of the wavelength range that is intensively absorbed by hemoglobin or other ocular pigments.

Indications

Laser photocoagulation is used for a variety of chorioretinal diseases such as diabetic retinopathy, retinal tears or holes, age-related macular degeneration, and tumors such as retinal capillary hemangioma, choroidal hemangioma, and retinoblastoma.

Transpupillary Thermotherapy

Similar to laser photocoagulation, transpupillary thermotherapy (TTT) is based on the concept of tissue hyperthermia (Chapter 40).[10]

Photodynamic Therapy

In PDT, light and light absorbing agents such as verteporfin are combined in an oxygen-rich environment.[11] Verteporfin is a special dye with a light absorption peak at 692 nm. It is prepared in a 30-mL glucose solution at a dose of 6 mg per m² of the body surface area. During the first step, the patient receives a verteporfin infusion over 10 minutes through a cubital vein. Fifteen minutes after the start of the infusion, the fundus lesion receives a diode laser application via a slit-lamp delivery system and a hand-held contact lens. A light dose of 50 J/cm² is delivered at an intensity of 600 mW/cm^2 for 83 seconds as one spot covering the lesion in its greatest linear diameter plus a safety zone of 500 μm. The currently recommended treatment protocol has been proven to be safe and effective in the TAP and VIP trials.[12]

REFERENCES

1. L'Esperance FJ. *Ophthalmic Lasers*. St Louis, MO: CV Mosby, 1983; 340-350.
2. Kohnen T. Laser in eye surgery. www.krager.com/gazette. 2005.
3. Fankhauser F, Kwasniewska S, eds. *Laser in Ophthalmology. Basic, Diagnostic and Surgical Aspects*. The Hague: Kugler Publications; 2003.
4. Peyman GA, Raichand M, Zeimer RC. Ocular effects of various laser wavelengths. *Surv Ophthalmol*. 1984;28:391-404.
5. Dewey D. Corneal and retinal energy density with various laser beam delivery systems and contact lenses. *SPIE*. 1991;1423:105-116.
6. Marshall J, Bird A. A comparative histopathologic study of argon and krypton laser irradiation of the human retina. *Br J Ophthalmol*. 1979;63:657-668.
7. L'Esperance F Jr. Clinical photocoagulation with the organic dye laser. A preliminary communication. *Arch Ophthalmol*. 1985;103:1312-1316.
8. Noyori K, Shimizu K, Trokel S. *Ophthalmic Laser Therapy*. Tokyo: Igaku-Shoin; 1992.
9. Folk JC, Pulido JS. *Laser Photocoagulation of the Retina and Choroid*. San Francisco, CA: American Academy of Ophthalmology; 1997.
10. Oosterhuis JA, Journee-de Korver HG, Kakebeeke-Kemme HM, Bleeker JC. Transpupillary thermotherapy in choroidal melanomas. *Arch Ophthalmol*. 1995;113:315-321.
11. Schmidt-Erfurth U, Michels S, Barbazetto I, et al. Photodynamic effects on choroidal neovascularization and physiological choroid. *Invest Ophthalmol Vis Sci*. 2002;43:830-841.
12. Treatment of Age-Related Macular Degeneration with Photodynamic Therapy (TAP) Study Group. Photodynamic therapy of subfoveal choroidal neovascularization in age-related macular degeneration with verteporfin: two-year results of 2 randomized clinical trials—TAP report 2. *Arch Ophthalmol*. 2001;119:198-207.

Principles of Radiation Therapy

Carryn Anderson, Peter Fleming, Allan Wilkinson, and Arun D. Singh

INTRODUCTION

Radioactivity was first described by Henri Becquerel and Pierre and Marie Curie in the late 1890s. Wilhelm Roentgen discovered X-rays in 1895, and subsequent physics and biology research revealed the therapeutic properties of radiation.

BASIC PRINCIPLES

Radiation therapy takes advantage of the energy created by the interaction of electrons, protons, and neutrons with each other. This energy can break chemical bonds and create ions such as oxygen radicals.

Dual Nature of Radiation

Radiation can be in the form of electromagnetic waves, particles, or both.

Radioactive Decay

Radioactive elements are in an unstable, high-energy state and emit radiation to return to a stable, low-energy state. This process of returning to stability is called decay. Three different types of radiation can be emitted from the nucleus during this process: α particles with a positive electrical charge (helium nucleus), β particles with a negative charge (electrons), and γ rays with no electrical charge. Radioactive decay is the process utilized in cobalt-60 machines, gamma-knife radiotherapy, and brachytherapy.

TELETHERAPY SOURCES

Teletherapy is the process of delivering radiation from a remote distance. In modern clinical practice, a cobalt-60 unit, linear accelerator, or cyclotron is used to generate and deliver external-beam photon therapy and particle radiotherapy.

Cobalt-60 Unit

A cobalt-60 unit holds a radioactive cobalt source that emits γ radiation as it decays to nickel-60. The average energy of the γ photon beam is 1.25 million electron volts (MeV), with the maximum dose being delivered to a depth of 0.5 to 1 cm.

Linear Accelerator

A linear accelerator uses high-frequency electromagnetic waves to accelerate electrons to high energies through a linear vacuum tube. The monoenergetic electron beam can be used to treat superficial tumors. Typical energies used range from 6 to 18 MeV, with 80% of the maximum dose delivered to a depth of 2 to 6 cm and a relatively steep dose drop-off beyond this. When deeper tumors need to be treated or the skin needs to be spared, the linear accelerator electron beam is directed at a target (usually tungsten). The resultant atomic interactions produce a range of high-energy X-rays, also called photons. Photons are characteristically more penetrating than electrons.

Cyclotron

This is a heavy particle accelerator capable of producing neutron and proton beams. Proton beams have a unique dose distribution characteristic called the Bragg peak. There is a steep peak of maximal dose deposit and a sharp distal drop-off. This Bragg peak can be directed accurately and precisely on the tumor.[1] The sharp distal drop-off and the minimal scatter from the proton beam translates into less dose to surrounding normal tissues. Proton beam radiotherapy is used for treatment of uveal melanoma and retinoblastoma.[2,3] Proton beam radiotherapy of uveal melanoma is discussed in detail elsewhere (Chapter 43).

RADIATION PARAMETERS

Radiation Dose

Radiation absorbed dose is defined in grays (Gy), which represent 1 J of energy absorbed per kg mass. Centigray (cGy) is also commonly used, and this is 1/100th of a gray.

Relative Biological Effectiveness

Relative biological effectiveness (RBE) is a measure of the efficiency of a specific radiation in producing a specific biologic response. This can be expressed in the equation RBE = Ds/Dr, where Ds and Dr are the doses of standard radiation (250 kVp X-rays) and a test radiation (r) is needed to produce an equivalent biologic response. Protons and neutrons have greater biological effectiveness than photons and electrons.

Cobalt Gray Equivalents

The amount of absorbed dose from neutron and proton beams is higher than with X-ray or γ-ray beams. In order to compare to standard doses, the term cobalt gray equivalents (CGE) was developed: CGE = dose in proton or neutron gray multiplied by the corresponding RBE value.

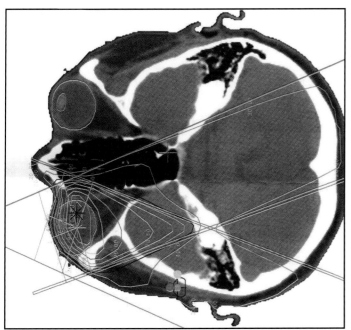

Figure 8-1. An example of external beam radiation planning with 6 MV photons to treat choroidal metastasis of the right eye. A right anterior oblique beam and a left anterior oblique beam are used.

TREATMENT PARAMETERS

Target Volume

Several target tissue volumes are considered when determining the prescription dose. Gross target volume (GTV) is the visible tumor extension. Clinical target volume (CTV) is the GTV plus margin to cover microscopic tumor extension. Planning target volume (PTV), the volume ultimately treated, is CTV plus a safety margin accounting for set-up variations and organ motion. The treatment margin beyond the CTV typically ranges from 0.5 to 2 cm, depending on the accuracy of the treatment machine, the immobilization device, and the tumor type.

Total Dose

The total dose given depends on tumor responsiveness, gross versus microscopic disease, the purpose of the radiation (curative or palliative), and limitations of surrounding normal tissues.

Fractionation

In general, the total dose is divided into fractions delivered over several weeks. Fractionation is used to minimize late radiation side effects. The larger fraction size (>200 cGy) is associated with a greater tendency for late side effects, such as severe dry eye, cataract, and optic neuropathy. On the other hand, reducing the fraction size diminishes the therapeutic effects of radiation (tumor kill). Conventional fractionation uses one treatment per day, at a dose of 180 to 200 cGy/fraction for 5 days a week. Recent data suggest that hyperfractionation (110 to 120 cGy/fraction twice daily) may reduce the risk of radiation retinopathy in patients treated for head and neck cancer.[4]

Tissue Tolerance

In treating ophthalmic tumors with external beam radiation, the exposure of several critical structures, such as the lens, optic nerve, opposite orbit, pituitary, and brain to radiation must be taken into account.[5]

TELETHERAPY TECHNIQUES

External Beam Therapy

When a patient is scheduled for external beam therapy, the first appointment is for simulation. During simulation, the patient is placed in the treatment position, including immobilization devices such as a mask. An MRI scanner, CT scanner, or fluoroscope is used to take images of the patient's anatomy in the treatment position. The tumor area and the surrounding normal structures are identified and contoured on the simulation images (Figure 8-1).

Conventional Radiation Therapy

Standard or conventional radiation therapy uses bony landmarks on fluoroscopy or external landmarks on physical examination to determine gross anatomical boundaries for field shapes and sizes.

Lens-Sparing Radiation Therapy

Several techniques of beam design and arrangements—so-called "lens-sparing radiation therapy"—have been developed to minimize exposure of the lens to radiation and to avoid radiation-induced cataract.[6]

Three-Dimensional Conformal Therapy

Three-dimensional conformal therapy (3D-CRT) is the technique of using CT or MRI simulation images to create a three-dimensional target.

Intensity-Modulated Radiation Therapy

In intensity-modulated radiation therapy, a process of inverse planning is often used, which means that the dose criteria are set before beam arrangements are designed. The computer generates a plan that best fits the specified criteria.

Stereotactic Radiosurgery

This procedure uses highly focused, precisely aimed radiation (usually within 0.5 mm of the specified isocenter) to treat small tumors (≤4 cm) at very high doses per fraction. Two forms of stereotactic radiosurgery exist: linac-based and gamma-knife (Chapter 44).[7,8]

BRACHYTHERAPY

Brachytherapy is the process of placing a radioactive source next to or within a tumor. Brachytherapy is used for the treatment of intraocular tumors such as choroidal metastases, uveal melanoma, and retinoblastoma (Chapter 44).

REFERENCES

1. Goitein M, Miller T. Planning proton therapy of the eye. *Med Phys.* 1983;10:275-283.
2. Gragoudas ES, Marie Lane A. Uveal melanoma: proton beam irradiation. *Ophthalmol Clin North Am.* 2005;18:111-118.
3. Krengli M, Hug EB, Adams JA, et al. Proton radiation therapy for retinoblastoma: comparison of various intraocular tumor locations and beam arrangements. *Int J Radiat Oncol Biol Phys.* 2005;61:583-593.

4. Monroe AT, Bhandare N, Morris CG, Mendenhall WM. Preventing radiation retinopathy with hyperfractionation. *Int J Radiat Oncol Biol Phys.* 2005;61:856-864.

5. Emami B, Lyman J, Brown A, et al. Tolerance of normal tissue to therapeutic irradiation. *Int J Radiat Oncol Biol Phys.* 1991;21:109-122.

6. Schipper J. An accurate and simple method for megavoltage radiation therapy of retinoblastoma. *Radiother Oncol.* 1983;1:31-41.

7. Zehetmayer M, Kitz K, Menapace R, et al. Local tumor control and morbidity after one to three fractions of stereotactic external beam irradiation for uveal melanoma. *Radiother Oncol.* 2000;55:135-144.

8. Rennie I, Forster D, Kemeny A, et al. The use of single fraction Leksell stereotactic radiosurgery in the treatment of uveal melanoma. *Acta Ophthalmol Scand.* 1996;74:558-562.

Ocular Complications of Radiotherapy

Mehran Taban, Mehryar Taban, James P. Bolling, and Arun D. Singh

INTRODUCTION

Ocular and orbital structures have a wide range of dose-dependent sensitivities to radiation exposure, and there is potential for functional, cosmetic, visual, and rarely lethal consequences.[1,2] Tissue tolerance to radiation is an important consideration in treatment planning.[3] In general, acute radiation effects (<4 weeks) manifest as the anterior segment changes and late complications (>4 weeks) involve the posterior segment and the orbital tissues.

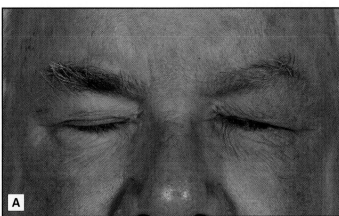

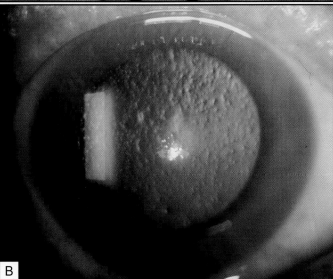

Figure 9-1. Acute complications of radiotherapy. Radiation dermatitis (A). Punctate keratitis (B).

EYELID/PERIORBITAL SKIN

Acute

Loss of eyelashes is one of the first and most common adverse effects that occur after radiotherapy; although, they usually grow back (Figure 9-1). Erythema may occur within hours of radiotherapy.[4] Desquamation and scaling of the skin can follow lower dose (10 Gy) radiation exposure, and more severe dermatitis occurs with higher doses of radiation (40 Gy).[4]

Late

Late sequelae include trichiasis, telangiectasia, hyperpigmentation, hyperkeratosis, entropion, ectropion, and punctal occlusion.[2,4]

CONJUNCTIVA

Acute

Conjunctivitis, chemosis, and a clear or purulent discharge may occur when radiotherapy doses of >5 Gy are used.[2,4]

Late

Late effects of radiotherapy to the conjunctiva include telangiectasia, symblepharon, and sequelae of loss of goblet cells (keratinization and scarring).[2,4] Dose of approximately 50 Gy leads to conjunctival scarring. Severe contracture occurs with doses of more than 60 Gy, and symblepharon is frequent with doses above 80 to 100 Gy.[5]

CORNEA

Acute

The corneal epithelium is affected with radiation doses of 10 to 20 Gy. Early effects include decreased corneal sensation, corneal epithelial defects, and punctate keratitis (Figure 9-1).[4]

Late

Late radiation effects to the cornea include keratinization, epithelial desquamation, corneal edema, corneal neovascularization, corneal ulceration, and corneal perforation.[2,4,5]

SCLERA

Sclera is the most radioresistant ocular structure, and it can tolerate radiation doses up to 900 Gy from radioactive plaques.[2,4]

IRIS

Acute iritis is dose related and occurs with at least a single dose of 20 Gy or a fractionated dose of >60 Gy.[4] The main long-term effects of irradiation to the iris include iris atrophy, posterior synechiae, rubeosis iridis, and neovascular glaucoma.[2,4]

LENS

The lens is the most radiosensitive structure of the eye, and cataract is a well-recognized long-term consequence of radiotherapy.[4] In most human studies, total fractionated doses less than 500 cGy have not produced visually significant lens opacities. Whereas a single dose as low as 2 Gy can induce cataract, higher doses of 10 to 15 Gy are required with fractionated radiotherapy to induce cataracts.[6] Radiation cataract usually presents 2 to 3 years later as posterior subcapsular opacification.[7] Prevention of cataract formation is best accomplished by fractionation of the radiation dose and by lens-shielding or lens-sparing techniques.[8]

ORBIT SOFT TISSUE, LACRIMAL GLAND, AND ORBITAL BONES

Orbit Soft Tissue

The late effects of radiation can induce enophthalmic socket.[9,10] Dry eyes are most commonly a result of radiation to the conjunctiva and only partially from delayed atrophy of the lacrimal gland associated with high doses (50 to 60 Gy) of radiation exposure.[2,11]

Lacrimal Gland

Effects of radiation on the orbital bones are most pronounced when external beam irradiation is applied to the growing facial bones of children.[9,10] Children with heritable retinoblastoma (bilateral or familial) are genetically predisposed to develop second malignant neoplasms later on in life (Chapter 71).

RADIATION RETINOPATHY

Radiation retinopathy is a delayed onset, slowly progressive occlusive retinal microangiopathy.[12] The median time to diagnosis of radiation retinopathy is about 2.6 years.[1,13,14]

Clinical Features

Doses of 40 to 60 Gy produced retinopathy only in 10% of the cases as compared with 30% of patients receiving more than 60 Gy (Figure 9-2). Hyperfractionation (two fractions/day) appears to reduce the risk of radiation retinopathy.[15-17] Following plaque radiotherapy (85 Gy apical dose), Kaplan-Meier estimates of nonproliferative and proliferative radiation retinopathy was 42% and 8% at 5 years, respectively.[18] The source of the radiation also influences the dose to other ocular structures.[19]

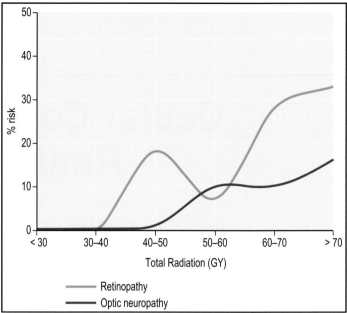

Figure 9-2. Total dose of radiation and risk of radiation retinopathy and radiation optic neuropathy. (This data was published in *Int J Radiat Oncol Biol Phys,* 61, Monroe AT, Bhandare N, Morris CG, Mendenhall WM, Preventing radiation retinopathy with hyperfractionation, 856-864, © Elsevier 2005 and *Int J Radiat Oncol Biol Phys,* 62, Bhandare N, Monroe AT, Morris CG, et al, Does altered fractionation influence the risk of radiation-induced optic neuropathy, 1070-1077, © Elsevier 2005.)

Nonproliferative Radiation Retinopathy

The earliest features of radiation retinopathy include discrete foci of occluded capillaries (cotton wool spots) and irregular dilatation of the neighboring retinal microvasculature (Figure 9-3).

Radiation Maculopathy

As the retinopathy progresses, microaneurysms, telangiectatic changes, exudation, and edema develop predominantly in the macular region.

Proliferative Radiation Retinopathy

Most patients who develop proliferative retinopathy develop the new vessels within 2 years of onset of radiation retinopathy.[20,21] Anterior segment neovascularization may also occur, leading to neovascular glaucoma.

Treatment

Extramacular radiation retinopathy (both nonproliferative and proliferative) responds well to sector laser photocoagulation and may even reduce the risk of developing radiation retinopathy if laser is applied prophylactically.[22]

However, it is the treatment of visually significant radiation maculopathy that has not been promising. The benefit of grid laser photocoagulation for the treatment of radiation maculopathy remains to be established.[23,24] Intravitreal triamcinolone provides only temporary resolution of retinal edema without any effect on underlying retinal ischemia.[25]

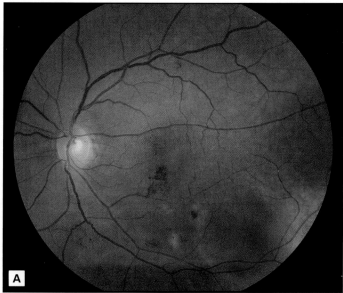

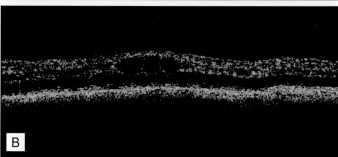

Figure 9-3. Characteristic features of nonproliferative radiation retinopathy such as cotton wool spots, telangiectasia, retinal hemorrhages, and macular edema following brachytherapy for choroidal melanoma (A). Cystoid macular edema on the optical coherent tomography (B).

RADIATION OPTIC NEUROPATHY

The diagnostic criteria of radiation optic neuropathy (RON) include acute loss of vision, visual field defects, onset of symptoms within 3 years of radiation therapy, and no evidence of visual pathway compression by neuroimaging.

Clinical Features

The incidence and latency of optic nerve injury after radiation is predominantly dose dependent (see Figure 9-2).[26] RON generally occurs with doses exceeding 50 Gy.[26] Shorter latency after plaque may be related to the higher dose and absence of fractionation with brachytherapy.[27] RON manifests acutely as disc swelling with surrounding exudates, hemorrhages, and subretinal fluid.[27] Optic atrophy may ensue in the later stages.

Treatment

As in the case of radiation retinopathy, there is as yet no effective treatment for visual loss after RON. High-dose steroids, anticoagulation, and hyperbaric oxygen have been tried without proven effectiveness.

Prognosis

The visual prognosis in RON is guarded.

REFERENCES

1. Monroe AT, Bhandare N, Morris CG, Mendenhall WM. Preventing radiation retinopathy with hyperfractionation. *Int J Radiat Oncol Biol Phys.* 2005;61:856-864.
2. Brady LW, Shields J, Augusburger J, et al. Complications from radiation therapy to the eye. *Front Radiat Ther Oncol.* 1989;23:238-250.
3. Emami B, Lyman J, Brown A, et al. Tolerance of normal tissue to therapeutic irradiation. *Int J Radiat Oncol Biol Phys.* 1991;21:109-122.
4. Servodidio CA, Abramson DH. Acute and long-term effects of radiation therapy to the eye in children. *Cancer Nurs.* 1993;16:371-381.
5. Hempel M, Hinkelbein W. Eye sequelae following external irradiation. *Recent Results Cancer Res.* 1993;130:231-236.
6. Merriam GR Jr, Szechter A, Focht EF. The effects of ionizing radiations on the eye. *Front Radiation Ther Onc.* 1972;6:346-385.
7. Cogan DG, Donaldson DD, Reese AB. Clinical and pathological characteristics of radiation cataract. *AMA Arch Ophthalmol.* 1952;47:55-70.
8. Hungerford JL, Toma NM, Plowman PN, et al. Whole-eye versus lens-sparing megavoltage therapy for retinoblastoma. *Front Radiat Ther Oncol.* 1997;30:81-87.
9. Heyn R, Ragab A, Raney RB Jr, et al. Late effects of therapy in orbital rhabdomyosarcoma in children. A report from the Intergroup Rhabdomyosarcoma Study. *Cancer.* 1986;57:1738-1743.
10. Larson DL, Kroll S, Jaffe N, et al. Long-term effects of radiotherapy in childhood and adolescence. *Am J Surg.* 1990;160:348-351.
11. Parsons JT, Fitzgerald CR, Hood CI, et al. The effects of irradiation on the eye and optic nerve. *Int J Radiat Oncol Biol Phys.* 1983;9:609-622.
12. Archer DB, Amoaku WM, Gardiner TA. Radiation retinopathy—clinical, histopathological, ultrastructural and experimental correlations. *Eye.* 1991;5:239-251.
13. Irvine AR, Wood IS. Radiation retinopathy as an experimental model for ischemic proliferative retinopathy and rubeosis iridis. *Am J Ophthalmol.* 1987;103:790-797.
14. Midena E, Segato T, Valenti M, et al. The effect of external eye irradiation on choroidal circulation. *Ophthalmology.* 1996;103:1651-1660.
15. Brown GC, Shields JA, Sanborn G, et al. Radiation retinopathy. *Ophthalmology.* 1982;89:1494-1501.
16. Gragoudas ES, Li W, Lane AM, et al. Risk factors for radiation maculopathy and papillopathy after intraocular irradiation. *Ophthalmology.* 1999;106:1571-1577.
17. Viebahn M, Barracks ME. Potentiating effect of diabetes in radiation retinopathy. *Int J Radiat Oncol Biol Phys.* 1993;25:379-380.
18. Gunduz K, Shields CL, Shields JA, et al. Radiation retinopathy following plaque radiotherapy for posterior uveal melanoma. *Arch Ophthalmol.* 1999;117:609-614.
19. Jaakkola A, Heikkonen J, Tommila P, et al. Strontium plaque brachytherapy for exudative age-related macular degeneration. *Ophthalmology.* 2005;112:567-573.
20. Kinyoun JL, Lawrence BS, Barlow WE. Proliferative radiation retinopathy. *Arch Ophthalmol.* 1996;114:1097-1100.
21. Amoaku WM, Archer DB. Fluorescein angiographic features, natural course and treatment of radiation retinopathy. *Eye.* 1990;4:657-667.
22. Finger PT, Kurli M. Laser photocoagulation for radiation retinopathy after ophthalmic plaque radiation therapy. *Br J Ophthalmol.* 2005;89:730-738.
23. Kinyoun JL, Zamber RW, Lawrence BS, et al. Photocoagulation treatment for clinically significant radiation macular oedema. *Br J Ophthalmol.* 1995;79:144-149.

24. Hykin PG, Shields CL, Shields JA, Arevalo JF. The efficacy of focal laser therapy in radiation-induced macular edema. *Ophthalmology.* 1998;105:1425-1429.

25. Sutter FK, Gillies MC. Intravitreal triamcinolone for radiation-induced macular edema. *Arch Ophthalmol.* 2003;121:1491-1493.

26. Bhandare N, Monroe AT, Morris CG, et al. Does altered fractionation influence the risk of radiation-induced optic neuropathy? *Int J Radiat Oncol Biol Phys.* 2005;62:1070-1077.

27. Brown GC, Shields JA, Sanborn G, et al. Radiation optic neuropathy. *Ophthalmology.* 1982;89:1489-1493.

Principles of Chemotherapy

Michael Levien, Jennifer Gravette, and Joanne Hilden

INTRODUCTION

The overall survival rate for cancer has improved dramatically since the institution of chemotherapy for the treatment of childhood leukemia in the 1940s.[1] The ultimate prognosis for each cancer is contingent on the histologic type, the extent of disease, and several other biologic parameters.[2] Recent progress in molecular biology, biochemistry, and genetics has provided new insights into the complex molecular changes associated with malignant transformation of a cell. These discoveries are offering new classes of drug that are being currently evaluated in clinical trials along with conventional agents.[3]

BASIC PRINCIPLES

Most conventional anti-cancer drugs have non-selective mechanisms of action that target DNA, RNA, or metabolic pathways in both malignant and normal cells. In the latter, undesirable and potentially severe toxic effects can result.

Mechanism of Action

Alkylating agents such as cyclophosphamide, cisplatinum, and carboplatinum damage DNA by covalently binding to and cross-linking nucleosides within the DNA.

Antimetabolites such as methotrexate block the synthesis of nucleotide precursors, or are incorporated directly into DNA as fraudulent bases. Topoisomerases are nuclear enzymes that maintain the three-dimensional structure of DNA, critical for DNA replication, transcription, and recombination. Etoposide (VP-16), anthracyclines (doxorubicin), and camptothecins (topotecan, irenotecan) interfere with the religation of DNA, resulting in DNA strand breaks.

A relatively new class of chemotherapy drugs, such as the monoclonal antibody rituxan (anti-CD 20), has been used successfully in the treatment of CD 20-positive non-Hodgkin's lymphomas. Other agents such as prednisone, cyclosporin, and interferons alter immune system function. Thalidomide, because of its anti-angiogenic effects, has become important in the treatment of chemotherapy-resistant brain tumors.

The Cell Generation Cycle

Drugs affect different stages of the cell cycle (Figure 10-1). Knowledge of the normal cell cycle and how different chemotherapeutic anti-cancer drugs disrupt this cycle is integral in helping to develop effective chemotherapy regimens. Agents that are cell-cycle phase specific will kill a fraction of cells passing through that phase of the cycle. On the other hand, agents that are not phase specific produce a continuous exponential decrease in cell survival because they affect all cells, regardless of their phase in the cycle.[4,5]

Tumor Cell Kinetic Model

Exposing a tumor to a drug at a predetermined concentration over an established period will result in a constant fraction of tumor cells being killed, regardless of tumor size.

This fractional cell kill hypothesis forms the rationale for repeated courses of therapy at maximum tolerated doses. The chemotherapy is given in cycles as soon as blood counts recover to achieve the goal of reducing tumor cells to zero.[5]

Combination Regimen

The use of combination chemotherapy with alternating regimens of non-cross-resistant drugs decreases the incidence of the development of drug resistance. The most successful combination chemotherapy uses agents that also have additive or synergistic mechanisms of action, with non-overlapping toxicities (if possible) to allow each agent to be used at optimal dosing.[4] This approach has contributed to the significant improvement in survival (90% cure rate) in acute lymphocytic leukemia.[6]

DRUG RESISTANCE

Resistance to anti-cancer drugs is the primary reason for treatment failure in cancer patients. Drug resistance can be present at diagnosis or can develop over time by exposure to chemotherapy. Cancer cells undergo spontaneous generation of drug-resistant clones by mutation, deletion, gene amplification, translocation, or chromosomal rearrangement. This is due to the inherent genetic instability of each cancer cell. Drug resistance can target a single drug or multiple drugs.

DRUG DEVELOPMENT

The initial critical step in the development of anti-cancer drugs is to identify new candidate drugs. The National Cancer Institute's Drug Screening Program uses a panel of 60 human tumor cell lines to identify new candidate drugs. The screening program identifies more than 10,000 new chemical agents per

Table 10-1. Multidisciplinary Treatment of Common Ophthalmic Tumors			
Tumor	Chemotherapy	Surgery	Radiotherapy
Orbital rhabdomyosarcoma (embryonal: non-metastatic)	Vincristine Actinomycin D	+	+
Optic nerve glioma	Vincristine + carboplatin Vincristine + actinomycin D Velban	±	+ (age >5 years)
Retinoblastoma (non-metastatic)	Vincristine + etoposide + carboplatin	+	+
Retinoblastoma (metastatic)	Vincristine + etoposide + carboplatin	+	+
Uveal melanoma (non-metastatic)	Multiagent	+	
Uveal melanoma (metastatic)	Multiagent	+	
Conjunctival melanoma (non-metastatic)	±	+	-
Conjunctival squamous cell carcinoma (non-metastatic)	±	+	-

year. New gene chip technology has now been incorporated into the NCI's drug screening program. Candidate compounds are then tested in mice and dogs to determine the maximum tolerated dose (MTD). Pharmacokinetic parameters are also studied in animals to establish a safe starting dose for human clinical trials.[3,5,7]

CLINICAL TRIALS

Phase I

A phase I trial is designed to determine the MTD for a specific dosing schedule, define the toxicity profile in humans, identify dose-limiting toxicities, and study the pharmacokinetics of a drug. Phase I studies are open to patients who have had relapse(s) and have exhausted standard and established therapies. Usually a small numbers of patients (15 to 30) are enrolled, and the dose is then escalated in successive cohorts of three to six patients until a dose-limiting toxicity is consistently observed.

Phase II

After the optimal dose and schedule for a new drug is determined, phase II trials are conducted to determine the spectrum of anti-tumor activity and the response rate of the drug against a number of different tumors. Patients who have failed standard therapy are eligible for phase II trials.[3,8]

Phase III

New chemotherapy agents that have successfully been tested in phase I and II trials enter into phase III trials. Phase III trials are randomized studies in which new agents are studied in previously untreated patients (standard therapy and new agent versus standard therapy alone). Additional factors that must be considered in the development of treatment protocols include the drug's mechanism of action, pharmacokinetics, toxicities, potential drug interactions, and mechanisms of drug resistance.[1,6]

SIDE EFFECTS

Anti-neoplastic drugs have the lowest therapeutic index of any class of drug. They therefore predictably produce significant, and at times life-threatening, toxicities. The oncologist must balance the risk of toxicities against the risk of relapse as a result

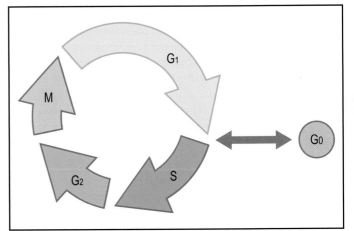

Figure 10-1. The cell generation cycle is divided into four phases. G1 begins immediately after mitosis. It is a period when the cell carries on its usual non-mitotic functions. It lasts until the beginning of the S phase. The S phase is the synthetic period when the genome is replicated. G2 is the period between the end of DNA synthesis and the beginning of cell division. M phase is the mitotic phase during which chromosome condensation occurs, the mitotic spindle appears, sister chromosomes separate, and the process of cell division occurs. G0 cells are those that have left the cycling pool. Cells that are temporarily in G0 can be recruited back into the proliferative cycle by appropriate growth factors. Some G0 cells may be terminally differentiated and cannot be recruited back into the proliferative cycle.

of inadequate treatment. Even a small reduction or delay in therapy to mitigate toxicities can result in tumor recurrence, which may lead to the death of the patient.

MULTIMODALITY THERAPY

At times, other treatment modalities, such as surgery and radiation therapy, are used in conjunction with chemotherapy for maximal clinical benefit.

Adjuvant Chemotherapy

Some patients receive local therapy at diagnosis (surgery and/or radiation therapy) to the primary tumor prior to chemotherapy (Table 10-1).

Neo-Adjuvant Chemotherapy

In the neo-adjuvant setting, patients receive chemotherapy at diagnosis to reduce the cancer burden prior to local measures being undertaken. In retinoblastoma, chemotherapy is used as a chemoreductive approach (neo-adjuvant therapy). Currently, six cycles of vincristine, etoposide (VP-16), and carboplatinum are given every 3 to 4 weeks. This is followed by local measures such as thermotherapy, cryotherapy, and plaque radiotherapy to treat intraocular tumors so as to avoid the use of external beam radiotherapy and enucleation.

REFERENCES

1. Balis F, Holcenberg J, Blaney S. General principles of chemotherapy. In: Pizzo P, Poplack D, eds. *Principles and Practice of Pediatric Oncology.* 4th ed. Philadelphia, PA: Lippincott, Williams & Wilkins; 2002.
2. Levien M. Clinical signs and prognostic factors in common pediatric malignancies. In: Sabella C, Cunningham R, Moodie D, eds. *Intensive Review of Pediatrics.* Philadelphia, PA: Lippincott, Williams & Wilkins; 2003.
3. Berg S, Poplack D. Pharmacology of antineoplastic agents and multidrug resistance. In: Nathan D, Orkin S, Ginsberg D, Look AT, eds. *Nathan and Oski's Hematology of Infancy and Childhood.* 6th ed. Philadelphia, PA: WB Saunders; 2003.
4. Berger N, Lazarus H. Medical therapy of hematologic malignancies. In: Handin R, Lux S, Stossel T, eds. *Blood, Principles and Practice of Hematology.* Philadelphia, PA: JB Lippincott; 1995.
5. Chabner B, Allegra C, Curt G, Calabresi P. Antineoplastic agents. In: Hardman J, Limbird L, Molinoff P, et al, eds. *Goodman and Gilman's The Pharmacologic Basis of Therapeutics.* 9th ed. New York, NY: McGraw-Hill; 1996:1233-1287.
6. Steinherz PG. Acute lymphoblastic leukemia of childhood. *Hematol Oncol Clin North Am.* 1987;1:549-566.
7. Newell DR. Pharmacologically based phase I trials in cancer chemotherapy. *Hematol Oncol Clin North Am.* 1994;8:257-275.
8. Chan HS, Gallie BL, Munier FL, Beck Popovic M. Chemotherapy for retinoblastoma. *Ophthalmol Clin North Am.* 2005;18:55-63.

Counseling Patients With Cancer

Sharon Cook and Bertil E. Damato

INTRODUCTION

Every oncology service should have systems for providing appropriate psychological support to patients and their relatives.

EMOTIONS AND FEARS

It is common for people with cancer to experience psychological distress, which is an understandable response to a traumatic and threatening life event. For the majority, this distress will be a short-lived experience, not causing lasting problems. In such cases, it can be understood as part of the patient's normal adjustment to his or her diagnosis. However, for some, the diagnoses and treatment for cancer increases the risk of developing depression, anxiety, and other forms of psychological morbidity such as adjustment disorder.

PATIENTS' NEEDS

Most patients want to be informed about their condition and its treatment, and are usually keen to be involved in decisions about their treatment and care.[1] However, it should be noted that patients vary in the amount of information they want and that this changes over time.[2] Above all, patients want to be treated as individuals, to have the opportunity to have their say and to feel understood.

COMMUNICATION

Effective communication is key to eliciting and addressing patients' psychological needs (Box 11-1). It also fosters good relationships between the patients and their caregivers. Patients' psychological well-being is greatly influenced by the way in which they are informed about their diagnosis and treatment. The manner in which health care staff respond to patients' concerns is also important.[3,4] If information is poorly communicated and

---

Box 11-1. Requirements for Effective Communication

- Quiet surroundings, free of interruptions and distractions
- Compassion and empathy
- Close friend or relative accompanying patient
- Respect for how much they wish to know
- Opportunity to ask questions and express opinions
- Help remembering what was said
- Chance to speak to previously treated patients

---

patients concerns are left undisclosed and unresolved, patients can become confused and resentful and have a high risk of developing clinical anxiety or depression.[3,5] If done well, communication can lessen distress and assist understanding and adaptation.[4,5] Increasingly in Britain, correspondence to the family doctor and general ophthalmologist is also sent to the patient.

REFERENCES

1. White CA. *Cognitive Behaviour Therapy for Chronic Medical Problems*. Chichester: Wiley; 2001.
2. Leydon GM, Boulton M, Moynihan C, Jones A, Mossman J, Boudioni M, et al. Cancer patients' information needs and information seeking behaviour: in depth interview study. *BMJ* 2000;320:909-913.
3. Maguire P. Breaking bad news. *Eur J Surg Oncol* 1998;24:188-191.
4. Brennan J. *Cancer in Context*. Oxford: Oxford University Press 2004.
5. Fallowfield L, Jenkins V. Communicating sad, bad, and difficult news in medicine. *Lancet*. 2004;363:312-319.

Chapter

12

Examination Techniques

Julian D. Perry

HISTORY

The history begins with a description of the symptoms and their severity, onset, and rate of progression.

Rate of onset and progression of symptoms helps characterize the pathology.

Past Medical History

Because the majority of eyelid neoplasia are epidermal in origin, the past medical history should focus on risk factors for epidermal malignancy. Information should be obtained regarding family history of cutaneous malignancy, skin type, freckle density, eye color, hair color, and prior history of skin cancer. The history should also describe tobacco use, prior radiotherapy, sun exposure, and similar growths elsewhere on the skin.

EXAMINATION

The physical examination should include a comprehensive inspection of the eyelid, ocular adnexa and orbit, eye, and other cutaneous lesions.

Eyelid Examination

The eyelid examination should characterize the appearance of the lesion as well as associated anatomical deformities and palpation. The dimensions should be measured using a ruler or slit-lamp beam. Areas of telangiectasia, nodularity, pearly translucency, ulceration, bleeding, crusting, irregularity of the eyelid margin, and loss of cilia should be particularly looked for, as these features are suggestive of malignancy (Figure 12-1).

Ocular Adnexal Examination

Eyelid tumors may spread directly to the lacrimal gland, orbit, or lacrimal outflow apparatus. Conversely, primary tumors of these areas can occasionally present with only eyelid signs and symptoms. The structure and function of the orbit and ocular adnexal tissues in proximity to the lesion should be evaluated. Cranial nerves V and VII should be tested carefully to assess for possible perineural spread of an eyelid malignancy.

Eye examination should focus on detecting findings caused by or associated with the eyelid lesion. The conjunctiva and

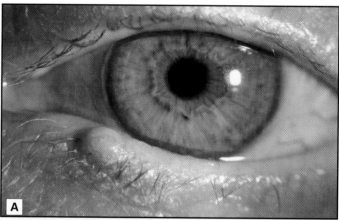

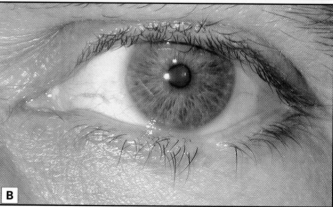

Figure 12-1. Lower eyelid showing a benign nodule without loss of lashes (A) and loss of eyelid tissue with cilia loss secondary to a malignant tumor (B).

cornea should be inspected for signs of mechanical or exposure keratoconjunctivitis using the slit lamp. The sclera and episclera should be observed for pigmentary changes during the evaluation of an eyelid nevus. Direct intraocular extension of eyelid tumors is extremely rare, but funduscopy should be performed to observe for signs of ocular or orbital involvement (choroidal folds, venous congestion) in suspected cases.

Chapter

13

Classification and Differential Diagnosis of Eyelid Tumors

Jacob Pe'er

INTRODUCTION

Despite being a small organ, the eyelid contains numerous histological elements that can be the origin of several types of benign or malignant tumors.

ANATOMICAL FEATURES

The eyelids are composed of four layers: skin and subcutaneous tissue, striated muscle (orbicular oculi), tarsus, and conjunctiva (Figure 13-1).[1] The rest of the orbital entrance, which clinically may be considered as part of the eyelids, is covered, behind the skin and the orbicularis muscle, by the orbital septum that holds back the orbital fat.

CLASSIFICATION OF EYELID TUMORS

Tumors of the eyelid may be classified according to their tissue or cell of origin and as benign or malignant. In most groups of tumors, unique histological subtypes behave differently in spite of having the same cell of origin (Table 13-1).[2] The vast majority of eyelid tumors, benign and malignant, are of epidermal origin. They are divided into nonmelanocytic and melanocytic tumors. Benign epithelial proliferations, basal cell carcinoma, cystic structures, and melanocytic nevi represent about 85% of all eyelid tumors.[3,4] Squamous cell carcinoma and melanoma are relatively rare.[4] Tumors arising from adnexal glands are very rare.

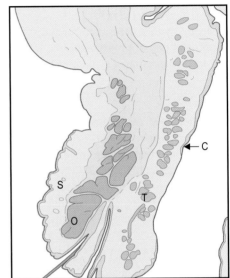

Figure 13-1. A cross-section through the eyelid. S-skin, O-orbicularis oculi muscle, T-tarsal plate, C-conjunctiva.

REFERENCES

1. Bedrossian EH. Embryology and anatomy of the eyelid. In: Tasman W, Jaeger EA. *Duane's Foundation of Clinical Ophthalmology.* Volume 1: Ocular anatomy, embryology and teratology. Philadelphia, PA: Lippincott Williams & Wilkins; 2004:1-24.
2. Campbell RJ, Sobin LH. Tumours of the eyelid. *Histological Typing of Tumours of the Eye and Its Adnexa.* 2nd ed. World Health Organization International Histological Classification of Tumors. Berlin: Springer Verlag; 1998:3-9.
3. Kersten RC, Ewing-Chow D, Kulwin DR, Gallon M. Accuracy of clinical diagnosis of cutaneous eyelid lesions. *Ophthalmology.* 1997;104:479-484.
4. Cook BE, Bartley GB. Epidemiologic characteristics and clinical course of patients with malignant eyelid tumors in an incidence cohort in Olmsted County, Minnesota. *Ophthalmology.* 1999;106:746-750.

Table 13-1. Major Types of Eyelid Tumors		
Category	Subtypes	
Epidermal tumors	Non-melanocytic tumors	Melanocytic tumors
Adnexal tumors	Sebaceous gland tumors	Hair follicle tumors
	Sweat gland tumors	Cystic lesions
Stromal tumors	Fibrous tissue tumors	Fibrohistiocytic tumors
	Lipomatous tumors	Neural tumors
	Smooth muscle tumors	Skeletal muscle tumors
	Vascular tumors	Perivascular tumors
	Lymphoid and plasmacytic	Cartilage and bone tumors
	Hamartoma	Choristoma
Secondary tumors		
Metastatic tumors		
Inflammatory and infectious lesions that simulate neoplasms		

Benign Epidermal Tumors

Edoardo Midena, Valentina de Belvis, Lynn Schoenfield, and Arun D. Singh

NON-MELANOCYTIC EPIDERMAL TUMORS

Squamous Cell Papilloma

This is a common benign tumor of the eyelid that occurs in middle-aged or older adults appearing as either a pedunculated or a sessile nodular growth with a convoluted surface (Table 14-1). Histopathologically, benign squamous epithelium with variable acanthosis and hyperkeratosis overlies a fibrovascular core (Figure 14-1).

Seborrheic Keratosis

This is a commonly acquired eyelid lesion affecting middle-aged and elderly patients. It usually appears as a lobulated, papillary or pedunculated mass with friable, cerebriform excrescences on the surface (Figure 14-2).[1]

Keratoacanthoma

The lesion begins as a small flesh-colored papule on the lower lid that develops rapidly over the course of a few weeks into a cup-shaped configuration with a central, keratin-filled crater with elevated rolled margins.[2]

Non-Specific Keratosis

Cutaneous horn is a clinically descriptive, non-diagnostic term for a non-specific keratosis (hyperkeratotic lesion, either benign or malignant).

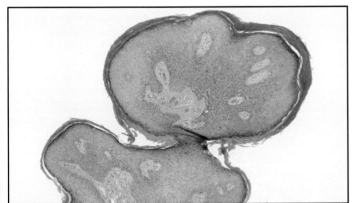

Figure 14-1. Squamous papilloma. Polypoid lesion consisting of benign squamous epithelium with variable acanthosis and hyperkeratosis overlying a fibrovascular core. (Hematoxylin and eosin; original magnification x4.)

Actinic (Solar) Keratosis

This is a result of damage to the epidermal cells of the skin and dermal collagen by ultraviolet radiation. Fair-skinned, older patients and those with a history of excessive sun exposure are typically affected.

Intraepithelial Neoplasia

High-grade squamous intraepithelial neoplasia is also considered equivalent to squamous carcinoma in situ. It occurs most commonly in fair-skinned elderly individuals who have a history of chronic sun exposure.[3]

MELANOCYTIC EPIDERMAL TUMORS

Melanocytic nevus is considered a benign tumor of neural crest-derived melanocytes.[4] An eyelid nevus can be congenital or acquired.

Congenital nevus is present in about 1% of newborns.[5] The congenital nevi are classified by their largest diameter as small (<1.5 cm), medium (1.5 to 19.9 cm), and large or giant congenital melanocytic nevi (>20 cm).[6]

Clinicopathologic Variants

- Neurocutaneous melanosis (NCM) is a rare association of multiple and large congenital cutaneous nevi and meningeal melanosis or melanoma.[7]
- Split nevus (kissing nevus) is a variant of congenital compound nevus involving both upper and lower eyelids.[8]
- Blue nevus arises from dermal, deeply located melanocytes that have been arrested in the dermis before reaching the epidermis.[9]
- Nevus of ota (oculodermal melanocytosis) occurs as a bluish discoloration of the eyelids, periorbital skin, and episclera.[10]

Acquired nevus develops between the ages of 5 and 10 years. Mild to moderate sun exposure in early life induces the development of nevi.[11] Atypical or dysplastic nevi are present in 2% to 5% of the white population. Such nevi are larger (>5 mm), with ill-defined borders, and are variegated in color.[12] Atypical nevi are associated with an increased risk for melanoma.

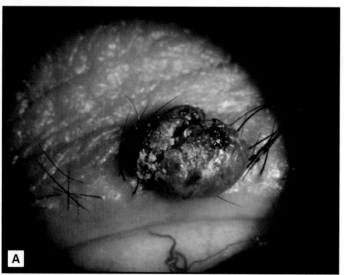
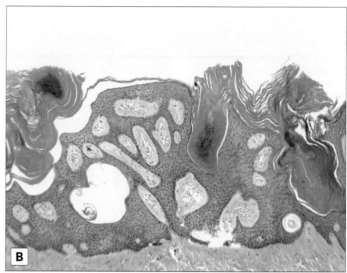

Figure 14-2. Seborrheic keratosis. Upper eyelid involvement in a 75-year-old man (A). Retiform pattern of squamous epithelium surrounding islands of connective tissue and composed of sheets of basaloid cells with keratin-filled horn pseudocysts (B). (Hematoxylin and eosin; original magnification x10.)

REFERENCES

1. Font RL. Eyelids and lacrimal drainage system. In: Spencer WH, ed. *Ophthalmic Pathology. An Atlas and Textbook*. Philadelphia, PA: WB Saunders; 1996:2229-2232.

2. Schwartz RA. Keratoacanthoma: a clinico-pathologic enigma. *Dermatol Surg.* 2004;30:326-333; discussion 333.

3. Lebwohl M. Actinic keratosis: epidemiology and progression to squamous cell carcinoma. *Br J Dermatol.* 2003;149(Suppl 66):31-33.

4. Krengel S. Nevogenesis—new thoughts regarding a classical problem. *Am J Dermatopathol.* 2005;27:456-465.

5. Tannous ZS, Mihm MC Jr, Sober AJ, Duncan LM. Congenital melanocytic nevi: clinical and histopathologic features, risk of melanoma, and clinical management. *J Am Acad Dermatol.* 2005;52:197-203.

6. Kopf AW, Bart RS, Hennessey P. Congenital nevocytic nevi and malignant melanomas. *J Am Acad Dermatol.* 1979;1:123-130.

7. Makkar HS, Frieden IJ. Neurocutaneous melanosis. *Semin Cutan Med Surg.* 2004;23:138-144.

8. McDonnell PJ, Mayou BJ. Congenital divided naevus of the eyelids. *Br J Ophthalmol.* 1988;72:198-201.

9. Gunduz K, Shields JA, Shields CL, Eagle RC Jr. Periorbital cellular blue nevus leading to orbitopalpebral and intracranial melanoma. *Ophthalmology.* 1998;105:2046-2050.

10. Singh AD, De Potter P, Fijal BA, et al. Lifetime prevalence of uveal melanoma in white patients with oculo(dermal) melanocytosis. *Ophthalmology.* 1998;105:195-198.

11. Wiecker TS, Luther H, Buettner P, Bauer J, Garbe C. Moderate sun exposure and nevus counts in parents are associated with development of melanocytic nevi in childhood: a risk factor study in 1,812 kindergarten children. *Cancer.* 2003;97:628-638.

12. NIH Consensus conference. Diagnosis and treatment of early melanoma. *JAMA.* 1992;268:1314-1319.

Table 14-1. Classification of Epidermal Tumors of the Eyelid

Types	Subtypes	
Non-melanocytic	Benign	Squamous cell papilloma
		Seborrheic keratosis
		Inverted follicular keratosis
		Reactive hyperplasia (pseudoepitheliomatous hyperplasia)
	Premalignant	Actinic (solar) keratosis
		Intraepithelial neoplasia
		Sebaceous nevus (of Jadassohn)
	Malignant	Basal cell carcinoma
		Squamous cell carcinoma
		Keratoacanthoma
Melanocytic	Epithelial pigmentation	Ephelis or freckles
		Lentigo simplex
		Solar lentigo
	Benign	Junctional nevus
		Intradermal nevus
		Compound nevus
		Spitz nevus
		Balloon cell nevus
		Blue nevus
		Cellular blue nevus
		Oculodermal nevus of Ota
	Premalignant	Congenital dysplastic nevus
		Lentigo maligna (melanotic freckle of Hutchinson)
	Malignant	Melanoma arising from nevi
		Melanoma arising in lentigo maligna
		Melanoma arising de novo

Basal Cell Carcinoma

Mordechai Rosner

INTRODUCTION

Basal cell carcinoma (BCC) is a malignant cutaneous neoplasm capable of extensive tissue destruction. It is often observed on the head and neck, and the eyelids are a common location.[1]

BCC is the most common human malignancy and accounts for nearly 90% of all non-melanoma skin cancers. It is also the most common skin cancer of the eyelid, accounting for 80% to 90% of cases. In the United States, the incidence of BCC is more than 500 per 100,000, and in parts of Australia it reaches 2400 per 100,000.[1-3]

ETIOLOGY

The risk factors for periocular BCC include ultraviolet (UV) irradiation, local and systemic immune dysfunction, previous ionizing radiation, and focal trauma.[1] Genetic or congenital diseases predisposing to BCC are Gorlin–Goltz syndrome, xeroderma pigmentosum, albinism, Basex–Dupré syndrome, Muir–Torre syndrome, Rombo syndrome, linear basocellular hamartoma, and sebaceous hamartoma of Jadassohn.

CLINICAL FEATURES

The average age at diagnosis for BCC of the eyelid is 60 years. However, rarely, a solitary BCC may arise in an adolescent or young adult who has no known risk factors (Figure 15-1).

HISTOPATHOLOGIC FEATURES

Histopathologically, BCC is characterized by a proliferation of cells with oval nuclei and scant cytoplasm that form infiltrative nests or strands (Figure 15-2). The neoplastic cells are relatively uniform in appearance and seldom display significant anaplasia or mitotic figures. At the periphery of the nests, they are usually arranged in a radial pattern called "palisading" (see Figure 15-2). Although this is not diagnostic, in its absence the diagnosis of BCC should be questioned. The two most important growth patterns are the circumscribed and the infiltrative.

DIFFERENTIAL DIAGNOSIS

BCC is by far the most common malignant lesion of the periocular skin; therefore, most periocular nodular or cystic skin lesions should be treated as suspicious. Challenging examples are trichoepithelioma and desmoplastic trichoepithelioma, metastatic carcinoma, sebaceous carcinoma, squamous cell carcinoma, and keratoacanthoma.

TREATMENT

The main treatment modality for BCC is surgical excision of the lesion with microscopic monitoring of its margins, or Mohs' microsurgery.[1,4] The other modalities include curettage and electrodessication, cryosurgery, radiotherapy, chemotherapy, photodynamic therapy, and immunotherapy. Selection of the appropriate therapy depends on the patient's age, anticipated life expectancy, and the location, size, and pattern of growth.

PROGNOSIS

Prognostic Factors

The morpheaform clinical pattern, the histologic finding of an infiltrative growth pattern, or metatypical (basosquamous carcinoma) differentiation have been correlated with deep invasion and greater recurrence after treatment.[1]

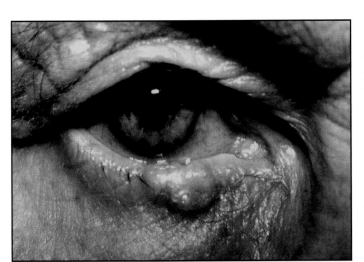

Figure 15-1. Nodular BCC of the lower lid margin, presenting as an irregular, pearly dome-shaped tumor.

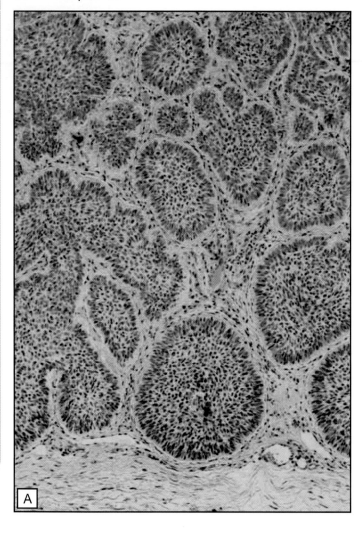

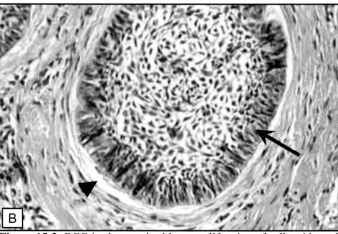

Figure 15-2. BCC is characterized by a proliferation of cells with oval nuclei and scant cytoplasm that form infiltrative nests or strands (A). At the periphery of the nests, the tumor cells are usually arranged in a radial pattern called "palisading" (arrow), and these are characteristically retracted from the stroma, creating a gap (arrowhead) (B).

Local Spread

The vast majority of BCC grow in a slow but relentless manner. BCC invades along the paths of least resistance followed by destruction of bone, cartilage, and muscle in the very late stages.

Recurrence rate of treated BCC of the eyelid averages 4.2% in the short term and 8.7% for more than 5 years.

Mortality from eyelid and medial canthal BCC is rare, and all deaths recorded were related to intracranial extension.

REFERENCES

1. Margo CE, Waltz K. Basal cell carcinoma of the eyelid and periocular skin. *Surv Ophthalmol.* 1993;38:169-192.
2. Allali J, D'Hermies F, Renard G. Basal cell carcinomas of the eyelids. *Ophthalmologica.* 2005;219:57-71.
3. Malhotra R, Huilgol SC, Huynh NT, Selva D. The Australian Mohs Database, Part I: periocular basal cell carcinoma. Experience over 7 years. *Ophthalmology.* 2004;111:624-630.
4. Cook BE Jr, Bartley GB. Treatment options and future prospects for the management of eyelid malignancies: an evidence-based update. *Ophthalmology.* 2001;108:2088-2098.

Squamous Cell Carcinoma

Mordechai Rosner

INTRODUCTION

Squamous cell carcinoma (SCC) is an invasive epithelial malignancy that arises from the prickle-squamous cell layers of the epidermis and shows keratinocytic differentiation. The terms *squamous cell epithelioma, epidermoid carcinoma, epithelioma spinocellular, prickle cell epithelioma,* and *spinalioma* have all been used in the literature, but *squamous cell carcinoma* is the preferred terminology.[1]

EPIDEMIOLOGICAL ASPECTS

SCC is the second most common malignant neoplasm of the eyelids after basal cell carcinoma (BCC), comprising 5% to 10% of all eyelid malignancies.[1-3]

CLINICAL FEATURES

SCC occurs most commonly in fair-skinned elderly individuals who have a history of chronic sun exposure.[1,2,4,5] The majority of patients with SCC are 60 years of age or older.[4,5] Periocular SCC occurs most frequently on the lower eyelid, followed by the medial canthus, the upper eyelid, and the lateral canthus, in that order of frequency.

Symptoms and Signs

SCC most often appears as a painless, elevated, nodular or plaque-like lesion with chronic scaling and fissuring of the skin. Pearly irregular borders and a tendency to develop ulceration with irregular rolled edges are also characteristic features (Figure 16-1).[1,5]

HISTOPATHOLOGIC FEATURES

In well-differentiated tumors, the cells are polygonal, with abundant acidophilic cytoplasm and prominent hyperchromatic nuclei that vary in size and staining properties. Characteristic findings are of abnormal keratinization with dyskeratotic cells and keratin pearls and intercellular bridges (Figure 16-2). Less common histologic variants include the spindle cell and adenoid (adenoacanthoma or pseudoglandular) squamous cell carcinoma.[1]

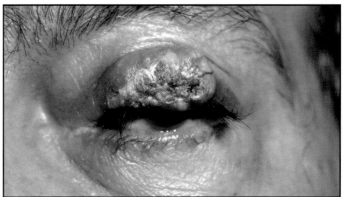

Figure 16-1. Squamous cell carcinoma of the upper lid presenting as an irregular, elevated lesion with masses of keratin.

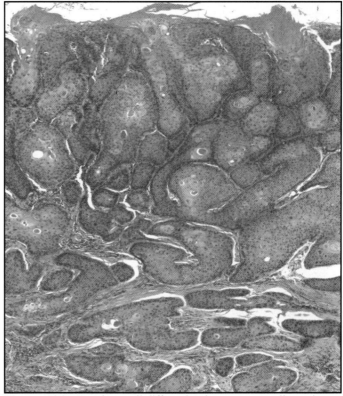

Figure 16-2. Invasive well-differentiated squamous cell carcinoma showing invasion of the dermis by tumor polygonal cells that vary in size and staining properties.

35

TREATMENT

Preventive

Minimizing sun exposure, especially in childhood and adolescence, is important.

Therapeutic

The main treatment modality used for eyelid SCC is surgical excision, with microscopic monitoring of the margins or Mohs' microsurgery. A variety of other forms of therapy, such as radiation therapy, cryotherapy, chemotherapy, curettage with carbon dioxide laser, photodynamic therapy, and treatment with retinoids or α-interferon are used. When used alone, these therapies have high recurrence rates, which are not acceptable for SCC of the eyelid, where recurrent tumors can be more aggressive and invasive. However, they may be appropriate for patients who cannot tolerate or who decline surgery.[5]

Sentinel Lymph Node Biopsy

Therapeutic value is questionable, and it may be associated with considerable morbidity.[5,6]

PROGNOSIS

Prognostic Factors

High-risk eyelid SCC lesions are those larger than 2 cm, with poor histological differentiation, deep invasion, and the presence of perineural invasion. Recurrent tumors and tumors developing in scars or in immunocompromised patients also imply a poor prognosis.[7]

Local Spread

Aggressive or neglected cases of eyelid SCC may spread into the lacrimal passages, the orbit, and the intracranial cavity. Orbital invasion of eyelid SCC may take years to occur, often preceded by several surgical interventions, irradiations, and recurrences of the tumor.[1]

Perineural Spread

The perineural infiltration of SCC of the eyelids along branches of the trigeminal nerve, the extraocular motor nerves, and the facial nerve facilitates its spread into the orbit, periorbital structures, and intracranial cavity.[8] Once clinical signs or symptoms of perineural spread have developed, the prognosis is poor, with an approximately 50% recurrence rate after simple excision.[8]

Local Recurrence

The 5-year local recurrence rate for SCC is about 23%. The 5-year metastatic rates vary between 5% and 45%.[7]

Metastasis

Unlike BCC, SCC has a tendency to metastasize to regional lymph nodes and distant sites through hematogenous and lymphatic pathways. The incidence of lymph node metastasis has ranged from 0% to as high as 21% and of distant metastasis varies from 1% to 21%.[1,9,10]

Mortality

The tumor-related mortality rates have been reported to be as high as 40%, and it is associated with lesions of the upper lid and medial canthus.[1] However, if detected early and treated adequately, the prognosis of SCC is generally excellent.[4]

REFERENCES

1. Reifler DM, Hornblass A. Squamous cell carcinoma of the eyelid. *Surv Ophthalmol.* 1986;30:349-365.
2. Malhotra R, Huilgol SC, Huynh N, Selva D. The Australian Mohs database: periocular squamous cell carcinoma. *Ophthalmology.* 2004;111:617-623.
3. Cook BE Jr, Bartley GB. Epidemiological characteristics and clinical course of patients with malignant eyelid tumors in an incidence cohort in Olmsted County, Minnesota. *Ophthalmology.* 1999;106:746-750.
4. Donaldson MJ, Sullivan TJ, Whitehead KJ, Williamson RM. Squamous cell carcinoma of the eyelids. *Br J Ophthalmol.* 2002;86:1161-1165.
5. Cook BE Jr, Bartley GB. Treatment options and future prospects for the management of eyelid malignancies: an evidence-based update. *Ophthalmology.* 2001;108:2088-2098.
6. Faustina M, Diba R, Ahmadi MA, et al. Patterns of regional and distant metastasis in patients with eyelid and periocular squamous cell carcinoma. *Ophthalmology.* 2004;111:1930-1932.
7. Rowe DE, Carroll RJ, Day CL Jr. Prognostic factors for local recurrence, metastasis, and survival rates in squamous cell carcinoma of the skin, ear, and lip. Implications for treatment modality selection. *J Am Acad Dermatol.* 1992;26:976-990.
8. Goepfert H, Dichtel WJ, Medina JE, et al. Perineural invasion in squamous cell carcinoma of the head and neck. *Am J Surg.* 1984;148:542-547.
9. Loeffler M, Hornblass A. Characteristics and behavior of eyelid carcinoma. *Ophthalmic Surg.* 1990;21:513-518.
10. Faustina M, Diba R, Ahmadi MA, et al. Patterns of regional and distant metastasis in patients with eyelid and periocular squamous cell carcinoma. *Ophthalmology.* 2004;111:1930-1932.

Sebaceous Gland Carcinoma

Mordechai Rosner

INTRODUCTION

Sebaceous gland carcinoma (SGC) is a malignant neoplasm capable of aggressive local behavior and metastasis to regional lymph nodes and distant organs. It originates from cells of the sebaceous glands and occurs most often in the periorbital area, usually in the eyelid.[1,2]

EPIDEMIOLOGICAL ASPECTS

In the United States, SGC accounts for only 5% of all malignant eyelid tumors.[3] A higher incidence of SGC has been observed in China, India, and other Asian countries, where it may be as prevalent as or even more common than periocular basal cell carcinoma (BCC) and squamous cell carcinoma (SCC).[1]

CLINICAL FEATURES

SGC is generally a disease of older individuals, with a mean age at diagnosis of 57 to 72 years.[4] Approximately 75% occur in the head and neck region.[5] About 65% of SGC occur in the upper eyelid, 25% in the lower eyelid, 5% involve both eyelids, and 5% arise in the caruncle.[2] The most common clinical variant of SGC is a solitary, firm, painless, sessile subcutaneous round nodule fixed to the tarsus. Unilateral diffuse thickening of the eyelid is the second most frequent presentation of SGC (Figure 17-1).

HISTOPATHOLOGIC FEATURES

SGC is an unencapsulated infiltrating mass composed of cells with finely vacuolated, frothy cytoplasm, pronounced nuclear pleomorphism, and, usually, high mitotic activity (Figure 17-2).[1] The presence of lipid can be demonstrated with the oil red-O stain (see Figure 17-2). SGC exhibits peculiar intraepithelial spread into the eyelid epidermis and the conjunctival epithelium in 44% to 80% of cases (pagetoid spread).[4] Immunohistochemistry may help to diagnose SGC. The central foamy cells of SGC express human milk fat globulin-1 (HMFG1) and epithelial membrane antigen (EMA). SGC also expresses Cam 5.2 and BRST-1, whereas BCC expresses neither EMA nor BRST-1, and SCC expresses EMA but not Cam 5.2.[6]

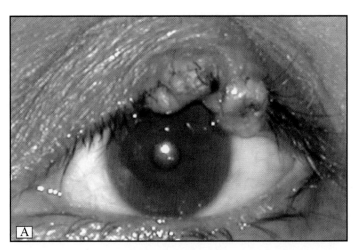

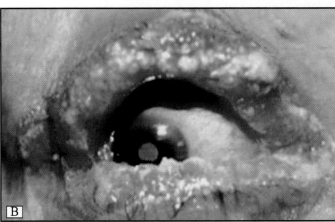

Figure 17-1. Sebaceous gland carcinoma. Local (A) and diffuse variants (B). (Courtesy of Dr. Santosh Honavar.)

TREATMENT

Surgery

The most acceptable management of periocular SGC is complete surgical removal. Either frozen section control or Mohs' microsurgery is usually used at the time of tumor excision. It has been suggested that wide margins, of at least 5 mm, should be taken in order to prevent recurrence.[1]

Cryotherapy by double freeze-thaw cycle is indicated for conjunctival involvement.[7] Topical chemotherapy[8] and radiotherapy[9] can also be used in advanced cases.

Systemic chemotherapy is used to treat regional lymph node spread and hematogenous metastasis.[10]

PROGNOSIS

Local Growth

Neglected or recurrent cases can invade the orbital soft tissues, lacrimal secretory system, lacrimal excretory system, and the cranial cavity.

Local Recurrence

The 5-year local recurrence rates following wide excision have ranged from 9% to 36%.[11]

Metastasis

The most common path of metastasis of eyelid SGC is via the lymphatic channels to regional lymph nodes, which occurs in about 30% of cases.

Mortality

Although the 5-year tumor-related death rate was estimated in the past to be as high as 30%, increased awareness and earlier aggressive treatment have markedly improved this to less than 10%.[12]

Prognostic Factors

Vascular, lymphatic, and orbital invasion, involvement of both upper and lower eyelids, poor differentiation, multicentric origin, pagetoid spread, and large tumor are poor prognostic factors.[1]

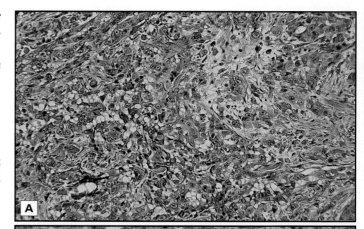

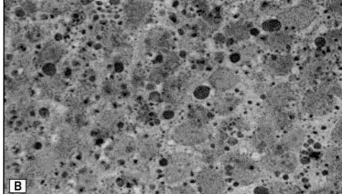

Figure 17-2. Histopathologically, sebaceous gland carcinoma is an unencapsulated infiltrating mass (A. Hematoxylin–eosin x100). Accentuation of the lipid using oil red-O stain. The lipid globules have a red color (B. Frozen section, oil red-O x250). (This figure was published in *Surv Ophthalmol,* 50, Shields JA, Demirci H, Marr BP, et al, Sebaceous carcinoma of the ocular region: a review, 103-122, © Elsevier 2005.)

REFERENCES

1. Shields JA, Demirci H, Marr BP, et al. Sebaceous carcinoma of the ocular region: a review. *Surv Ophthalmol.* 2005;50:103-122.
2. Kass LG, Hornblass A. Sebaceous carcinoma of the ocular adnexa. *Surv Ophthalmol.* 1989;33:477-490.
3. Margo CE, Mulla ZD. Malignant tumors of the eyelid: a population-based study of non-basal cell and non-squamous cell malignant neoplasms. *Arch Ophthalmol.* 1998;116:195-198.
4. Rao NA, Hiadayat AA, McLean IW, et al. Sebaceous carcinomas of the ocular adnexa: a clinicopathologic study of 104 cases, with five-year follow-up data. *Hum Pathol.* 1982;13:113-122.
5. Wick MR, Goellner JR, Wolfe JT et al. Adnexal carcinomas of the skin. II. Extraocular sebaceous carcinomas. *Cancer.* 1985;56:1163-1172.
6. Sinard JH. Immunohistochemical distinction of ocular sebaceous carcinoma from basal cell and squamous cell carcinoma. *Arch Ophthalmol.* 1999;117:776-783.
7. Lisman RD, Jakobiec FA, Small P. Sebaceous carcinoma of the eyelids. The role of adjunctive cryotherapy in the management of conjunctival pagetoid spread. *Ophthalmology.* 1989;96:1021-1026.
8. Rosner M, Hadar I, Rosen N. Successful treatment with mitomycin C eye drops for conjunctival diffuse intraepithelial neoplasia with sebaceous features. *Ophthalm Plast Reconstr Surg.* 2003;19:477-479.
9. Yen MT, Tse DT, Wu X, et al. Radiation therapy for local control of eyelid sebaceous cell carcinoma: report of two cases and review of the literature. *Ophthalm Plast Reconstr Surg.* 2000;16:211-215.
10. Murthy R, Honavar SG, Burman S, et al. Neoadjuvant chemotherapy in the management of sebaceous gland carcinoma of the eyelid with regional lymph node metastasis. *Ophthalm Plast Reconstr Surg.* 2005;21:307-309.
11. Callahan EF, Appert DL, Roenigk RK, Bartley GB. Sebaceous carcinoma of the eyelid: a review of 14 cases. *Dermatol Surg.* 2004;30:1164-1168.
12. Muqit MM, Roberts F, Lee WR, Kemp E. Improved survival rates in sebaceous carcinoma of the eyelid. *Eye.* 2004;18:49-53.

Melanoma of the Eyelid

Jacob Pe'er and Robert Folberg

INTRODUCTION

Cutaneous melanoma of the eyelid is a rare tumor, representing fewer than 1% of all malignant neoplasms of the eyelid skin,[1] 1% of all skin melanomas,[2] and 7% of cutaneous malignant melanomas of the head and neck region.[3] Many primary melanomas of the eyelid involve the mucosal surfaces of the palpebral and bulbar conjunctiva.

EPIDEMIOLOGICAL ASPECTS

Cutaneous melanoma of the eyelid is a tumor of adults and the elderly, with a peak incidence in the sixth and seventh decades of life. The vast majority of reported cases are of white patients from North America and Europe.[4] Sunlight exposure (ultraviolet radiation) most likely contributes to the etiology of eyelid melanoma.

Precursor Lesions

Eyelid cutaneous melanoma arises most frequently from a pre-existing long-standing pigmented lesion that shows a gradual increase in size.[5]

Lentigo

Lentigo is a slowly developing non-palpable pigmented macule, usually on exposed cutaneous surfaces in elderly patients. When there is transformation to lentigo maligna melanoma, the invasive areas are usually marked by small nodular formations and are usually dark brown or black.

Dysplastic Nevus

Eyelid melanomas may also evolve from a dysplastic nevus that affects the eyelid.

Oculodermal Melanocytosis

This may rarely lead to cutaneous melanoma.[6]

CLINICAL FEATURES

Eyelid cutaneous melanoma arises most frequently in the lower eyelid and can often involve the eyelid margin (Figure 18-1).[5] Documented growth, ulceration, hemorrhage, irregular borders, and variegated shades of brown, red, white, blue, or dark black are suspicious of melanoma.

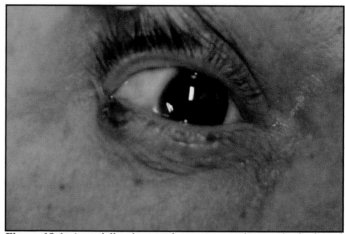

Figure 18-1. A partially pigmented cutaneous melanoma in the lateral aspect of the lower eyelid of the right eye, near the lateral canthus, that shows recent changes in its shape. (Photograph courtesy of Peter A. Martin, MD.)

HISTOPATHOLOGIC FEATURES

Lentigo maligna is remarkable for epidermal atrophy in the context of effacement of the rete and solar elastosis. Upon this background, atypical melanocytes populate the basal layers of the epidermis and may be identified along adnexal structures such as the pilar units of the eyelash. The term *melanoma in situ* is roughly equivalent to *primary acquired melanosis (PAM) with atypia* in the conjunctiva.

Malignant Melanoma

Any breach of the epidermal basement membrane by atypical melanocytes renders the lesion a malignant melanoma. Should the invasive component arise in the context of an intradermal melanocytic lesion featuring melanocytes in a pagetoid distribution, one might then state that the melanoma is of a superficial spreading type. The type of melanoma (lentigo maligna melanoma or superficial spreading melanoma) does not influence the clinical behavior of the lesion.

Prognostic Factors

Clark's microstaging of melanoma does not apply to the eyelid skin because in this location the dermis is not stratified into papillary and reticular zones, and there is no subcutaneous fat in the eyelid. The major prognostic parameter is the depth of invasion, as measured by a calibrated ocular micrometer from the top of the granular layer of the epidermis to the point of deepest invasion into the dermis.[7] Cell type, so significant among the histological characteristics of uveal melanoma, does not appear to play an independent role in the histological prognosis of eyelid melanoma.

TREATMENT

Surgical Excision

There is a general consensus that complete surgical excision with clear surgical margins is the treatment of choice.

Mohs' Surgery

Use of frozen tissue sections for melanoma is controversial because of freeze artifacts that make accurate interpretation difficult.

Other Methods of Treatment

The primary use of destructive treatment such as cryotherapy, radiotherapy, topical treatment with azelaic acid, and curettage is associated with high recurrence rates, and, therefore, is not recommended. Cryotherapy and external beam radiation can be used as adjuvant therapy.

Sentinel Lymph Node Biopsy

The issue of elective lymph node dissection in patients with periocular melanoma is controversial. The procedure is probably not indicated for lesions less than 1.0-mm thick and may offer little advantage for lesions thicker than 4.0 mm. It is currently recommended to perform elective lymph node dissection for melanomas of intermediate thickness (1 to 4 mm) that may have occult nodal metastases.

PROGNOSIS

Local recurrence of eyelid cutaneous melanoma is common with incompletely excised tumors.[5]

Prognostic factors such as age, gender, and histologic type are not of prognostic significance. Location of the tumor in the upper or lower lid and in the canthi also does not affect prognosis. However, involvement of the eyelid margin and the mucocutaneous junction is associated with a higher mortality.[8]

Mortality rate from eyelid cutaneous melanoma varies significantly in different series, ranging from 6% to 58%.[8] The late recurrence in a significant number of patients reinforces the need for long-term follow-up of patients treated for cutaneous eyelid melanoma.

REFERENCES

1. Cook BE Jr, Bartley GB. Treatment options and future prospects for the management of eyelid malignancies: an evidence-based update. *Ophthalmology.* 2001;108:2088-2100.
2. Rodriguez-Sains RS, Jakobiec FA, Iwamoto T. Lentigo maligna of the lateral canthal skin. *Ophthalmology.* 1981;88:1186-1192.
3. Batsakis J. *Tumors of the Head and Neck.* Baltimore, MD: Williams & Wilkins; 1974.
4. Naidoff MA, Bernardino VB, Clark WH. Melanocytic lesions of the eyelid skin. *Am J Ophthalmol.* 1976;82:371-382.
5. Vaziri M, Buffam FV, Martinka M, et al. Clinicopathologic features and behavior of cutaneous eyelid melanoma. *Ophthalmology.* 2002;109:901-908.
6. Patel BC, Egan CA, Lucius RW, et al. Cutaneous malignant melanoma and oculodermal melanocytosis (nevus of Ota): report of a case and review of the literature. *J Am Acad Dermatol.* 1998;38:862-865.
7. Breslow A. Thickness, cross-sectional areas and depth of invasion in the prognosis of cutaneous melanoma. *Ann Surg.* 1970;172:902-908.
8. Garner A, Koornneef L, Levene A, et al. Malignant melanoma of the eyelid skin: histopathology and behaviour. *Br J Ophthalmol.* 1985;69:180-186.

Chapter

19

Eyelid Adnexal Tumors

Karin U. Loeffler

INTRODUCTION

Eyelid adnexal tumors are frequent and comprise a large variety of different entities, because the lid is an organ rich in adnexal structures such as hairs (lashes) and glands. Overall, benign adnexal lesions of the eyelids are much more frequent than the malignant lesions.[1,2]

CLASSIFICATION

Eyelid adnexal tumors may be classified as cystic lesions and benign and malignant tumors arising from sweat glands, hair follicles, and sebaceous glands (Table 19-1).

CYSTIC LESIONS

Epidermal Inclusion Cysts

Epidermal inclusion cysts usually occur as smooth dome-shaped nodules of varying size, frequently revealing a punctum or pore. The characteristic feature is a cystic space filled with keratin, lined by regular keratinizing stratified squamous epithelium.

Sebaceous Cyst

"Sebaceous" cyst is a clinical misnomer, as despite the yellowish color of many cysts, histologic findings do not qualify any of them as sebaceous. Clinically, the term is used most often for epidermoid or trichilemmal cysts.

Retention Cyst

All glands can lead to retention cysts, particularly in cases of duct obstruction. The most frequent of these is the so-called sudoriferous cyst, originating from sweat glands.

SWEAT GLAND TUMORS

There are two types of sweat gland, eccrine and apocrine. Eccrine sweat glands are widely distributed in the body, and each consists of a single duct with a coiled deeper component.[3] By contrast, the apocrine sweat glands are limited to particular regions, such as the axilla, nipple, external ear, external genitalia, and the eyelids.[3] The apocrine glands and their ductal openings are closely associated with eyelashes.[4]

Table 19-1. Classification of Cystic and Adnexal Tumors		
Types		Subtypes
Cystic lesions	Benign	Epidermal inclusion cyst
		Sebaceous cyst
		Retention cyst
		Trichilemmal cyst
Sweat gland tumors	Benign	Apocrine hidrocystoma
		Eccrine hidrocystoma
		Syringoma
		Eccrine spiradenoma
		Pleomorphic adenoma (benign mixed tumor)
		Eccrine acrospiroma
		Eccrine cylindroma
		Apocrine adenoma
		Other benign tumors
	Malignant	Sweat gland adenocarcinoma
		Mucinous sweat gland adenocarcinoma
		Apocrine gland adenocarcinoma
		Porocarcinoma
Hair follicle tumors	Benign	Trichoepithelioma
		Trichofolliculoma/ trichoadenoma
		Trichilemmoma
		Pilomatrixoma (calcifying epithelioma of Malherbe)
	Malignant	Carcinoma of hair follicles
Sebaceous gland tumors	Benign	Sebaceous gland hyperplasia
		Sebaceous gland adenoma
	Malignant	Sebaceous gland carcinoma

Benign Tumors

Apocrine hidrocystoma (cyst of Moll, Figure 19-1) and eccrine hidrocystoma represent the majority of benign sweat gland tumors. In contrast to apocrine hidrocystoma, the eccrine hidrocystoma does not involve the eyelid margin. Syringoma usually present as multiple small nodules 2 to 3 mm in diameter but show a wide variety of clinical pictures (Figure 19-2).

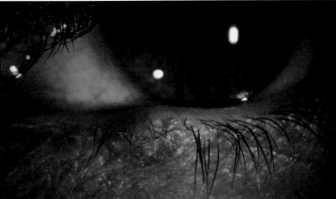

Figure 19-1. Apocrine hidrocystoma. Note bluish color of the cystic lesion involving the eyelid margin.

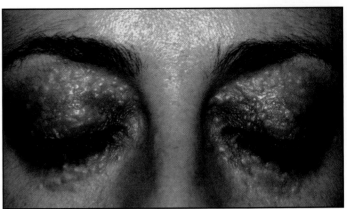

Figure 19-2. Multiple bilateral syringomas of upper and lower eyelids in a young woman. (Reproduced with permission from Wolff K, Johnson RA, Suurmond D, eds. *Fitzpatrick's Color Atlas and Synopsis of Clinical Dermatology.* 5th ed. © 2001 The McGraw-Hill Companies Inc.)

Malignant Tumors

Malignant tumors such as sweat gland adenocarcinoma (malignant syringoma), mucinous sweat gland adenocarcinoma, and apocrine gland adenocarcinoma (carcinoma of the glands of Moll) are rare.

TUMORS OF THE HAIR FOLLICLE

Benign Tumors

Trichoepithelioma is a hamartomatous lesion that may be solitary, multiple, or even familial.[5] Trichofolliculoma is a dome-shaped papule with a central pore and presence of one or more silky white thread-like hairs growing out of this opening.[6]

Trichoadenoma is a solitary, soft or firm nodule of varying size and is yellowish in color.

Trichilemmoma may be solitary or multiple and presents as a small warty or smooth skin-colored papule on the face of older adults. Associated with the presence of multiple trichilemmomas is the rare autosomal dominant condition called Cowden's (multiple hamartoma) disease.[7]

Pilomatrixoma (calcifying epithelioma of Malherbe) usually presents as a solitary lesion.[8]

Malignant Tumors

Carcinoma of hair follicles (trichilemmal carcinoma) is found predominantly on sun-exposed skin in the elderly.

SEBACEOUS GLAND TUMORS

Benign Tumors

Sebaceous gland hyperplasia usually presents as a yellowish umbilicated papule 1 to 2 mm in size on the face of older adults.

Sebaceous gland adenoma is a tan, yellow, or reddish papule/nodule most frequently located on the face. These can be an indication for Muir-Torre syndrome (Chapter 22).[9]

Nevus sebaceus of Jadassohn is a complex choristoma comprising abnormalities of the epidermis and adnexal glands (Chapter 64).[10]

Malignant Tumors

Sebaceous epithelioma is a variant of basal cell carcinoma with sebaceous differentiation. Sebaceous gland carcinoma is discussed in Chapter 17.

REFERENCES

1. Kersten RC, Ewing-Chow D, Kulwin DR, Gallon M. Accuracy of clinical diagnosis of cutaneous eyelid lesions. *Ophthalmology.* 1997;104:479-484.
2. Margo CE. Eyelid tumors: accuracy of clinical diagnosis. *Am J Ophthalmol.* 1999;128:635-636.
3. Warwick R, Williams PL. *Gray's Anatomy.* 35th ed. Edinburgh: Longman; 1973:1168-1169.
4. Warwick R. *Eugene Woll's Anatomy of the Eye and Orbit.* 7th ed. London: HK Lewis; 1976:195-197.
5. Aurora AL. Solitary trichoepithelioma of the eyelid. *Indian J Ophthalmol.* 1974;22:32-33.
6. Carreras B Jr, Lopez-Marin I Jr, Mellado VG, Gutierrez MT. Trichofolliculoma of the eyelid. *Br J Ophthalmol.* 1981;65:214-215.
7. Bardenstein DS, McLean IW, Nerney J, Boatwright RS. Cowden's disease. *Ophthalmology.* 1988;95:1038-1041.
8. Boniuk M, Zimmerman LE. Pilomatrixoma (benign calcifying epithelioma) of the eyelids and eyebrow. *Arch Ophthalmol.* 1963;70:399-406.
9. Singh AD, Mudhar H, Bhola R, Rundle PA, Rennie IG. Sebaceous adenoma of the eyelid in Muir-Torre syndrome. *Arch Ophthalmol.* 2005;123:562-565.
10. Traboulsi EI, Zin A, Massicotte SJ, et al. Posterior scleral choristoma in the organoid nevus syndrome (linear nevus sebaceus of Jadassohn). *Ophthalmology.* 1999;106:2126-2130.

Eyelid Stromal Tumors

Geeta K. Vemuganti and Santosh G. Honavar

INTRODUCTION

Eyelid stromal tumors can be divided into several distinct categories based on the tissue of origin: fibrous tissue tumors, fibrohistiocytic tumors, lipomatous tumors, smooth muscle tumors, skeletal muscle tumors, vascular tumors, perivascular tumors, neural tumors, lymphoid, plasmacytic, and leukemic tumors, cartilage and bone tumors, secondary tumors, metastatic tumors, and hamartomas, choristomas, and other miscellaneous lesions. Some of the inflammatory and infective conditions, such as chalazion, pyogenic granuloma, verruca vulgaris, and molluscum contagiosum, may manifest with features that clinically simulate a tumor.

FIBROHISTIOCYTIC TUMORS

Xanthelasma is a common bilateral, yellowish-tan subcutaneous lesion of the eyelid seen in normolipemic individuals and in those with primary hyperlipemia (type II and III) or secondary hyperlipemia (Figure 20-1).

Xanthogranuloma is an idiopathic inflammatory granuloma with juvenile and adult variants.

LIPOMATOUS TUMORS

The lipomatous tumors that affect the eyelid are lipoma, lipoma variants, and liposarcoma.

MYOGENIC TUMORS

Smooth muscle tumors of the eyelid are very rare and may be benign (leiomyoma, angiomyoma) or malignant (leiomyosarcoma). Rhabdomyoma and rhabdomyosarcoma are the skeletal muscle tumors (Chapter 97).

VASCULAR TUMORS

Nevus flammeus (port wine stain) is a diffuse congenital vascular malformation of the face that involves the periocular area and eyelid (Chapter 64).

Pyogenic Granuloma

Papillary endothelial hyperplasia or pyogenic granuloma is the most common acquired vascular lesion of the eyelid. It is neither pyogenic, nor is it a granuloma (Figure 20-2).

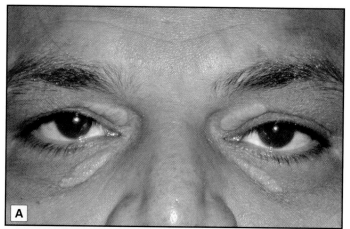

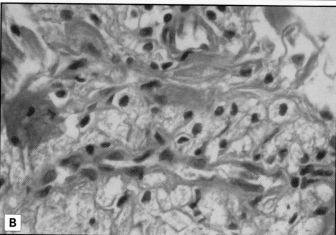

Figure 20-1. Xanthelasma. (A) Bilateral yellowish placoid lesions clinically diagnostic of xanthelasma. (B) Sheets of large foamy lipid laden cells on histopathology. (Hematoxylin and eosin, original magnification x400.)

Capillary Hemangioma

Capillary hemangioma of the eyelid is the most common vascular tumor of the eyelid in children (Figure 20-3). It is usually congenital and is often sporadic. Newborns of mothers who have undergone amniocentesis and premature infants are at risk of developing capillary hemangioma.[1]

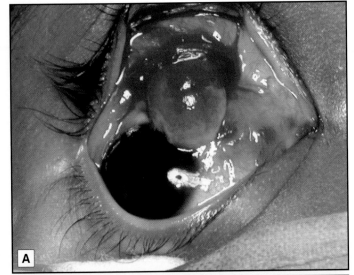

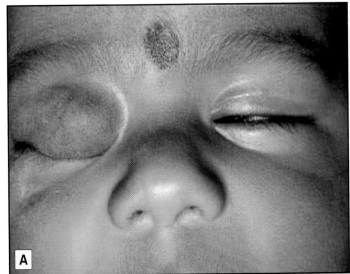

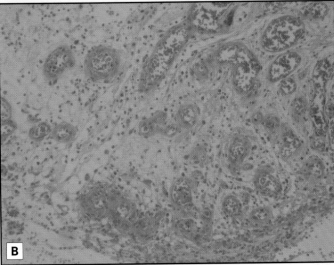

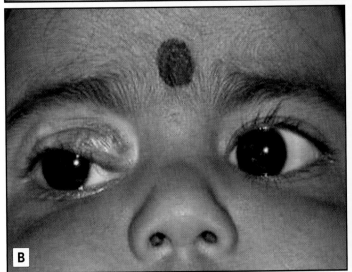

Figure 20-2. Pyogenic granuloma. (A) The tarsal conjunctiva of the upper eyelid shows a vascular polypoidal reddish pink mass with superficial ulceration. (B) Histopathologically a loose edematous stroma with surface necrosis, proliferating blood vessels, and mixed inflammatory infiltrates, characteristic of inflammatory granulation tissue, are present. (Hematoxylin and eosin, original magnification x200.)

Clinical Features

Congenital capillary hemangioma usually manifests at birth or within the first months of life. The superficial variant, better known as strawberry hemangioma, appears as a bright red soft eyelid mass that typically blanches on pressure. The superficial variant is localized to the epidermis and dermis, whereas the deep variant lies in the subcutaneous tissue and is bluish or blue-gray in color. Congenital capillary hemangioma grows rapidly in size and reaches its final size by 6 to 12 months of age. It then becomes stable and slowly involutes by 4 to 7 years of age.[2]

Systemic Association

In most instances, congenital capillary hemangioma is a sporadic condition, but in approximately 20% of patients, the central nervous system, the liver, and the gastrointestinal tract may be involved. Systemic lesions, especially those found in association with Kasabach–Merritt syndrome, may proliferate aggressively and lead to hemorrhage, platelet consumption, disseminated intravascular coagulation, cardiac failure, and death.

Figure 20-3. (A) Capillary hemangioma of the upper eyelid manifesting as a bright red, spongy, soft mass causing total ptosis. (B) It resolved following treatment with intralesional triamcinolone injection.

Treatment

The main ocular complications are amblyopia and strabismus. Amblyopia may be meridional because of induced astigmatism or because of stimulation deprivation secondary to mechanical ptosis. Because most lesions regress spontaneously, observation, refractive correction, and appropriate amblyopia management is the standard treatment. Active intervention in the form of intralesional, local, or systemic corticosteroids is indicated if the lesion extensively involves the face or is ulcerated with episodes of bleeding, if there is mechanical ptosis with obscuration of the pupillary axis, or induced astigmatism with amblyopia. Extensive lesions are treated with oral prednisolone 1 to 2 mg/kg body weight tapered over 4 to 6 weeks. Alternative treatment modalities include interferon, laser sclerotherapy, and excision of circumscribed anterior lesions (Figure 20-4).[3,4]

Cavernous hemangioma of the eyelid is rare and is generally seen in adults. It may be associated with blue rubber bleb nevus syndrome.[5]

Lymphangioma commonly manifests in the orbit rather than in the eyelid (Chapter 90).

Kaposi's sarcoma is a malignant vascular tumor that most often presents in the setting of acquired immunodeficiency syndrome (AIDS).[5]

Treatment

An improvement in immunological status and highly active antiretroviral therapy may result in spontaneous regression of Kaposi's sarcoma. Treatment modalities include local methods such as excision, cryotherapy, and radiotherapy. Systemic chemotherapy is indicated for widespread disease.[5]

Perivascular tumors of the eyelid are very rare and include benign or malignant hemangiopericytoma and glomus tumor (Chapter 90).

NEUROGENIC TUMORS

Neurogenic tumors of the eyelid include a variety of benign (neurofibroma, schwannoma, and neuroglial choristoma) and malignant tumors (malignant peripheral nerve sheath tumor and Merkel cell tumor) (Chapter 91).

INFLAMMATORY AND INFECTIVE LESIONS

Some common inflammatory and infective lesions such as chalazion, pyogenic, and molluscum contagiosum can simulate an eyelid tumor.

REFERENCES

1. Shields CL, Shields JA, Minzter R, Singh AD. Cutaneous capillary hemangiomas of the eyelid, scalp, and digits in premature triplets. *Am J Ophthalmol.* 2000;129:528-531.
2. Jackson R. The natural history of strawberry naevi. *J Cutan Med Surg.* 1998;2:187-189.
3. Kushner BJ. Local steroid therapy in adnexal hemangioma. *Ann Ophthalmol.* 1979;11:1005-1009.
4. McCannel CA, Hoenig J, Umlas J, et al. Orbital lesions in the blue rubber bleb nevus syndrome. *Ophthalmology.* 1996;103:933-936.
5. Brun SC, Jakobiec FA. Kaposi's sarcoma of the ocular adnexa. *Int Ophthalmol Clin.* 1997;37:25-38.

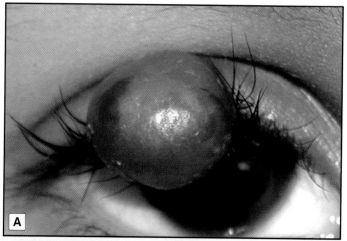

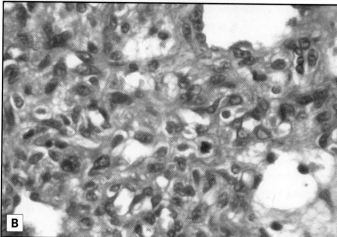

Figure 20-4. An older child with a large red vascular mass in the upper eyelid (A) that was excised. (B) Histopathology shows a lobulated appearance with vascular channels lined by plump endothelial cells. The presence of a few mitotic figures can be seen in proliferating lesions. (Hematoxylin and eosin original magnification x400.)

Surgical Techniques

Jennifer I. Hui and David T. Tse

INTRODUCTION

The treatment of malignant eyelid lesions includes complete excision of the tumor as well as reconstruction to provide optimum function, globe protection, and esthetics.[1] Mohs' micrographic surgery technique is the preferred method of excision of periocular malignancies, as it allows for clearance of the tumor margin while maximally conserving normal tissues (Figure 21-1). Repair of the eyelid depends on the size of the defect and whether or not the lid margin is involved. Most importantly, either the reconstructed anterior or the posterior lamella must have its own inherent blood supply (pedicle flap), as this will ensure tissue survival and an optimal surgical outcome for the patient.

Eyelid Reconstruction

General principles of eyelid reconstruction are as follows.[2]

- The eyelid is a bilamellar structure; the anterior lamella consists of the skin and orbicularis oculi muscle, and the posterior lamella consists of the tarsal plate and conjunctiva.
- The anterior or posterior lamella must have its own blood supply.
- Provision must be made for maximal horizontal stabilization with minimal vertical tension, proper canthal fixation, and an epithelialized internal surface.[3]

- Undermining should be sufficient to allow for tension-free closure.
- Identification of the transverse edge of the levator aponeurosis and a knowledge of facial nerve anatomy are essential in maintaining the opening and closing functions of the eyelid.

LOWER EYELID DEFECTS (FIGURE 21-2)

Anterior Lamellar Deficit, Lid Margin Intact

Primary Closure

In general, anterior lamellar defects without lid margin involvement may be closed primarily if this does not induce dis-

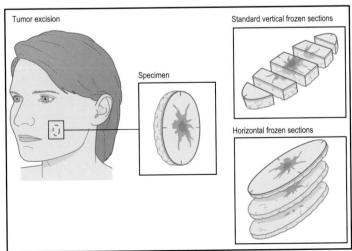

Figure 21-1. Mohs' micrographic surgery. Frozen sections are obtained from the undersurface and skin edges of the excised lesion. Locations of residual tumor are marked on a map for subsequent second-stage excision.

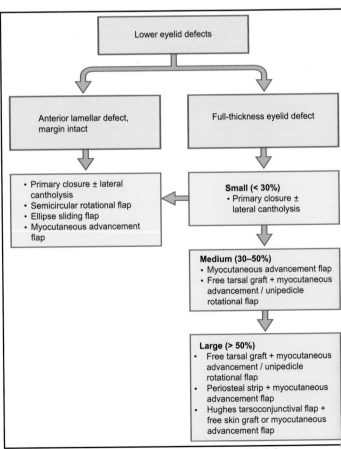

Figure 21-2. Algorithm for the repair of lower eyelid defects.

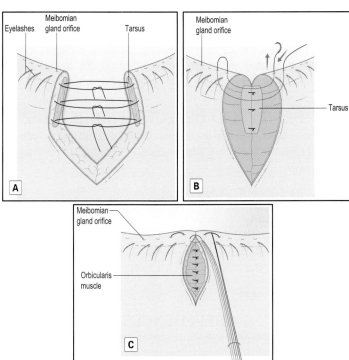

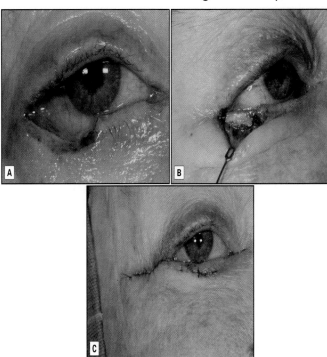

Figure 21-3. Lid margin repair, full-thickness defect. The eyelid margin defect may be closed primarily if less than one third of the margin is involved. An important step in primary closure of a full-thickness lid margin defect is precise approximation of the tarsal edges. Accurate vertical alignment provides the tension-bearing support of the wound. (A) Three interrupted 5-0 Vicryl sutures are placed at partial thickness through the tarsal plate. (B) The lid margin is closed with a vertical mattress suture using 6-0 silk sutures, which provide proper anteroposterior alignment. A vertical lid margin suture induces puckering of the wound edges to avoid notching after healing. (C) Two additional sutures, one posterior and another inferior to the lashes, are placed to align the lid margin. The three 6-0 silk sutures should be left long and secured away from the wound on to the lower lid skin with a suture.

Figure 21-4. Free tarsal graft plus myocutaneous advancement flap. (A) A full-thickness lower eyelid defect may be repaired with a free tarsal graft for posterior lamella replacement and an overlying myocutaneous advancement flap to provide vascular support. (B) The free tarsal graft, harvested from either the ipsilateral or the contralateral upper eyelid, provides posterior lamellar replacement. (C) The myocutaneous advancement flap, fashioned in the manner of a lower eyelid blepharoplasty, provides an inherent blood supply to the underlying free tarsal graft. This figure demonstrates the key principle that either the reconstructed anterior or posterior lamella must have its own inherent vascular supply (pedicle flap), thus ensuring tissue survival and optimum surgical outcome for the patient.

tortion. The wound is closed in two layers using deep, interrupted 6-0 Vicryl sutures and interrupted, superficial 6-0 or 7-0 nylon or silk sutures in the skin.

Skin Graft

For defects that are too large to close primarily, full-thickness skin grafts may be employed. Possible donor sites include the ipsilateral or contralateral upper eyelid, preauricular or retroauricular skin, and less commonly the supraclavicular fossa and the upper inner arm. In general, split-thickness skin grafts are not recommended in eyelid reconstruction.[1]

Ellipse Sliding Flap

This flap, however, should not be used to reconstruct anterior lamellar defects near the lid margin because ectropion or retraction may be induced.

Myocutaneous Advancement Flap

This is an ideal method to address a large anterior lamellar deficit because it provides the best tissue match with an independent blood supply.

Full-Thickness Eyelid Defect

Primary Closure

For small defects involving less than one-third of the lower eyelid margin, primary closure without lateral cantholysis is the best option (Figure 21-3). Primary layered closure provides the best tissue match. If tension is present and precludes proper lid margin reapproximation, a lateral canthotomy with inferior cantholysis may be performed to yield 5 to 6 mm of the temporal eyelid margin.

Semicircular Rotational Flap

This type of flap may be used to reconstruct up to two-thirds of a central lower lid defect if there is a sufficient temporal tarsal remnant.

Free Tarsal Graft and
Myocutaneous Advancement Flap

For larger defects where primary closure is not possible, a free tarsal graft from the ipsilateral or contralateral upper eyelid can be used for posterior lamella replacement (Figure 21-4).

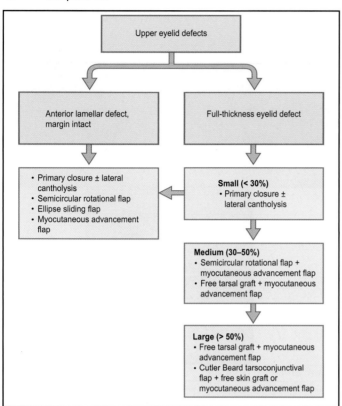

Figure 21-5. Algorithm for the repair of upper eyelid defects.

Periosteal Strip and
Myocutaneous Advancement Flap

This is an alternative to the free tarsal graft.[2]

Free Tarsal Graft and Unipedicle Flap
From the Upper Eyelid

A free tarsal graft with a unipedicle flap from the upper eyelid is another method used to close full-thickness lower eyelid defects.

UPPER EYELID DEFECTS (FIGURE 21-5)

Techniques for closure of upper eyelid defects and defects in special circumstances[4] are summarized in Figures 21-5 and 21-6, respectively.

Full-Thickness Eyelid Defect

Primary Closure

Central upper lid defects—up to 30% in younger patients and 50% in older patients—may be closed using the same technique as in the lower lid. The levator aponeurotic attachments should not be disturbed.

REFERENCES

1. Cook BE Jr, Bartley GB. Treatment options and future prospects for the management of eyelid malignancies: an evidence-based update. *Ophthalmology.* 2001;108:2088-2098; quiz 2099-2100, 2121.
2. Kronish J. Eyelid reconstruction. In: Tse DT, ed. *Color Atlas of Ophthalmic Surgery: Oculoplastic Surgery.* Philadelphia, PA: JB Lippincott; 1992.
3. Nerad JA. The requisites in ophthalmology oculoplastics surgery: eyelid reconstruction. In: Krachmer JH, ed. *Requisites in Ophthalmology: Oculoplastic Surgery.* St Louis, MO: Mosby; 2001.
4. Tse DT, Goodwin WJ, Johnson T, et al. Use of galeal or pericranial flaps for reconstruction of orbital and eyelid defects. *Arch Ophthalmol.* 1997;15:932-937.

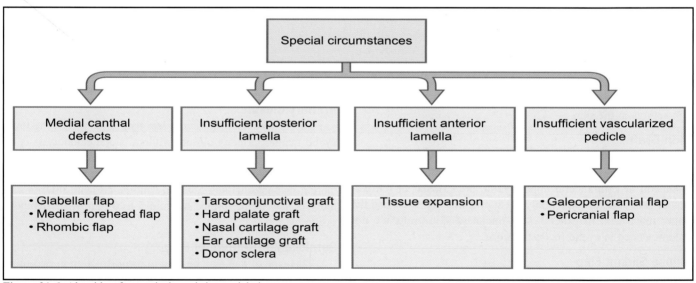

Figure 21-6. Algorithm for surgical repair in special circumstances.

Systemic Associations of Eyelid Tumors

Arun D. Singh and Elias I. Traboulsi

INTRODUCTION

There are several rare eyelid tumors that may be manifestations of a systemic disease (Table 22-1). Patients with an inherited predisposition for tumors tend to develop them at an earlier age, have multiple tumors with bilateral involvement, and may have a positive family history of similar lesions.[1] The majority of eyelid tumors in the setting of an inherited predisposition are benign, but some malignant tumors are also known to have a syndromic association (Gorlin–Goltz syndrome).

NEUROFIBROMA

Neurofibroma is the hallmark finding of neurofibromatosis type 1 (Chapter 65).

NEVUS FLAMMEUS

In general, only about 10% of all patients with nevus flammeus or port-wine stain of the eyelid are associated with Sturge–Weber syndrome (Chapter 65).[2]

GARDNER SYNDROME

Extracolonic manifestations of Gardner syndrome include orbital osteoma, soft tissue tumors of the brows or eyelids, and epidermoid cysts of the eyelid (Chapter 65).[3]

Table 22-1. Various Eyelid Tumors That Are Markers of a Syndromic Association

Entity	Eyelid Tumor	Associated Features	Locus/Gene
Neurofibromatosis type 1	Neurofibroma	Lisch nodules	17q
		Café au lait spots	NF1 gene
		Pheochromocytoma	
Sturge-Weber syndrome	Diffuse hemangioma	Leptomeningeal hemangioma	Sporadic
Gardner syndrome	Epidermoid cyst	CHRPE	5q21
	Fibroma	Colorectal polyps/carcinoma	APC gene
	Orbital osteoma		
Gorlin-Goltz syndrome	Basal cell carcinoma	Odontogenic cysts	9q 22
		Bifid ribs	PTC gene
		Palmar pits	
		Ovarian tumor	
Cowden syndrome	Trichilemmoma	Oral papilloma	10q23
		Breast tumor	PTEN gene
		Thyroid tumor	
Carney complex	Myxoma	Spotty mucocutaneous pigmentation	17q PRKAR1A
		Schwannoma	gene
		Endocrine overactivity	chromosome 2
		Testicular tumor	
Muir-Torre syndrome	Sebaceous adenoma	Keratoacanthoma	2p
		Basal cell carcinoma	hMLH1
		Colorectal adenocarcinoma	hMSH2

CHRPE, congenital hypertrophy of retinal pigment epithelium.

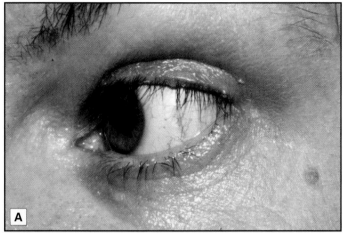

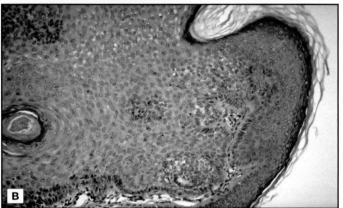

Figure 22-1. (A) Clinical photograph of flesh-colored papular lesions at the eyelid margin. (B) High-power photomicrograph of trichilemmoma with basal palisading and bland-looking cells with more cytoplasm than basal cell carcinoma cells. (Hematoxylin and eosin, original magnification x200.) (This figure was published in *Ophthalmology,* 95, Bardenstein DS, McLean IW, Nerney J, Boatwright RS, Cowden disease, 1038-1041, © Elsevier 1988.)

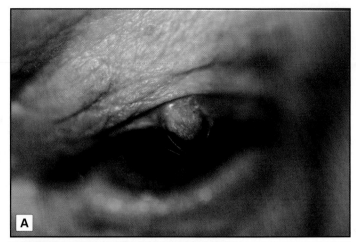

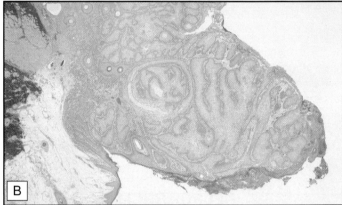

Figure 22-2. Sebaceous adenomas on the face in a patient with Muir–Torre syndrome. Note a yellowish pink warty growth arising from anterior lamella of the left upper eyelid (A). Both eyelid and facial biopsies revealed sebaceous adenomas (B). (Reproduced with permission from Singh AD, Mudhar H, Bhola R, et al. Sebaceous adenoma of the eyelid in Muir–Torre syndrome. *Arch Ophthalmol.* 2005;123:562-565. Copyright © 2005 American Medical Association. All rights reserved.)

NEVOID BASAL CELL CARCINOMA SYNDROME (GORLIN–GOLTZ SYNDROME)

Nevoid basal cell carcinoma syndrome (NBCCS) is also referred to as basal cell nevus syndrome, Gorlin syndrome, or Gorlin–Goltz syndrome.[4] The risk of multiple basal cell carcinoma and developmental anomalies characterizes NBCCS.

MULTIPLE HAMARTOMA SYNDROME (COWDEN SYNDROME)

Eyelid trichilemmomas are the hallmark manifestation of Cowden syndrome (Figure 22-1).[5]

CARNEY COMPLEX

Carney complex is characterized by cutaneous pigmentary abnormalities, myxomas, endocrine tumors, and schwannomas.

MUIR–TORRE SYNDROME

Muir–Torre syndrome is characterized by sebaceous adenoma and sebaceous carcinoma, keratoacanthoma, basal cell carcinoma, and internal malignancy (Figure 22-2).[6]

REFERENCES

1. Ponder BAJ. Inherited cancer syndromes. In: Carney D, Sikora K, eds. *Genes and Cancer.* New York, NY: John Wiley & Sons; 1990.
2. Tallman B, Tan OT, Morelli JG, et al. Location of port-wine stains and the likelihood of ophthalmic and/or central nervous system complications. *Pediatrics.* 1991;87:323-327.
3. Gardner EJ, Richards RC. Multiple cutaneous and subcutaneous lesions occurring simultaneously with hereditary polyposis and osteomatosis. *Am J Hum Genet.* 1953;5:139-147.
4. Gorlin RJ. Nevoid basal-cell carcinoma syndrome. *Medicine (Baltimore).* 1987;66:98-113.
5. Bardenstein DS, McLean IW, Nerney J, Boatwright RS. Cowden's disease. *Ophthalmology.* 1988;95:1038-1041.
6. Singh AD, Mudhar HS, Bhola R, et al. Sebaceous adenoma of the eyelid in Muir-Torre syndrome. *Arch Ophthalmol.* 2005;123:562-565.

Examination Techniques, Classification, and Differential Diagnosis of Conjunctival and Corneal Tumors

Jacob Pe'er

INTRODUCTION

The conjunctiva is a translucent vascularized mucous membrane. It may be divided into three portions: the bulbar conjunctiva, including the corneoconjunctival limbus, which covers the sclera in the anterior part of the eyeball; the superior, inferior, and lateral conjunctival fornices; and the palpebral conjunctiva, including the mucocutaneous transitional zone in the lid margin, which covers the back surface of the upper and lower eyelids.

HISTOLOGY

The conjunctiva is composed of the non-keratinized stratified squamous epithelium and the subepithelial stroma—the substantia propria. Goblet cells appear to be present in the middle and superficial layers of the epithelium and are most numerous in the lower forniceal portion. Melanocytes are scattered in the basal layer of the epithelium.

Specialized Regions

Plica semilunaris is a vertical fold of conjunctiva lying lateral to the caruncle. The caruncle is a fleshy prominence located in the medial canthus that contains both conjunctival and cutaneous structures. Tumors of the caruncle can be of both mucosal and skin origin.

EXAMINATION TECHNIQUES

The conjunctiva and cornea are readily visible tissues; thus, tumors and related lesions that occur on the ocular surface are usually recognized and diagnosed at a relatively early stage. External ocular examination and detailed slit-lamp examination are vital to diagnose conjunctival and corneal tumors correctly.

Ancillary Studies

Drawings/Photography

The lesion should be drawn (or preferably photographed) externally or via the slit lamp in order to document the tumors accurately, particularly their margins.

High-Frequency Ultrasonography

When the tumor is thick or adheres to its surroundings, high-frequency ultrasonography can be used to determine its depth and its extension into the sclera, cornea, or rarely into intraocular structures.

Histopathologic Evaluation

The definite diagnosis of conjunctival and corneal tumors is by histopathology. However, benign-looking asymptomatic tumors are often managed by periodic observation, and only when there is evidence of growth or malignant changes is a biopsy taken.

Excisional Biopsy

If a small tumor does require a biopsy, it is preferable to remove the lesion completely.

Incisional Biopsy

In large conjunctival lesions, where complete removal of the tumor may severely compromise the ocular surface, or when it is impossible to perform total excision, it is appropriate to perform an incisional biopsy, sampling the tumor by wedge or punch biopsy. Incisional biopsy is also appropriate when complete excision is not the treatment of choice and in tumors that are preferably treated by radiotherapy, chemotherapy, and local means such as cryotherapy and topical chemotherapy.

Exfoliative Cytology

This provides information only on the superficial layers of the lesion and does not show the invasiveness of the tumor.

CLASSIFICATION OF CONJUNCTIVAL AND CORNEAL TUMORS

Most conjunctival tumors are epithelial or melanocytic in origin (Table 23-1). Most of the other tumors are of various elements of the conjunctival stroma and include vascular, fibrous, neural, histiocytic, myogenic, myxoid, lipomatous, and lymphoproliferative tumors.[1-3]

Three unique groups of conjunctival tumors are the hamartomas and choristomas, the caruncular tumors, and metastatic and secondary tumors.

Epithelial tumors are usually classified into non-melanocytic and melanocytic, based on the clinical presence or absence of brown pigmentation and the histological presence of melanocytes (Table 23-2).

Stromal tumors are similar in variety to the stromal tumors of the eyelid (Chapter 20).

Congenital epibulbar tumors diagnosed in infancy and childhood are usually hamartomatous or choristomatous.

Table 23-1. Major Types of Conjunctival Tumor

Type	Subtypes	
Epidermal	Non-melanocytic	Melanocytic
Stromal	Vascular	Fibrous tissue
	Neural	Histiocytic
	Myxoid	Myogenic
	Lipomatous	Lymphoproliferative
Congenital	Hamartoma	Choristoma
Caruncular		
Metastatic		
Secondary		
Simulating lesions		

In cases of metastatic and secondary tumors, there is usually a history of primary malignancy in the surrounding structures or elsewhere.

Simulating lesions—although not neoplastic in origin, drug and metallic deposits, mascara deposits, foreign body, inflammatory, and infectious lesions should be included in the differential diagnosis.

REFERENCES

1. Campbell RJ, Sobin LH. Tumors of the conjunctiva and caruncle. In: *Histological Typing of Tumours of the Eye and Its Adnexa*. 2nd ed. World Health Organization International Histological Classification of Tumours. Berlin: Springer Verlag; 1998:9-15.
2. Shields CL, Shields JA. Tumors of the conjunctiva and cornea. *Surv Ophthalmol.* 2004;49:3-24.
3. Grossniklaus HE, Green WR, Luckenbach M, Chan CC. Conjunctival lesions in adults. A clinical and histopathologic review. *Cornea.* 1987;6:78-116.

Table 23-2. Classification of Epidermal Tumors of the Conjunctiva

Type		Subtypes
Non-melanocytic	Benign	Squamous papilloma
		Keratotic plaque
		Keratoacanthoma
		Reactive hyperplasia (pseudoepitheliomatous hyperplasia)
		Inverted follicular keratosis
		Hereditary intraepithelial dyskeratosis
		Oncocytoma
		Dacryoadenoma
	Premalignant and malignant	Actinic (solar) keratosis
		Conjunctival intraepithelial neoplasia (CIN)
		Squamous cell carcinoma
		Xeroderma pigmentosum
Melanocytic	Benign	Junctional nevus
		Compound nevus
		Spitz nevus
		Blue nevus
		PAM without atypia
		Congenital melanosis
		Racial melanosis
	Premalignant and malignant	PAM with atypia
		Melanoma arising from nevi
		Melanoma arising in PAM
		Melanoma arising de novo

PAM, primary acquired melanosis.

Chapter

24

Benign Conjunctival Tumors

Jacob Pe'er

INTRODUCTION

Benign tumors of the conjunctiva are much more common than malignant tumors. In this chapter, benign tumors of epithelial and melanocytic origin, which comprise the majority of the conjunctival tumors, are described. Benign stromal tumors are described in Chapter 28.

Squamous Cell Papilloma

This more commonly occurs in young adults.[1] In children, the papillomas have been documented to be associated with human papilloma virus (mostly types 6, 11, and 16) infection of the conjunctiva (Figure 24-1).[2] Cryotherapy is often used in conjunction with surgical excision, either to the conjunctiva around the excised lesion or to the lesion itself that is then excised in frozen state. Sometimes, cryotherapy may be performed without excision. Recurrent lesions may be treated by adjuvant interferon alpha-2B locally or systemically[3,4] or topical mitomycin C.[5]

Inverted Papilloma (Inverted Follicular Keratosis)

The lesions derive their name from the propensity to invaginate inward into the underlying conjunctival substantia propria, instead of growing in an exophytic manner outward.[6]

Reactive Epithelial Hyperplasia (Pseudoepitheliomatous Hyperplasia)

This may be secondary to irritation by concurrent or pre-existing stromal inflammation.[1]

Hereditary Benign Intraepithelial Dyskeratosis

Hereditary benign intraepithelial dyskeratosis (HBID) is an autosomal dominant disorder with a high degree of penetrance occuring in descendants of an inbred isolate of European, African-American, and Native American (Haliwa Indian) origin in northeastern North Carolina. Using genetic linkage analysis, the HBID gene was localized to chromosome 4 (4q35).[7] HBID is characterized by bilateral elevated fleshy plaques on the nasal or temporal perilimbal bulbar conjunctiva, with dilated conjunctival vessels around it.

Epithelial Cysts

Common cysts are epithelial inclusion cyst and ductal cysts, usually of accessory lacrimal gland origin.

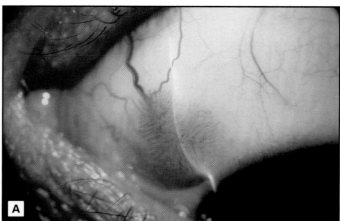

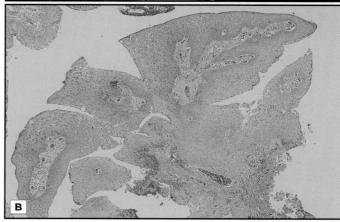

Figure 24-1. Solitary sessile squamous papilloma of the bulbar conjunctiva. Clinical appearance (A). Histopathology shows papillomatous fronds of acanthotic non-keratinized squamous epithelium with central fibrovascular cores (B). (Hematoxylin and eosin, original magnification x4.)

BENIGN MELANOCYTIC TUMORS

Conjunctival Nevus

The circumscribed nevus is the most common melanocytic conjunctival tumor. It appears in all races, although is more common in Caucasians (Figure 24-2). Most acquired conjunctival nevi will appear during the first two decades of life. Melanocytic conjunctival lesions that appear later in life are suspicious for PAM or melanoma.

In childhood and adolescence, conjunctival nevi may become more pink and congested, due to inflammatory infiltration.[8] The presence of cystic structures can help in differentiating nevi from other possible amelanotic conjunctival lesions. The overall risk of malignant transformation is about 1%.[9]

Congenital Melanosis Oculi (Congenital Ocular Melanocytosis)

This pigmentary condition of the sclera and uvea usually involves the periocular skin, orbit, meninges, and soft palate. The conjunctiva is usually not pigmented; it is included here because it is often considered in the clinical differential diagnosis of conjunctival pigmented lesion. When the periocular skin is involved, the condition is called "oculodermal melanocytosis" or "nevus of Ota."

TUMORS OF THE CARUNCLE

The caruncle contains both conjunctival and cutaneous elements. Consequently, any tumor of the conjunctiva and skin may occur in the caruncle. The vast majority of tumors in this location are benign, led by squamous papillomas and nevi. Only about 5% of the tumors are malignant.

REFERENCES

1. Sjo N, Heegaard S, Prause JU. Conjunctival papilloma. A histo-pathologically based retrospective study. *Acta Ophthalmol Scand.* 2000;78:663-666.

2. Lass JH, Jenson AB, Papale JJ, et al. Papillomavirus in human conjunctival papillomas. *Am J Ophthalmol.* 1983;95:364-368.

3. Schechter BA, Rand WJ, Velazquez GE, et al. Treatment of conjunctival papillomata with topical interferon Alfa-2b. *Am J Ophthalmol.* 2002;134:268-270.

4. Lass JH, Foster CS, Grove AS, et al. Interferon-alpha therapy of recurrent conjunctival papillomas. *Am J Ophthalmol.* 1987;103:294-301.

5. Hawkins AS, Yu J, Hamming NA, et al. Treatment of recurrent conjunctival papillomatosis with mitomycin C. *Am J Ophthalmol.* 1999;128:638-640.

6. Streeten BW, Carrillo R, Jamison R, et al. Inverted papilloma of the conjunctiva. *Am J Ophthalmol.* 1979;88:1062-1066.

7. Allingham RR, Seo B, Rampersaud E, et al. A duplication in chromosome 4q35 is associated with hereditary benign intraepithelial dyskeratosis. *Am J Hum Genet.* 2001;68:491-494.

8. Zamir E, Mechoulam H, Micera A, et al. Inflamed Juvenile Conjunctival Naevus: clinicopathological characterisation. *Br J Ophthalmol.* 2002;86:28-30.

9. Shields CL, Fasiudden AF, Mashayekhi A, et al. Conjunctival nevi: clinical features and natural course in 410 consecutive patients. *Arch Ophthalmol.* 2004; 122:167-175.

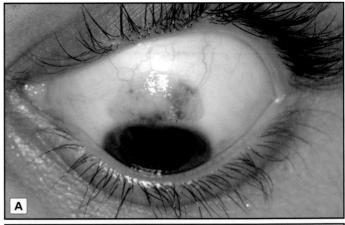

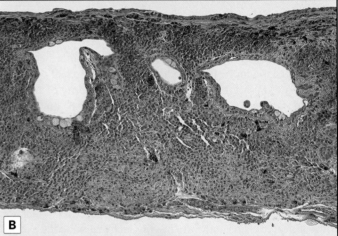

Figure 24-2. A partially pigmented compound conjunctival nevus with cystic elements is typically located near the limbus (A). Histopathology of a compound nevus of the conjunctiva with cystic structures lined by conjunctival epithelium (B). (Hematoxylin and eosin, original magnification x10.)

Ocular Surface Squamous Neoplasia

Jacob Pe'er and Joseph Frucht-Pery

INTRODUCTION

Ocular surface squamous neoplasia (OSSN) is the currently used term for the precancerous and cancerous epithelial lesions of the conjunctiva and cornea that previously had various names.[1,2] Other terms for the intraepithelial ocular surface neoplasia are conjunctival intraepithelial neoplasia[3] or corneal intraepithelial neoplasia (CIN), or both together (CCIN).

EPIDEMIOLOGICAL ASPECTS

OSSN is common in countries that are closer to the equator and in those where exposure to sunlight is more frequent.

Sunlight Exposure

Exposure to solar ultraviolet radiation has been identified in many studies as a major etiologic factor.[3-5]

Human Papillomavirus

In recent years, human papillomavirus (HPV), mainly type 16, has been demonstrated in tissue of OSSN.[6] However, HPV was detected also in uninvolved eyes with apparently healthy conjunctiva, suggesting that other factors are involved in causation.

Acquired Immunodeficiency Syndrome (AIDS)

The incidence of OSSN has increased significantly since the eruption of the AIDS epidemic, especially in sub-Saharan African countries.[7] OSSN tends to occur in younger people and is more aggressive in the presence of AIDS.[7]

CLINICAL FEATURES

In addition to the presence of the lesion on the ocular surface, other symptoms include ocular redness and irritation. Clinically, it may be difficult to distinguish among conjunctival epithelial dysplasia, carcinoma in situ, and invasive squamous cell carcinoma. These lesions arise commonly within the interpalpebral fissure, mostly at the limbus, although they may be found in any part of the conjunctiva and cornea (Figure 25-1). OSSN may appear gelatinous, with superficial vessels, or papilliform or leukoplakic, with a white keratin plaque covering the lesion.[3] It may also appear as a nodular lesion, especially when it is invasive SCC, or as a diffuse lesion masquerading as chronic conjunctivitis.

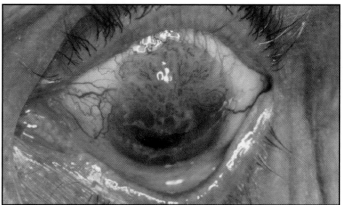

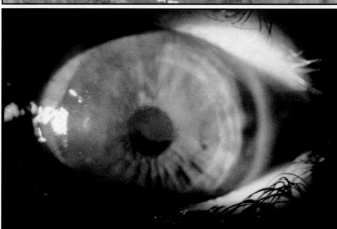

Figure 25-1. Elevated CIN at the upper limbal area with irregular papillary surface (bottom figure) and diffuse corneal involvement.

HISTOPATHOLOGIC FEATURES

Only histological evaluation of excised lesions, from either incisional or excisional biopsy, can differentiate between the three lesions within the spectrum of OSSN.[1,2]

Dysplastic lesions exhibit mild, moderate, or severe degrees of cellular atypia that may involve various thicknesses of the epithelium, starting from the basal layer outwards (Figure 25-2). Usually, the most superficial layers are uninvolved. Severe dysplastic change is the same as carcinoma in situ.

Carcinoma in situ may exhibit all the histological features of SCC but it remains confined to the epithelium, respecting the basement membrane.

Invasive squamous cell carcinoma shows features similar to carcinoma in situ, but the basement membrane of the epithelium is breached and the subepithelial tissue of the conjunctiva is invaded. Most conjunctival SCC are well differentiated and often show surface keratinization.

Histopathologic variants with aggressive behavior are spindle cell squamous carcinoma, mucoepidermoid carcinoma, and adenoid squamous cell carcinoma.

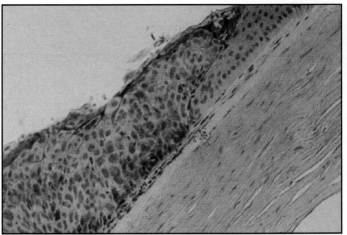

Figure 25-2. Acanthotic conjunctival epithelium with dysplastic changes involving most of the epithelial thickness. The epithelium lost its normal cellular polarity. Normal conjunctival epithelium is seen on the right side. (Hematoxylin and eosin, original magnification x100.)

TREATMENT

Surgery

Surgical excision is the traditional method of treatment for OSSN lesions. To avoid recurrence, it is recommended to excise the tumor tissue with wide surgical margins of 2 to 3 mm. When the deep cornea or sclera is involved, deep lamellar keratectomy or sclerectomy is performed (Chapter 29).

Cryotherapy

Combining surgical excision and cryosurgery reduces the recurrence rates.[8]

Brachytherapy

The most commonly used radioactive material has been strontium-90, with a recommended dose of 20 to 180 Gy to the tumor surface.[9]

Topical Chemotherapy

Because of the possible complications of surgical excision, cryotherapy and brachytherapy, topical chemotherapy using mitomycin C drops, 5-fluorouracil, or interferon alpha 2b have been advocated. Our protocol included treatment with 0.02% (0.2 mg/mL) mitomycin C drops four times daily for 2 weeks, repeated as necessary.[10] The main adverse reaction to the mitomycin C drops is hyperemia, and some patients experienced pain or a burning sensation due to corneal epithelial toxicity. The side effects disappeared within 2 weeks of stopping the topical mitomycin C, with or without the addition of topical steroids. Because of the superficial effects of mitomycin C drops, we do not recommend using them in invasive SCC as primary treatment.

PROGNOSIS

Local recurrence OSSN is considered to be a low-grade malignancy.[3,5] Recurrences after surgical excision depend on the surgical margins (5% when margins are free and 50% when margins are involved).[5]

Intraocular invasion is rare.

Metastasis of conjunctival SCC is extremely rare.[11] Sites of metastasis include preauricular, submandibular and cervical lymph nodes, parotid gland, lungs, and bones. The main cause of metastasis is delay in diagnosis and treatment.

REFERENCES

1. Lee GA, Hirst LW. Ocular surface squamous neoplasia. *Surv Ophthalmol.* 1995;39:429-450.
2. Pe'er J. Ocular surface squamous neoplasia. *Ophthalmol Clin North Am.* 2005;18:1-13.
3. Pizzarello LD, Jakobiec FA. Bowen's disease of the conjunctiva: a misnomer. In: Jakobiec FA, ed. *Ocular and Adnexal Tumors.* Birmingham, AL: Aesculapius; 1978:553-571.
4. Sun EC, Fears TR, Goedert JJ. Epidemiology of squamous cell conjunctival cancer. *Cancer Epidemiol Biomarkers Prev.* 1997;6:73-77.
5. Erie JC, Campbell RJ, Liesegang J. Conjunctival and corneal intraepithelial and invasive neoplasia. *Ophthalmology.* 1986;93:176-183.
6. McDonnell JM, Mayr AJ, Martin WJ. DNA of human papillomavirus type 16 in dysplastic and malignant lesions of the conjunctiva and cornea. *N Engl J Med.* 1989;320:1442-1446.
7. Goedert JJ, Cote TR. Conjunctival malignant disease with AIDS in USA. *Lancet.* 1995;346:257-258.
8. Fraunfelder FT, Wallace TR, Farris HE, et al. The role of cryosurgery in external ocular and periocular disease. *Trans Am Acad Ophthalmol Otolaryngol.* 1977;83:713-724.
9. Lommatzsch P. Beta-ray treatment of malignant epithelial tumors of the conjunctiva. *Am J Ophthalmol.* 1976;81:198-206.
10. Zehetmayer M, Menapace R, Kulnig W. Combined local excision and brachytherapy with Ruthenium-106 in the treatment of epibulbar malignancies. *Ophthalmologica.* 1993;207:133-139.
11. Frucht-Pery J, Sugar J, Baum J, et al. Mitomycin C treatment for conjunctival-corneal intraepithelial neoplasia: a multicenter experience. *Ophthalmology.* 1997;104:2085-2093.

Primary Acquired Melanosis

Jacob Pe'er and Robert Folberg

INTRODUCTION

The term primary acquired melanosis (PAM) represents flat, brown, intraepithelial conjunctival lesions. "Primary" denotes that the lesion is not the result of generalized (racial) dark pigmentation, systemic disease (eg, Addison's disease), or local factors (foreign body, injury, inflammation, medication, etc); "acquired" distinguishes these lesions from those that are congenital; "melanosis" indicates that the pigment in the lesion is derived specifically from the production of melanin rather than another pigment or a drug deposit.[1]

EPIDEMIOLOGICAL ASPECTS

PAM is more prevalent in fair-complexioned individuals than in those with dark skin tones and is almost always unilateral. If bilateral conjunctival pigmentation is encountered, the ophthalmologist should first consider either complexion-associated conjunctival pigmentation or a systemic condition associated with bilateral conjunctival pigmentation.

CLINICAL FEATURES

PAM occurs typically in middle-aged or elderly white patients and appears as a flat and variably brown conjunctival lesion, ranging from golden brown to dark chocolate in color (Figure 26-1).[1] However, there are no published size criteria for the clinical diagnosis of PAM.[2] PAM develops most commonly at the limbus and epibulbar interpalpebral region and may extend into the corneal epithelium. The lesion may involve any area of the conjunctiva in a contiguous or multispotted pattern, necessitating eversion of the eyelids to examine both the upper and lower palpebral zones. Parts of or, rarely, the entire lesion can be amelanotic (sine pigmento).[3]

HISTOPATHOLOGIC FEATURES

Histologically, PAM is divided into two major groups: PAM without atypia and PAM with atypia (Figures 26-2 and 26-3). Most conjunctival melanomas arise in the context of PAM with atypia. PAM with atypia is confined to the epithelium and is called *melanoma in situ* by some pathologists.[4]

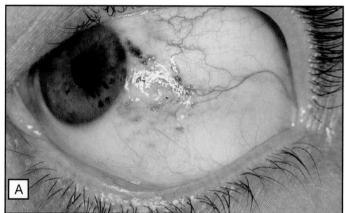

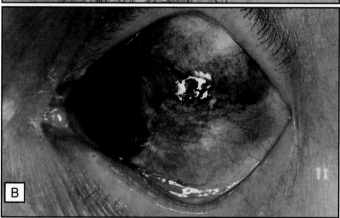

Figure 26-1. Localized (A) and diffuse variants of PAM (B).

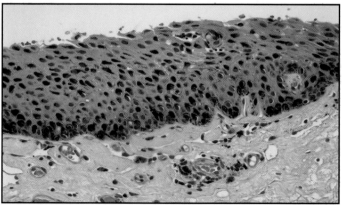

Figure 26-2. PAM without atypia. Melanin pigmentation is distributed throughout the conjunctival epithelium without melanocytic hyperplasia or atypia. (Hematoxylin and eosin, x20.)

TREATMENT

The appropriate management approach to PAM remains controversial.

Observation

A small subtle PAM lesion may be observed by periodic follow-up, which should include a thorough examination of the bulbar and palpebral conjunctiva and documentation of location, size, and appearance of each lesion.[2]

Surgery

The overwhelming consensus among ophthalmic oncologists and pathologists endorses biopsy of all conjunctival lesions that meet the clinical criteria for PAM.[3] Small lesions should be completely excised, whereas in widespread lesions, incisional biopsy should be performed from various sites of the affected conjunctiva. The specimen should be examined to determine the presence or absence of cytologic atypia and for the involvement of surgical margins.

Cryotherapy

Because of recurrences of PAM with atypia and the development of melanoma in these lesions, adding cryotherapy to the surgical excision is recommended (Chapter 29).[5]

Topical Mitomycin Chemotherapy

In order to cover the entire conjunctival and corneal surface, treating hidden areas of the PAM and preventing the complications of cryotherapy, we recommended a protocol of 0.04% (0.4 mg/mL) mitomycin C drops four times daily for 2 weeks with a pause of 2 weeks between courses. This regimen is repeated as necessary, until the remnants of the pigmentation disappear or stabilize. At least three courses are recommended. It is important to note that treatment with mitomycin C should be applied only to intraepithelial lesions and should not be used in invasive conjunctival melanoma.[6]

PROGNOSIS

The incidence of recurrence of PAM depends on the presence or absence of atypia.[3] Recurrence after excision is rare in PAM without atypia. On the other hand, about 60% of lesions designated as PAM with atypia recur after excision alone; half of them recur initially as malignant melanoma. No mortality has been reported from PAM without transformation to melanoma.

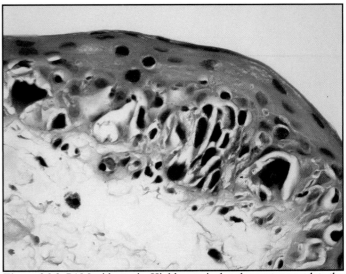

Figure 26-3. PAM with atypia. Highly atypical melanocytes populate the conjunctival epithelium singly and in nests. Note the lack of contact between these cells and the epithelium. (Hematoxylin and eosin, x40.)

REFERENCES

1. Jakobiec FA, Folberg R, Iwamoto T. Clinicopathologic characteristics of premalignant and malignant melanocytic lesions of the conjunctiva. *Ophthalmology.* 1989;96:147-166.
2. Gloor P, Alexandrakis G. Clinical characterization of primary acquired melanosis. *Invest Ophthalmol Vis Sci.* 1995;36:1721-1729.
3. Folberg R, McLean IW, Zimmerman LE. Primary acquired melanosis of the conjunctiva. *Hum Pathol.* 1985;16:129-135.
4. Ackerman AB, Sood R, Koenig M. Primary acquired melanosis of the conjunctiva is melanoma in situ. *Mod Pathol.* 1991;4:253-263.
5. Jakobiec FA, Rini FJ, Fraunfelder FT, et al. Cryotherapy for conjunctival primary acquired melanosis and malignant melanoma. Experience with 62 cases. *Ophthalmology.* 1988;95:1058-1070.
6. Pe'er J, Frucht-Pery J. The treatment of primary acquired melanosis (PAM) with atypia by topical mitomycin C. *Am J Ophthalmol.* 2005;139:229-234.

27

Conjunctival Melanoma

Jacob Pe'er and Robert Folberg

INTRODUCTION

Conjunctival nevi, conjunctival primary acquired melanosis (PAM), and conjunctival melanomas all arise from melanocytes that migrate from the neural crest to reside in the conjunctival epithelium. Conjunctival melanoma may arise de novo or in the context of conjunctival nevus, PAM, or both.[1,2]

EPIDEMIOLOGY

According to several studies, conjunctival melanoma accounts for 2% to 5% of ocular malignant melanomas[1] and less than 3% of excisional biopsies of conjunctival lesions.[3,4] Cutaneous melanoma was found to be 450 to 900 times more common than conjunctival melanoma, a ratio that is increasing. Conjunctival melanoma is more common in middle-aged and older persons, between the fourth and seventh decades of life.[4,5] Conjunctival melanomas are much less common in the black population and in other non-white individuals.[1]

CLINICAL FEATURES

Conjunctival melanoma usually affects one eye, and although these tumors are typically pigmented, amelanotic conjunctival melanomas do occur and can be mistaken for squamous cell carcinomas and lymphomas. It may arise in any region of the conjunctiva, including the bulbar, palpebral, and forniceal conjunctiva, and in the caruncle and plica semilunaris (Figures 27-1 and 27-2). Most conjunctival melanomas develop at the limbus. Multifocal conjunctival melanomas have been reported, and most of these originated from PAM with atypia (Figure 27-3).[6] The definite diagnosis of conjunctival melanoma is made by histopathologic examination. Most cases can be diagnosed with confidence by light microscopic features. If in doubt, pathologists can apply immunohistochemical stains such as HMB-45 or Melan-A, either individually or in a cocktail, to demonstrate melanocytes.

DIFFERENTIAL DIAGNOSIS

Any new, elevated pigmented conjunctival lesion that develops in adulthood should be viewed with suspicion. Conjunctival nevi almost always arise in the bulbar conjunctiva and caruncle. Therefore, any pigmented lesion presenting in the palpebral conjunctiva or fornix is suspicious for melanoma.[6]

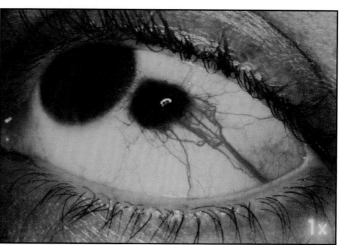

Figure 27-1. Melanoma of the perilimbal bulbar conjunctiva with "feeder vessels" entering the tumor.

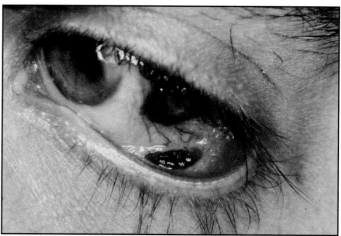

Figure 27-2. Multifocal melanoma arising from PAM with atypia, with a tumor in the bulbar conjunctiva and a tumor in the lower fornix.

Epithelial lesions such as squamous papilloma, conjunctival intraepithelial neoplasia, and invasive squamous cell carcinomas may acquire melanin pigment in darkly complexioned individuals.[7] Staphylomas, subconjunctival hematomas, foreign bodies, and hematic cysts may also be confused clinically with conjunctival melanoma.[1] The rare occurrence of metastatic cutaneous melanoma to the conjunctiva has been reported.[8] Epibulbar extension of uveal melanoma or melanocytoma should also be considered in the differential diagnosis.

TREATMENT

The primary treatment of conjunctival melanoma is excision of the entire tumor with wide surgical margins of 3 to 5 mm. When deep limbal and scleral involvement is suspected, scleroconjunctivectomy should be considered.[9] Most surgeons will add an adjuvant treatment with cryotherapy to the surgical margins and/or the surgical bed. Others advocate supplemental brachytherapy, usually using β irradiation. Some surgeons use absolute alcohol to devitalize corneal epithelial cells adjacent to a limbal melanoma before excision. Exenteration of the orbit, including the eyelids in order to include the palpebral and forniceal conjunctiva, is currently reserved only as a palliative treatment for advanced stages of conjunctival melanoma.

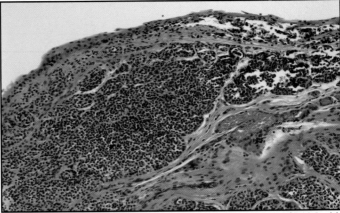

Figure 27-3. Conjunctival melanoma arising in the context of PAM with atypia. Note the lack of maturation or architectural organization from top to bottom, and the presence of atypical intraepithelial melanocytes that do not appear to be cohesive or to have any architectural relationship with the epithelial cells. (Hematoxylin and eosin, original magnification x20.)

CLINICAL COURSE

Local recurrence of conjunctival melanoma has been reported in 56% to 65% of patients.[1] Adjuvant treatment reduces the risk of recurrences. The most common location of metastases is regional: the preauricular and submandibular lymph nodes. Other common locations are the brain, liver, and lung.[10] The conjunctival melanoma- related mortality rate is 12% to 19% in 5 years and 23% to 30% in 10 years.[10] Regional metastases can be treated by lumpectomy and adjuvant radiotherapy.[10] Most patients with disseminated conjunctival melanoma are treated with systemic chemotherapy.

REFERENCES

1. Seregard S. Conjunctival melanoma. *Surv Ophthalmol.* 1998;42:321-350.
2. Folberg R, McLean IW, Zimmerman LE. Malignant melanoma of the conjunctiva. *Hum Pathol.* 1985;16:136-143.
3. Grossniklaus HE, Green WR, Luckenbach M, et al. Conjunctival lesions in adults. A clinical and histopathologic review. *Cornea.* 1987;6:78-116.
4. De Woolf-Rouendaal D. Conjunctival melanoma in the Netherlands: a clinicopathological and follow-up study. [Thesis] Katwijk, All in BV, 1990.
5. Yu GP, Hu DN, McCormick S, et al. Conjunctival melanoma: is it increasing in the United States? *Am J Ophthalmol.* 2003;135:800-806.
6. Jakobiec FA, Folberg R, Iwamoto T. Clinicopathologic characteristics of premalignant and malignant melanocytic lesions of the conjunctiva. *Ophthalmology.* 1989;96:147-166.
7. Folberg R, Jakobiec FA, Bernardino VB, et al. Benign conjunctival melanocytic lesions. Clinicopathologic features. *Ophthalmology.* 1989;96:436-461.
8. Kiratli H, Shields CL, Shields JA, et al. Metastatic tumours to the conjunctiva: report of 10 cases. *Br J Ophthalmol.* 1996;80:5-8.
9. Shields JA, Shields CL, DePotter P. Surgical management of conjunctival tumors. *Arch Ophthalmol.* 1997;115:808-815.
10. Tuomaala S, Kivela T. Metastatic pattern and survival in disseminated conjunctival melanoma: implications for sentinel lymph node biopsy. *Ophthalmology.* 2004;111:816-821.

Conjunctival Stromal Tumors

Jacob Pe'er

INTRODUCTION

The conjunctival stroma contains various tissue elements, such as vascular, fibrous, neural, and others. Naturally, benign and malignant tumors may originate from these types of tissue (Table 28-1). However, conjunctival stromal tumors are rare.

Pyogenic Granuloma

The term *pyogenic granuloma* is a misnomer, as it is neither pyogenic nor granulomatous. It is granulation tissue, fibrovascular response to a tissue insult, such as surgical or nonsurgical trauma, or inflammation, although spontaneous pyogenic granulomas have also been reported (Figure 28-1).[1]

Lymphangiectasia

When lymphatic channels in the conjunctiva are dilated and prominent, the condition is called lymphangiectasia.

Fibrous Histiocytoma

Fibrous histiocytoma (FH) of the conjunctiva can be benign, locally aggressive, or malignant. FH generally occurs in adults. Conjunctival FH appears as an amelanotic mass that can range from well-circumscribed to diffuse. It often presents at the limbus.[2] It is composed of a mixture of spindle-shaped fibroblasts, often arranged in a storiform pattern, with lipid-laden histiocytes. Conjunctival FH with benign histological appearance may show a malignant clinical course. Malignant FH of the conjunctiva is extremely rare and shows marked pleomorphism, many mitotic figures, and multinucleated giant cells.[3]

Neurofibroma

Neurofibroma is a peripheral nerve sheath tumor that can occur in the conjunctival stroma as a solitary circumscribed diffuse or plexiform mass.

CHORISTOMA

Choristomas are congenital lesions representing normal tissue in an abnormal location. When the lesion is composed of one type of tissue, it is considered to be a simple choristoma; when combinations of displaced tissue are involved, it is termed *complex choristoma*. Epibulbar choristomas are the most common epibulbar tumors in children.[4] Among them, dermoids and dermolipomas are very common. Epibulbar choristomas may be associated

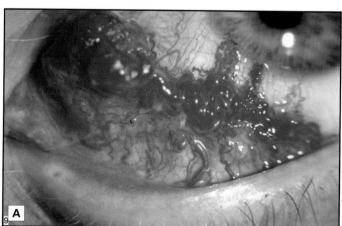
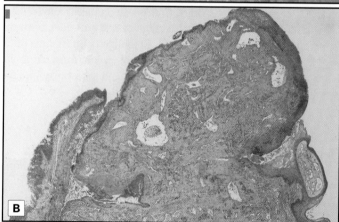

Figure 28-1. Pyogenic granuloma. A 31-year-old man with a 3-week history of a rapidly growing recurrent conjunctival vascular growth in the inferonasal conjunctival fornix. Note prominent vascularity (A). Polypoid lesion with lobular pattern of capillary proliferation. The vessels are variably dilated (B). (Original magnification x4.)

with coloboma, Goldenhar syndrome, or organoid nevus syndrome.

Dermoid

Epibulbar dermoid is a well-circumscribed, firm, solitary, congenital mass that involves the bulbar conjunctiva and often the corneoscleral limbus (Figure 28-2).

Table 28-1. Classification of Stromal Tumors of the Conjunctiva

Category	Subtypes	
Vascular tumors	Capillary hemangioma	Cavernous hemangioma
	Varix	Racemose malformation
	Hemangiopericytoma	Kaposi's sarcoma
	Lymphangiectasia	Lymphangioma
	Malignant hemangioendothelioma	
Fibrous tumors	Fibroma	Nodular fasciitis
	Benign fibrous histiocytoma	Malignant fibrous histiocytoma
Neural tumors	Neurofibroma (localized)	Neurofibroma (diffuse)
	Schwannoma (neurilemmoma)	Granular cell tumor
Histiocytic tumors	Xanthoma	Juvenile xanthogranuloma
	Reticulohistiocytoma	
Myxoid tumors	Myxoma	
Myogenic tumors	Rhabdomyosarcoma	
Lipomatous tumors	Lipoma	Herniated orbital fat
	Liposarcoma	
Lymphoproliferative tumors	Benign reactive lymphoid hyperplasia	Lymphoma
	Leukemic infiltrates	
Choristomas	Dermoid	Dermolipoma
	Osseous choristoma	Lacrimal gland choristoma
	Complex choristoma	
Metastatic tumors		
Secondary tumors		

Dermolipoma

This is a yellowish-tan, soft, fusiform tumor, usually localized to the temporal or superotemporal aspect of the conjunctiva, near the lateral canthus. Although it is congenital, it may remain asymptomatic for years until detected when it protrudes from the superotemporal conjunctival fornix. Epibulbar dermolipoma often extends between the lateral and superior rectus muscles to lie close to the lacrimal gland. It may also extend posteriorly into the orbit or anteriorly toward the limbus.

Lacrimal Gland Choristoma

Lacrimal gland choristoma (ectopic lacrimal gland) is a simple choristomatous congenital lesion that presents as an asymptomatic pink stromal mass, typically in the superotemporal or temporal part of the conjunctiva.

Complex Choristoma

Complex choristoma is a congenital, unilateral lesion that contains tissue derived from two germ layers, ectoderm and mesoderm.[4]

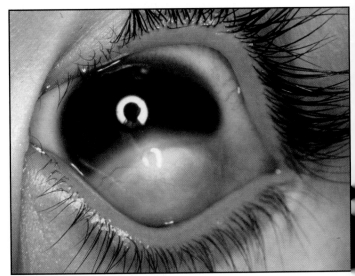

Figure 28-2. Epibulbar dermoid.

REFERENCES

1. Ferry AP. Pyogenic granulomas of the eye and ocular adnexa: a study of 100 cases. *Trans Am Ophthalmol Soc.* 1989;87:327-343.
2. Jakobiec FA. Fibrous histiocytoma of the corneoscleral limbus. *Am J Ophthalmol.* 1974;78:700-706.
3. Pe'er J, Levinger S, Ilsar M, Climenhaga H, Okon E. Malignant fibrous histiocytoma of the conjunctiva. *Br J Ophthalmol.* 1990;74:624-628.
4. Mansour AM, Barber JC, Reinecke RD, Wang FM. Ocular choristomas. *Surv Ophthalmol.* 1989;33:339-358.

Chapter

29

Surgical Techniques

Anat Galor, Bennie H. Jeng, and Arun D. Singh

INTRODUCTION

A detailed slit-lamp examination is not only vital to diagnose conjunctival and corneal tumors correctly, but is also critical for planning the appropriate surgery. A drawing or photograph clearly depicting the extent of involvement that can be readily viewed during surgery is helpful for obtaining adequate surgical margins.

ANESTHESIA

Local anesthesia can be used for most procedures, depending on patient cooperation. Most authors recommend retrobulbar anesthesia with sedation to avoid disruption of the conjunctival architecture.[1]

GENERAL SURGICAL TECHNIQUE

The surgical procedure can be divided into four sequential steps: corneal excision (if corneal involvement is present), conjunctival excision, supplemental cryotherapy (if needed), and wound closure.

Corneal Excision

Corneal excision is usually limited to the removal of corneal epithelium (corneal epitheliectomy). Care must be taken not to disrupt Bowman's layer, as it is thought to serve as a natural ocular barrier to invasion. Deeper invasion of the cornea, if present, necessitates lamellar keratectomy. Prior to scraping off the affected epithelium with a no. 57 Beaver blade, absolute alcohol is applied with a cotton-tipped applicator to denature the involved corneal epithelium.

Conjunctival Excision

Simple

Benign lesions that do not penetrate the sclera can be removed by a simple excisional biopsy with 1- to 2-mm margins of non-affected tissues.[2]

Complex

For potentially malignant tumors, a wider margin of excision of clinically non-affected tissue (4 to 5 mm) and lamellar sclerectomy are necessary. The conjunctiva and Tenon's fascia are incised with scissors, exposing the underlying sclera (Figure 29-1). A partial sclerectomy is performed with no. 57 Beaver blade to approximately 20% of the depth of the sclera.

Supplemental Cryotherapy

A flat-tipped nitrous oxide probe is placed on the underside of the conjunctival edge, lifting the conjunctiva to avoid damage to the sclera.[2] The tissue is allowed to thaw spontaneously and is refrozen for a "double freeze–thaw" cycle.

Wound Closure

To prevent the possibility of planting tumor cells on unaffected tissue, it is important to use a different set of instruments to close the conjunctiva than were used to remove the lesion. If a simple excisional biopsy is performed, the surrounding conjunctiva can be left to re-epithelialize. For larger defects, the conjunctiva can be primarily closed by undermining the surrounding conjunctivae. A large defect can be closed with a conjunctival graft harvested from the opposite eye, or with an amniotic membrane.[3]

SPECIFIC SURGICAL TECHNIQUES

Prior discussion with a pathologist is important to identify the proper fixative agent; most commonly, 10% formalin is used. For suspected lymphoid tumors, tissue should be transported fresh in a small amount of saline for flow cytometric analysis. Specimens are prepared by laying the tissue flat, epithelial side up, on sterile paper wetted with balanced salt solution. Orientation is drawn with a graphite pencil.

COMPLICATIONS

Infection, bleeding, delayed epithelial healing, pyogenic granuloma, Tenon's cyst, conjunctival and corneal scarring, and restrictive strabismus are uncommon.

REFERENCES

1. Shields JA, Shields CL, De Potter P. Surgical management of conjunctival tumors. *Arch Ophthalmol.* 1997;115:808-815.
2. Peksayar G, Altan-Yaycioglu R, Onal S. Excision and cryosurgery in the treatment of conjunctival malignant epithelial tumours. *Eye.* 2003;17:228-232.
3. Paridaens D, Beekhuis H, van Den Bosch W, et al. Amniotic membrane transplantation in the management of conjunctival malignant melanoma and primary acquired melanosis with atypia. *Br J Ophthalmol.* 2001;85:658-661.

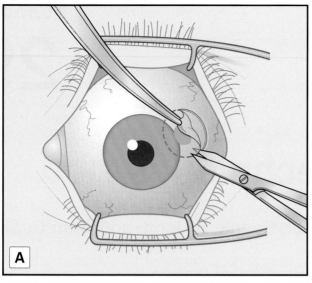

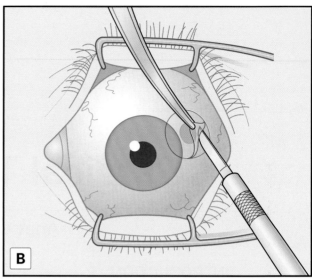

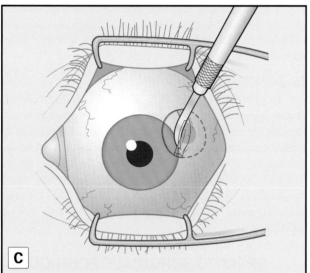

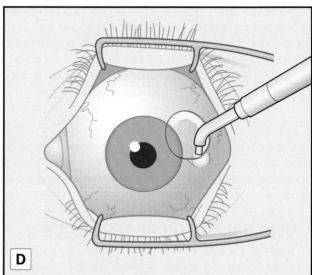

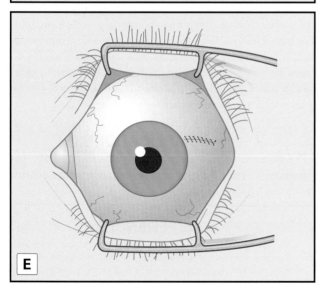

Figure 29-1. Complex conjunctival excision. Large conjunctival lesion being excised with a 4-mm margin of unaffected conjunctiva. (A) Conjunctival flap being fashioned. (B) Partial-thickness scleral incision with a no. 57 Beaver blade. (C) Lamellar scleral dissection with a crescent blade. (D) Cryotherapy to the edges of the conjunctival wound. (E) Closure of the wound.

Systemic Associations of Conjunctival and Corneal Tumors

Arun D. Singh and Elias I. Traboulsi

INTRODUCTION

Conjunctival tumors and tumor-like conditions with syndromic association can be considered under the categories of pigmented lesions (Peutz–Jeghers syndrome), benign tumors (Goldenhar syndrome), malignant tumors (xeroderma pigmentosum), and amyloidosis (Table 30-1).

Goldenhar Syndrome (Oculoauriculovertebral Dysplasia)

Goldenhar described a triad of epibulbar dermoids, pre-auricular appendages, and pretragal fistula (Figure 30-1).[1]

Table 30-1. Various Conjunctival Tumors That Are Markers of Syndromic Association

Pattern		Entity	Conjunctival Features	Associated Features	Locus/Gene
Pigmentation		Carney complex	Conjunctival pigmentation	Spotty mucocutaneous pigmentation Schwannoma Endocrine overactivity Testicular tumor	17q PRKAR1A gene chromosome 2
		Peutz-Jeghers	Conjunctival pigmentation	Mucocutaneous pigmentation Gastrointestinal polyposis	19p13.3 STK11
Benign tumors	Dermoid	Organoid nevus syndrome	Epibulbar dermoid Coloboma	Cutaneous sebaceus nevus	Sporadic
		Goldenhar syndrome	Epibulbar dermoid	Preauricular appendages Pretragal fistula Vertebral anomalies	Sporadic
		Proteus	Epibulbar dermoid Strabismus Orbital exostoses	Connective tissue nevi Lipoma Vascular malformations Epidermal nevi	Sporadic
	Neuroma	MEN-2B	Conjunctival neuroma	Thickened corneal nerves Mucocutaneous neuroma Endocrine tumor	10q11.2 RET protooncogene
Malignant tumors		Xeroderma pigmentosum	Conjunctiva xerosis Keratitis Ocular surface neoplasms	Skin atrophy with pigmentary changes Neurological abnormalities	Variable
Amyloidosis			Conjunctival nodule Conjunctival hemorrhage	Variable	Sporadic Familial

MEN, multiple endocrine neoplasia.

Proteus Syndrome

This is a severe and highly variable disorder characterized by asymmetric and disproportionate overgrowth of body parts and hamartomas.[2] Epibulbar and eyelid dermoids, strabismus, nystagmus, high myopia, orbital exostoses, and posterior segment hamartoma are most commonly observed.

Multiple Endocrine Neoplasia

Multiple endocrine neoplasia (MEN) refers to a genetic predisposition to develop benign and malignant tumors of various endocrine glands. MEN 2B is also called mucosal neuroma syndrome or Wagenmann-Froboese syndrome and is the only MEN subgroup that is of ophthalmic interest. MEN 2B is inherited as an autosomal dominant trait. About half the cases are due to de novo mutations. Common ophthalmic manifestations include prominent corneal nerves (100%), eyelid neuroma or thickening (88%), subconjunctival neuroma (79%) (Figure 30-2), and dry eyes (48%).[3]

Xeroderma Pigmentosum

This is a genetic disorder characterized by extreme sensitivity to sunlight and a constellation of cutaneous, ophthalmic, and neurological findings.[4] The cutaneous findings are the defining features of this entity. Eyelid skin atrophy with pigmentary changes and loss of lashes is common. Corneal complications include keratitis, pterygium, vascularization, and corneal ulceration. Most significant is the predisposition to develop multiple eyelid and ocular surface neoplasms including basal cell carcinoma, squamous cell carcinoma, and melanoma.

REFERENCES

1. Goldenhar M. Associations malformatives de l'oeil et de l'oreille: en particulier, le syndrome: dermoid epibulbaire-appendices auriculaires-fistula auris congenita et ses relations avec la dysostose mandibulo-faciale. *J Genet Hum.* 1952;1:243-282.
2. Wiedemann HR, Burgio GR, Aldenhoff P, et al. The proteus syndrome. Partial gigantism of the hands and/or feet, nevi, hemihypertrophy, subcutaneous tumors, macrocephaly or other skull anomalies and possible accelerated growth and visceral affections. *Eur J Pediatr.* 1983;140:5-12.
3. Robertson DM, Sizemore GW, Gordon H. Thickened corneal nerves as a manifestation of multiple endocrine neoplasia. *Trans Sect Ophthalmol Am Acad Ophthalmol Otolaryngol.* 1975;79:OP772-787.
4. Kraemer KH, Lee MM, Scotto J. Xeroderma pigmentosum. Cutaneous, ocular, and neurologic abnormalities in 830 published cases. *Arch Dermatol.* 1987;123:241-250.

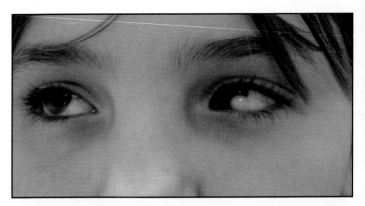

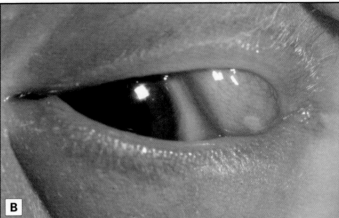

Figure 30-1. (A) Epibulbar dermoid and facial pit and (B) dermolipoma in Goldenhar syndrome.

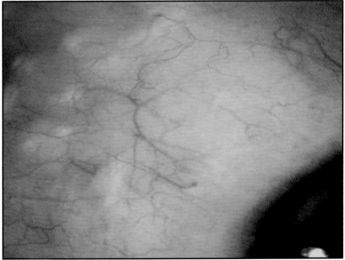

Figure 30-2. Plexiform subconjunctival neuroma. (Reproduced with permission from Eter N, Klingmuller D, Hoppner W, Spitznas M. Typical ocular findings in a patient with multiple endocrine neoplasia MEN-2B syndrome. *Graefes Arch Clin Exp Ophthalmol.* 2001;239:391-394. © Springer-Verlag 2001.)

Examination Techniques

Nikolaos Trichopoulos and Bertil E. Damato

INTRODUCTION

This chapter highlights procedures that are specific to the assessment of a patient with a uveal tumor (Box 31-1).

HISTORY TAKING

The history can sometimes provide diagnostic clues, for example if the patient has been a heavy smoker for many years or if a previous mastectomy has been performed. Although such information might suggest the source of an intraocular metastasis, it should not be relied upon to distinguish between a metastasis and other types of tumor, such as melanoma and hemangioma. The history also provides an understanding of the patient's visual needs, which may help in the selection of the most appropriate form of treatment. The duration of the visual loss can have prognostic significance, for example in patients with choroidal hemangioma in whom visual loss is irreversible if long-standing.

VISUAL ACUITY

If possible, visual acuity should be measured using a LogMAR chart, which overcomes the limitations of the Snellen test and which also facilitates statistical analysis of vision in any outcomes analysis.

SLIT-LAMP EXAMINATION

It is necessary to define the primary tumor, recognizing any secondary effects, predisposing factors, and concurrent disease.

INDIRECT OPHTHALMOSCOPY

It is essential to examine the entire fundus, with indentation if necessary, to identify any other pathology and to exclude any other tumors. Both eyes should be examined, ideally with mydriasis. The senior author has devised the mnemonic MELANOMA to alert the clinician to the presence of an intraocular tumor in situations where the pupils are not routinely dilated (Box 31-2).

It is necessary to describe the primary tumor, any secondary effects, and any predisposing factors, as follows:

- Tissue of origin (choroid, retina, retinal pigment epithelium)
- Quadrant (superotemporal, superior, superonasal, etc)
- Shape (flat, dome, collar-stud)
- Margins (discrete, diffuse)

Box 31-1. Examination Techniques

- These include history taking, slit-lamp examination, and ophthalmoscopy
- Drawings can complement photography
- Tumor dimensions can be estimated both using charts and ophthalmoscopically
- Three-mirror examination is useful in selected cases
- Transillumination gives an approximate indication of tumor extent

Box 31-2. Symptoms and Signs Indicating the Presence of an Intraocular Tumor

- Melanoma or other tumor visible externally in the iris or episclera
- Eccentric visual phenomena, such as photopsia, floaters, and field loss
- Lens abnormalities, such as cataract, astigmatism, and coloboma
- Afferent pupillary defect, mostly caused by secondary retinal detachment
- No optical correction with spectacles because of blurring or metamorphopsia
- Ocular hypertension, especially if asymmetrical
- Melanocytosis, predisposing to melanoma
- Asymmetrical episcleral vessels, indicating a ciliary body tumor

- Color (pink, white, yellow, red, orange, tan, brown, black, etc)
- Vascularity (vascular, avascular)
- Posterior extent, including distances to optic disc margin and fovea
- Anterior extent (post-equatorial, pre-equatorial, pars plana, pars plicata, etc)
- Circumferential involvement

- Internal spread (subretinal space, retina, vitreous)
- Secondary effects (eg, RPE changes such as drusen and orange pigment over the tumor[1]; RPE changes adjacent to the tumor[2]; exudative retinal detachment; and hemorrhage[3,4])
- Predisposing factors (ocular melanocytosis)[5]

FUNDUS DRAWING

Fundus drawings complement any photography in several ways, for example allowing important features to be highlighted by means of notes and markers.

ESTIMATION OF INTRAOCULAR TUMOR BASAL DIMENSIONS

Schematic diagrams have been prepared to facilitate the estimation of ocular dimensions on clinical examination. In addition, indirect ophthalmoscopy can be used to estimate the basal dimensions of intraocular tumors. The chord length tumor basal diameters (anteroposterior or longitudinal and circumferential or latitudinal) are estimated while performing indirect ophthalmoscopy by assessing the proportion of a specific condensing lens field that is filled by the tumor's image. During this assessment, a 20 D lens is considered to have a field diameter of approximately 12 mm, whereas a 28 D lens is regarded to have a field diameter of 13 mm. For example, a tumor that fills half of the 20 D lens field would be judged to have a diameter of approximately 6 mm, whereas one that fills two thirds of a 28 D lens field would be considered to be about 8.5 mm in diameter. The indications for three-mirror examination are to identify the cause of raised intraocular pressure; determine whether a lesion behind the iris is solid or cystic; find a small retinal angioma; determine the anterior extent of a pre-equatorial tumor; and measure the circumferential extent of ciliary body or angle involvement by a tumor, aligning in turn each lateral tumor margin with the center of the mirror.

TRANSILLUMINATION

Transillumination can be used to locate tumor margins. In general, pigmented tumors and intraocular hemorrhage would block the transmission of light. It must be realized that not all pigmented tumors are melanoma and, conversely, not all melanomas are pigmented. Different techniques are possible (Figure 31-1).

ANCILLARY TESTS

Tumor thickness is best estimated by ultrasonography. Ancillary investigations such as photography, angiography, and ultrasonography are discussed in detail elsewhere (Chapter 32).

REFERENCES

1. Damato BE, Foulds WS. Tumour-associated retinal pigment epitheliopathy. *Eye.* 1990;4:382-387.
2. Haut J, Sobel-Martin A, Dureuil J, Larricart P, Sarnikowski C. Atrophies "like flows" of the retinal pigment epithelium: a neuroepithelium-draining method of the posterior pole. *Ophthalmologica.* 1984;189:121-127.
3. Lee J, Logani S, Lakosha H, et al. Preretinal neovascularization associated with choroidal melanoma. *Br J Ophthalmol.* 2001;85:1309-1312.
4. el Baba F, Hagler WS, De la Cruz A, Green WR. Choroidal melanoma with pigment dispersion in vitreous and melanomalytic glaucoma. *Ophthalmology.* 1988;95:370-377.
5. Shetlar DJ, Folberg R, Gass JD. Choroidal malignant melanoma associated with a melanocytoma. *Retina.* 1999;19:346-349.

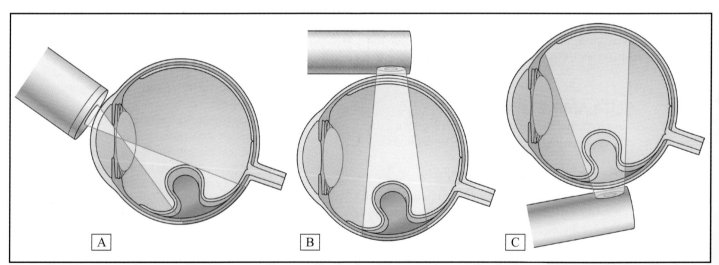

Figure 31-1. Tumor extension assessed by (A) transpupillary transillumination; (B) transocular transillumination; and (C) transscleral transillumination. Note the exaggeration of posterior tumor extension with transpupillary transillumination. (This figure was published in Damato B. *Ocular Tumours: Diagnosis and Treatment.* © Elsevier 1999.)

Diagnostic Techniques

Sophie Bakri, LuAnne Sculley, and Arun D. Singh

INTRODUCTION

In uveal melanoma, the diagnostic accuracy is more than 99% based on indirect ophthalmoscopy, ultrasonography, and angiography.[1] However, in atypical cases, a variety of other imaging modalities can be used to establish the diagnosis.

PHOTOGRAPHY

Anterior segment photography is used to document the size, shape, and surface features of iris lesions such as cysts, nevi, and melanomas.

Fundus photography is particularly useful when evaluating indeterminate choroidal tumors for growth, the response of choroidal melanoma to therapy, and assessing for recurrences (Figure 32-1A).

FLUORESCEIN ANGIOGRAPHY

The characteristic angiographic features of choroidal melanomas include intrinsic tumor circulation ("double circulation"), hot spots, and late leakage (Figure 32-1B, C). Intrinsic tumor circulation is evident in medium and large choroidal melanoma in early phases representing abnormal vessels within the choroidal tumor. The hot spots are caused by pinpoint leaks from the retinal pigment epithelium that enlarge minimally and stain late. An absence of late diffuse leakage within the choroidal tumor goes against the diagnosis of choroidal melanoma.[2]

INDOCYANINE GREEN ANGIOGRAPHY

Indocyanine green angiography allows better visualization of the tumor vasculature than fluorescein angiography because of several physicochemical properties of indocyanine green (ICG) (Figure 32-1D).[3] Choroidal melanomas achieve maximal fluorescence at an average of 18 minutes after injection of the dye.[4] In general, non-pigmented choroidal melanomas show an earlier onset of fluorescence (<1 minute) than the pigmented variety (3 minutes).

Overall, the pattern of fluorescence within a choroidal melanoma is heterogeneous and varies from hypofluorescent to isofluorescent and hyperfluorescent, depending on the extent of tumor pigmentation. In contrast, choroidal metastases tend to have a homogeneous and diffuse fluorescence with late isofluorescence.

Choroidal hemangiomas have a unique pattern of fluorescence on ICG angiography, characterized by early onset of fluorescence with early maximal fluorescence (within 5 minutes), followed by "washout" of the dye in the late phases of the angiogram.[5]

ULTRASONOGRAPHY

A/B scan ultrasonography imaging with A and B scan techniques is currently the most important test in the diagnosis of choroidal melanoma.[4] It not only provides clues to the diagnosis, but also defines the intraocular extent of the tumor. Extraocular extension of the tumor is also readily detected by ultrasonography (Figure 32-2). There may be vascular pulsations in a highly vascularized tumor. A mushroom-like configuration, indicating that the tumor has broken through Bruch's membrane, is almost pathognomonic of choroidal melanoma (see Figure 32-2).[5,6] On A-scan ultrasonography, choroidal melanoma shows characteristic low to medium internal reflectivity, with a high initial spike "positive-angle κ sign" (see Figure 32-2). Ultrasonography can be a useful tool to differentiate melanomas from a variety of simulating lesions. However, there are no pathognomonic features that differentiate a choroidal nevus from a small choroidal melanoma. Choroidal metastases have medium-high reflectivity with a "negative angle κ" sign (the back portion of the tumor climbs toward the sclera). Choroidal hemangiomas have high reflectivity. A choroidal osteoma shows calcification on B scan, with shadowing in the orbit and high surface reflectivity.

Color Doppler imaging is an ultrasound technique that displays color-encoded Doppler flow information, thereby detecting intrinsic circulation[7] supportive of a choroidal melanoma.

Ultrasound biomicroscopy allows quantitative measurements of tumor size, tumor extension, as well as differentiation of solid and cystic lesions (Figure 32-3).[8]

OPTICAL COHERENCE TOMOGRAPHY

Anterior segment optical coherence tomography is an alternative modality to ultrasound biomicroscopy for the assessment of iris and ciliary body lesions.[9]

Posterior segment optical coherence tomography is useful for detecting subtle changes in the vitreoretinal interface, retina, and retinal pigment epithelium.[10]

Figure 32-1. Fundus appearance of a choroidal melanoma (A). Fluorescein angiogram showing characteristic ill-defined leakage in the early phase (B), which progresses with angiogram into the late phase (C). Indocyanine green angiography allows better visualization of the intrinsic tumor vasculature (D). (Reproduced with permission from Bakri SJ, Sculley L, Singh AD. Imaging techniques for uveal melanoma. *Int Ophthalmol Clin.* 2006;46:1-13.)

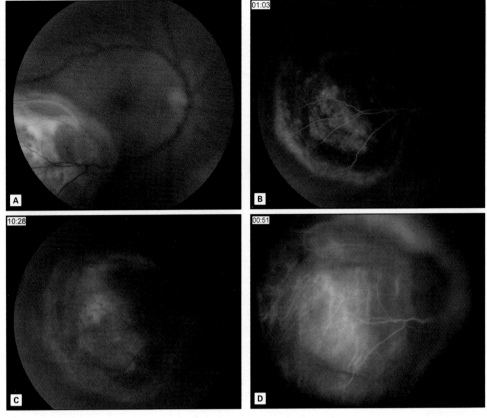

Figure 32-2. Ultrasonographic features of a choroidal melanoma. Acoustic quiet zone within the tumor on B-scan ultrasonography (A). (B) The mushroom-like configuration is almost pathognomonic. (C) Low internal reflectivity on A-scan. (D) Extrascleral extension (arrow). (Reproduced with permission from Bakri SJ, Sculley L, Singh AD. Imaging techniques for uveal melanoma. *Int Ophthalmol Clin.* 2006;46:1-13.)

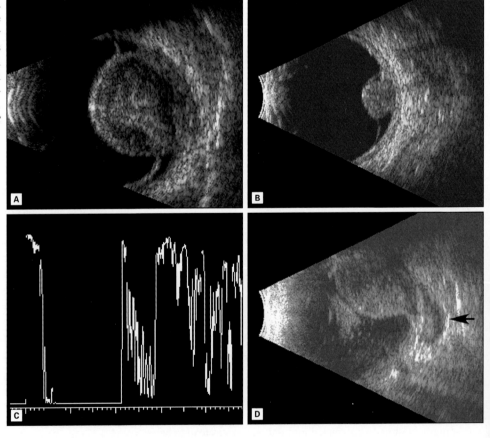

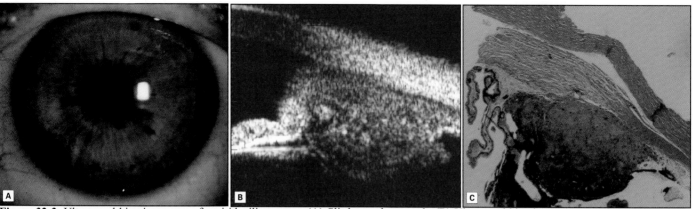

Figure 32-3. Ultrasound biomicroscopy of an iridociliary mass. (A) Slit-lamp photograph. (B) Ultrasound biomicroscopy revealed a ciliary body mass with anterior extension into the iris root. (C) Note the close correlation between histopathological appearance (after iridocyclectomy) and biomicroscopic findings. (Reproduced with permission from Bakri SJ, Sculley L, Singh AD. Imaging techniques for uveal melanoma. *Int Ophthalmol Clin.* 2006;46:1-13.)

COMPUTERIZED TOMOGRAPHY, MAGNETIC RESONANCE IMAGING, POSITRON EMISSION TOMOGRAPHY

These imaging modalities are less reliable than ultrasonography in differentiating between uveal masses.

REFERENCES

1. Group COMS. Accuracy of diagnosis of choroidal melanomas in the Collaborative Ocular Melanoma Study. COMS report no. 1. *Arch Ophthalmol.* 1990;108:1268-1273.
2. Char DH, Stone RD, Irvine AR, et al. Diagnostic modalities in choroidal melanoma. *Am J Ophthalmol.* 1980;89:223-230.
3. Sallet G, Amoaku WM, Lafaut BA, et al. Indocyanine green angiography of choroidal tumors. *Graefes Arch Clin Exp Ophthalmol.* 1995;233:677-689.
4. Shields CL, Shields JA, De Potter P. Patterns of indocyanine green videoangiography of choroidal tumours. *Br J Ophthalmol.* 1995;79:237-245.
5. Arevalo JF, Shields CL, Shields JA, et al. Circumsbribed choroidal hemangioma: characteristic features with indocyanine green video-angiography. *Ophthalmology.* 2002;107:344-350.
6. Verbeek AM, Thijssen JM, Cuypers MH, et al. Echographic classification of intraocular tumours. A 15-year retrospective analysis. *Acta Ophthalmol (Copenh).* 1994;72:416-422.
7. Lieb WE, Shields JA, Cohen SM, et al. Color Doppler imaging in the management of intraocular tumors. *Ophthalmology.* 1990;97:1660-1664.
8. Marigo FA, Finger PT, McCormick SA, et al. Iris and ciliary body melanomas: ultrasound biomicroscopy with histopathologic correlation. *Arch Ophthalmol.* 2000;118:1515-1521.
9. Radhakrishnan S, Rollins AM, Roth JE, et al. Real-time optical coherence tomography of the anterior segment at 1310 nm. *Arch Ophthalmol.* 2001;119:1179-1185.
10. Muscat S, Srinivasan S, Sampat V, et al. Optical coherence tomography in the diagnosis of subclinical serous detachment of the macula secondary to a choroidal nevus. *Ophthalmol Surg Lasers.* 2001;32:474-476.

Chapter

33

Classification of Uveal Tumors

Bertil E. Damato, Sarah E. Coupland, and Paul Hiscott

Uveal tumors can be classified according to their location, etiopathology, histopathology, histogenesis, genotype, and various other ontological methods. Each approach has its advantages and limitations. A classification based on tumor location within the uvea would need to mention some tumors more than once if these can arise at different sites, and, furthermore, it can be impossible to locate the origin of an extensive tumor. The World Health Organization (WHO) classification is essentially based on histology and is therefore not ideal for the clinician.[1]

We prefer an alternative pathological classification of uveal tumors (Table 33-1).

REFERENCES

1. Campbell RJ. *Histological Typing of Tumours of the Eye and Its Adnexa.* Berlin: Springer Verlag; 1998:15-20.

Table 33-1. Pathological Classification of Uveal Tumors

Category	Subtype		
	Benign	Malignant	
		Primary	Secondary
Uvea			
Melanocytes	Melanocytosis	Melanoma	Conjunctival melanoma
	Melanocytoma		
	Melanocytic nevus		
	Diffuse melanocytic hyperplasia		
Blood vessels	Hemangioma		
	Hemangiopericytoma		
Nerves	Schwannoma		
	Glioneuroma		
Smooth muscle	Leiomyoma	Leiomyosarcoma	
	Mesectodermal leiomyoma		
Striated muscle		Rhabdomyosarcoma	
Fibroblasts	Neurofibroma		
Histiocytes	Juvenile xanthogranuloma		
Lymphocytes	Lymphocytic proliferation	Lymphoma	Lymphoma
Leukocytes			Leukemia
Epithelium			
Non-pigmented	Adenoma	Adenocarcinoma	Conjunctival carcinoma
	Adenomatous hyperplasia		
	Reactive epithelial hyperplasia		
	Cyst		
	Stromal cyst		
Pigmented	Congenital hypertrophy of the RPE		
	Cyst		
	Combined hamartoma of the RPE & retina		
	Adenoma	Adenocarcinoma	
	Cyst		
	Medulloepithelioma	Medulloepithelioma	
Ectopic tissue	Lacrimal gland choristoma		Metastatic carcinoma
	Osteoma		Metastatic sarcoma

Tumors of the Uvea: Benign Melanocytic Tumors

Arun D. Singh

INTRODUCTION

Nevus is a Latin word that means birthmark or mole and is a general term for a congenital mark on the skin. In ophthalmology, the term *nevus* refers to an abnormal, hamartomatous cluster of melanocytes. Uveal melanocytes are of neural crest origin and share embryologic origin with cutaneous melanocytes.[1]

IRIS NEVUS

Iris nevus is a stromal lesion and is therefore quite different from an iris freckle, in which melanocytes collect only superficially, without stromal involvement. Iris freckles can be seen in up to 60% of the population, whereas nevi are less common (4% to 6%).[2] Both iris freckles and nevi are more frequent in light-colored irides.[2] Patients with dysplastic nevus syndrome may have a tendency to develop iris nevi.[3,4]

Clinical Features

Iris nevus is typically solitary and circumscribed (Figure 34-1). Most are located in the lower quadrants of the iris and vary in color from tan to dark brown. A nevus that is very dark and almost black is more likely to be a melanocytoma. Intrinsic vasculature may be visible if the tumor is lightly pigmented.

Pupillary changes such as corectopia, irregularity of the margin, and ectropion iridis may occur with nevi involving the pupillary margin and do not imply malignancy. Similarly, extension into the trabecular meshwork does not signify malignant change.

Clinical Variants

Tapioca iris nevus is a multinodular, amelanotic, or lightly pigmented iris nevus that resembles tapioca grains.

Diffuse iris nevus, usually observed in association with ocular melanocytosis, may be sectoral or may involve the whole iris (Figure 34-2).

Iris Nevus Syndrome

A rare variant of iridocorneal endothelial syndrome, the iris nevus syndrome (Cogan–Reese syndrome), is the result of corneal endothelial overgrowth across the angle and over the iris surface, which gives rise to multiple small iris nodules and secondary glaucoma.[5]

Iris mammillations are multiple, dark brown nodular elevations on the iris seen commonly in darkly pigmented races or in association with oculo(dermal) melanocytosis.[6]

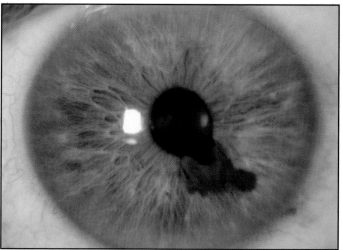

Figure 34-1. Slit-lamp photograph of a circumscribed iris nevus demonstrating localized iris thickening, pupillary distortion, and ectropion irides.

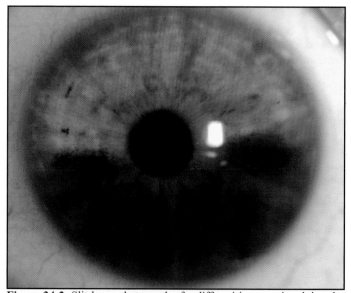

Figure 34-2. Slit-lamp photograph of a diffuse iris nevus involving the lower half of the iris in association with oculo(dermal) melanocytosis.

Lisch nodules occur in patients with neurofibromatosis type 1. They consist of small collections of melanocytes and are histologically indistinguishable from common nevi, except that they are perhaps more superficial.[7]

Aggressive Nevi of Childhood

As with similar lesions in other parts of the body, iris nevi in children can enlarge rapidly.[8]

Treatment

Observation as initial management is widely recommended. In the presence of features suspicious for melanoma (Box 34-1) or documented rapid growth, prompt excision may be considered.

Prognosis

Less than 5% of iris nevi exhibit clinical evidence of enlargement.[9]

Box 34-1. Clinical Features Suspicious of Iris Melanoma

- Symptoms
- Tumor size (ie, basal diameter >3 mm)
- Prominent tumor vascularity
- Pigment dispersion
- Secondary glaucoma
- Local spread (ie, seeding, ciliary body or extraocular extension)
- Documented rapid growth

CHOROIDAL NEVUS

Although a strict clinical definition of typical choroidal nevus is lacking, the Collaborative Ocular Melanoma Study Group defined it as a choroidal melanocytic lesion that is 5 mm or smaller in largest basal dimension and not more than 1 mm in height.[10] The reported prevalence rates vary from 0.2% to 30% because of differences in study designs.[11]

Terminology

In contrast to a choroidal nevus, a choroidal freckle is composed of an increased density of normal melanocytes, which do not disturb the normal architecture so that it is always flat, often with visible, normal choroidal vessels passing undisturbed through the lesion (Figure 34-3). In addition to typical choroidal nevi, larger choroidal lesions have been variously categorized as suspicious nevi, intermediate lesions, indeterminate lesions, and even small melanomas.[12]

Clinical Features

Choroidal nevi do not usually cause any symptoms. A macular nevus can cause visual loss from photoreceptor atrophy. Subretinal fluid in association with nevus may induce symptoms of metamorphopsia or photopsia. Choroidal nevus appears as a slate-gray to brown lesion with minimal thickness (see Figure 34-3). The margins are usually ill defined.

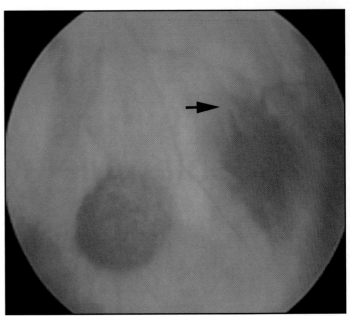

Figure 34-3. Choroidal nevus and a choroidal freckle (arrow). Note normal choroidal vessels passing undisturbed through the choroidal freckle.

Treatment

At present, only periodic observation is recommended for choroidal nevi. Associated subretinal fluid has been treated with surface and surrounding laser photocoagulation. Photodynamic therapy may be effective in rare cases when associated choroidal neovascularization is present.

Prognosis

With the assumption that all melanomas arise from pre-existing nevi, the risk of malignant transformation is estimated to be 1 in 8845.[11] The estimated risk stated above applies only to typical choroidal nevi, and it is expected that it would be higher for indeterminate lesions. Choroidal freckles are not known to undergo malignant transformation.

Risk Factors for Growth

In addition to recording the size (largest basal diameter and thickness) and location of the choroidal nevus, it is important to evaluate associated features such as drusen, subretinal fluid, orange pigment, and retinal pigment epithelial atrophy/proliferation, as these are statistically significant predictive factors of growth (Figure 34-4).[12]

CILIARY BODY NEVUS

Nevi of the ciliary body have been rarely reported in the literature but they are suspected to occur more frequently.[13,14] A ciliary body nevus usually appears as a dome-shaped mass with a smooth surface. Intrinsic vascularity is usually not present. Unexplained sentinel vessels, sectoral cataract, or localized shallowing of the anterior chamber should prompt evaluation of the ciliary body (Figure 34-5).

Treatment

There is no consensus as to whether ciliary body tumors should be observed or excised. Before undertaking complex excisional surgery, there may be scope for incisional or fine needle aspiration biopsy.[15] However, the detection of benign cells does not entirely exclude malignancy, because of the risk of sampling error.[16] Excision under a lamellar scleral flap is the treatment of choice for small, circumscribed ciliary body tumors (involving no more than three clock hours) without extrascleral extension.[16] En bloc excision with simultaneous full-thickness corneoscleral resection is indicated when extraocular extension is present.[16] Another approach is to treat ciliary body tumors with plaque or proton beam radiotherapy, perhaps excising any extraocular tumor nodule if necessary.

MELANOCYTOSIS

Ocular melanocytosis is a congenital condition characterized by hyperpigmentation of the episclera and uvea (Figure 34-6). Associated cutaneous hyperpigmentation in the distribution of the trigeminal nerve is called oculodermal melanocytosis (nevus of Ota). The orbit and meninges can also be involved.

Association With Uveal Melanoma

Overall, it is estimated that the lifetime risk of developing uveal melanoma in a Caucasian with oculo(dermal) melanocytosis is about 1 in 400.[17] Although ocular and oculodermal melanocytosis is common in Asians, the occurrence of uveal melanoma in this population is rare.[18]

Treatment

It is generally recommended that patients with oculo(dermal) melanocytosis be monitored annually.

OPTIC DISC MELANOCYTOMA

Melanocytoma is a benign pigmented ocular tumor that predominantly involves the optic disc and uvea.[19] Optic disc and uveal melanocytomas are considered to be congenital hamartomas, arising from dendritic uveal melanocytes scattered throughout the uvea.[19]

Clinical Features

Most patients are asymptomatic, and the condition is detected on routine ophthalmoscopy. On ophthalmoscopy, optic disc melanocytoma is a dark-brown or black, flat or slightly elevated mass, usually located inferotemporally (Figure 34-7).

Prognosis

A large majority of optic disc melanocytomas remain stable over many years.[20] Subtle growth over several years is observed in about 10% of cases.[21] Rapid enlargement, indicative of malignant transformation into melanoma, is observed in about 2% of cases.[22]

UVEAL MELANOCYTOMA

Uveal melanocytomas are clinically indistinguishable from uveal nevus and melanoma, and most are probably managed as such. As with optic disc melanocytoma, uveal melanocytoma can give rise to melanoma.[23]

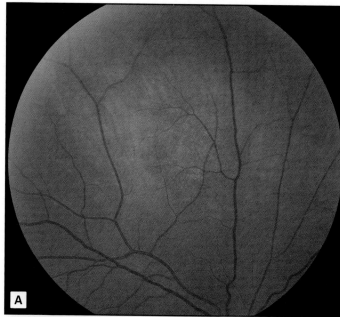

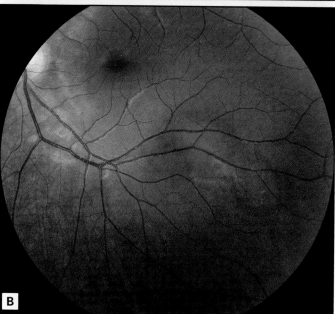

Figure 34-4. A choroidal nevus with fine drusen (A) and with orange pigment (B). Note localized shallow subretinal fluid along the temporal margin.

REFERENCES

1. Johnston MC. A radioautographic study of the migration and fate of cranial neural crest cells in the chick embryo. *Anat Rec.* 1966;156:143-155.

2. Harbour JW, Brantley MA Jr, Hollingsworth H, Gordon M. Association between posterior uveal melanoma and iris freckles, iris naevi, and choroidal naevi. *Br J Ophthalmol.* 2004;88:36-38.

3. Rodriguez-Sains RS. Ocular findings in patients with dysplastic nevus syndrome. An update. *Dermatol Clin.* 1991;9:723-728.

4. Toth-Molnar E, Olah J, Dobozy A, Hammer H. Ocular pigmented findings in patients with dysplastic naevus syndrome. *Melanoma Res.* 2004;14:43-47.

5. Cogan DG, Reese AB. A syndrome of iris nodules, ectopic Descemet's membrane, and unilateral glaucoma. *Doc Ophthalmol.* 1969;26:424-433.

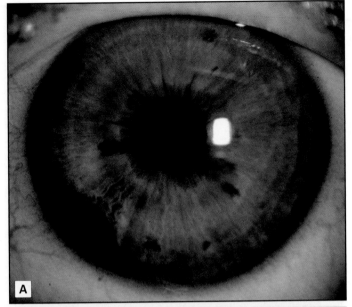

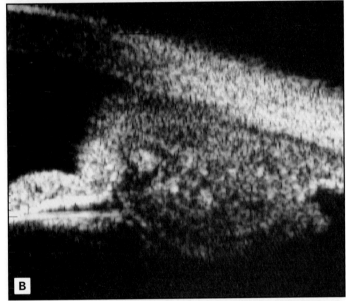

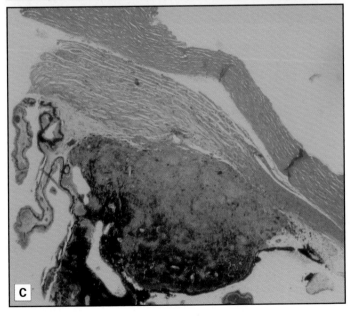

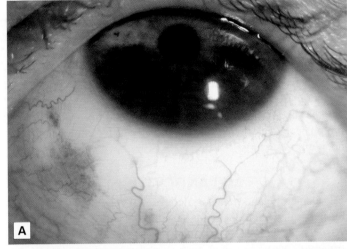

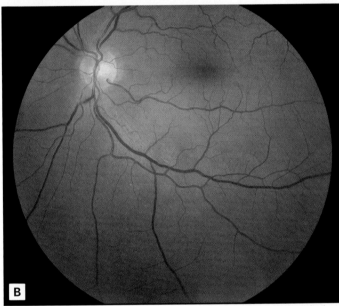

Figure 34-6. Oculo(dermal) melanocytosis. Note slate-gray episcleral pigmentation, diffuse iris nevus (A), and corresponding inferior sectoral choroidal hyperpigmentation (B).

Figure 34-5. Ultrasound biomicroscopy of an iridociliary mass. (A) Slit-lamp photograph. (B) Ultrasound biomicroscopy revealed a ciliary body mass with anterior extension into the iris root. (C) Note the close correlation between histopathological appearance (after iridocyclectomy) and biomicroscopic findings. (Reproduced with permission from Bakri SJ, Sculley L, Singh AD. Imaging techniques for uveal melanoma. *Int Ophthalmol Clin.* 2006;46:1-13.)

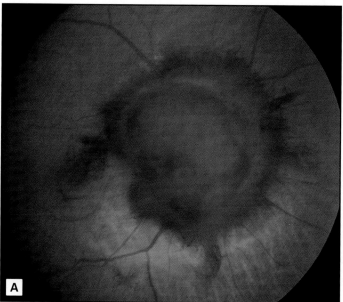 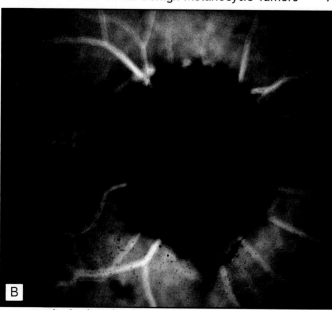

Figure 34-7. Fundus photograph of the right eye showing a large melanocytoma completely obscuring the optic disc. Note its feathery margins (A). Fluorescein angiography shows an area of dense hypofluorescence that persists through all the phases of the angiogram (B). (This figure was published in Singh AD. Optic disc melanocytoma. In: Huang D, Kaiser P, Lowder, CY, Traboulsi EI, eds. *Retinal Imaging*, 556-558. © Elsevier 2006.)

6. Ragge NK, Acheson J, Murphree AL. Iris mammillations: significance and associations. *Eye*. 1996;10:86-91.

7. Ragge NK, Falk RE, Cohen WE, Murphree AL. Images of Lisch nodules across the spectrum. *Eye*. 1993;7:95-101.

8. Paridaens D, Lyons CJ, McCartney A, Hungerford JL. Familial aggressive nevi of the iris in childhood. *Arch Ophthalmol*. 1991;109:1552-1554.

9. Territo C, Shields CL, Shields JA, et al. Natural course of melanocytic tumors of the iris. *Ophthalmology*. 1988;95:1251-1255.

10. Group COMS. *COMS manual of procedures: accession no. PBS 179693*. Springfield, VA: National Technical Information Service, 1995.

11. Singh AD, Kalyani P, Topham A. Estimating the risk of malignant transformation of a choroidal nevus. *Ophthalmology*. 2005;112:1784-1789.

12. Singh AD, Mokashi AA, Bena JF, et al. Small choroidal melanocytic lesions: features predictive of growth. *Ophthalmology*. 2006;113:1032-1039.

13. Cogan DG, Kuwabara T. Tumors of the ciliary body. *Int Ophthalmol Clin*. 1971;11:27-56.

14. Gordon E. Nevus of the choroid and pars plana. Enucleation for suspected malignant melanoma. *Surv Ophthalmol*. 1963;123:507-511.

15. El-Harazi SM, Kellaway J, Font RL. Melanocytoma of the ciliary body diagnosed by fine-needle aspiration biopsy. *Diagn Cytopathol*. 2000;22:394-397.

16. Rummelt V, Naumann GO, Folberg R, Weingeist TA. Surgical management of melanocytoma of the ciliary body with extrascleral extension. *Am J Ophthalmol*. 1994;117:169-176.

17. Singh AD, De Potter P, Fijal BA, et al. Lifetime prevalence of uveal melanoma in white patients with oculo(dermal) melanocytosis. *Ophthalmology*. 1998;105:195-198.

18. Infante de German-Ribon R, Singh AD, Arevalo JF, et al. Choroidal melanoma with oculodermal melanocytosis in Hispanic patients. *Am J Ophthalmol*. 1999;128:251-253.

19. Zimmerman LE, Garron LK. Melanocytoma of the optic disc. *Int Ophthalmol Clin*. 1962;2:431-440.

20. Reidy JJ, Apple DJ, Steinmetz RL, et al. Melanocytoma: nomenclature, pathogenesis, natural history and treatment. *Surv Ophthalmol*. 1985;29:319-327.

21. Shields JA, Demirci H, Mashayekhi A, Shields CL. Melanocytoma of optic disc in 115 cases: the 2004 Samuel Johnson Memorial Lecture, part 1. *Ophthalmology*. 2004;111:1739-1746.

22. Apple DJ, Craythorn JM, Reidy JJ, et al. Malignant transformation of an optic nerve melanocytoma. *Can J Ophthalmol*. 1984;19:320-325.

23. Roth AM. Malignant change in melanocytomas of the uveal tract. *Surv Ophthalmol*. 1978;22:404-412.

Uveal Malignant Melanoma: Epidemiologic Aspects

Arun D. Singh, Louise Bergman, and Stefan Seregard

INTRODUCTION

Approximately 5% of all melanomas arise in ocular and adnexal structures.[1] Most (85%) ocular melanomas are uveal in origin, whereas primary conjunctival and orbital melanomas are very rare.[1,2] Uveal melanoma is the most common primary intraocular malignant tumor. In this chapter, the incidence of uveal melanoma and various etiological factors implicated in the pathogenesis of uveal melanoma are briefly outlined (Box 35-1).

INCIDENCE

The reported incidence of uveal melanoma has ranged from 4.3 to 10.9 cases per million population because of variations in methodology. In a recent study from the United States, based on data derived from the Surveillance and Epidemiology and End Result (SEER) program of the National Institutes of Health (Maryland, USA), the overall mean incidence of uveal melanoma was 4.3 per million, with a higher rate in males (4.9 per million) than in females (3.7 per million).

Global Incidence

The incidence of uveal melanoma has been reported in several countries (Table 35-1). The incidence in the United States and European countries is similar to that in Australia[3] and New Zealand,[4] where the population is exposed to a higher intensity of ultraviolet light.

Age- and Gender-Specific Incidence

Uveal melanoma is more commonly seen in the older age group, with a progressively rising age-specific incidence rate, which peaks at the age of 70 years (24.5 per million in males and 17.8 per million in females) (Figure 35-1).[2]

Temporal Stability

Unlike global trends indicating a rising incidence of cutaneous melanoma, the incidence of uveal melanoma has either remained stable or declined slightly during the past several decades (Figure 35-2).[2,5]

ETIOLOGICAL FACTORS: HOST FACTORS

Several host factors, such as race, association with choroidal nevi, and genetic predisposition, have been investigated. Various

---

Box 35-1. Important Epidemiological Features of Uveal Melanoma

- 5% of all melanomas arise from the ocular and adnexal structures
- 85% of ocular melanomas are uveal in origin
- The incidence of uveal melanoma in the United States is 4.3 per million (males 4.9 per million; females 3.7 per million)
- The incidence of uveal melanoma has remained stable for the past 50 years
- There are strong racial variations in the incidence, with white populations most commonly affected
- Clinical, epidemiological, physiological, and genetic evidence argues against a major role of UV light in the causation of uveal melanoma
- Oculo(dermal) melanocytosis predisposes to uveal melanoma

---

environmental factors such as sunlight exposure and occupational association have also been investigated in case–control studies.

Race seems to be the most significant factor as uveal melanoma is about 150 times more common in whites than in blacks.[6] This tumor is also less common in Asians.[6] Light skin color, blond hair, and blue eyes are also specific host risk factors.[6]

Genetic Predisposition

Uveal melanomas usually occur sporadically, but there have been rare instances indicative of an inherited predisposition, such as familial uveal melanoma, uveal melanoma in young individuals, bilateral primary uveal melanoma, and multifocal primary uveal melanoma.[7]

Familial Uveal Melanoma

A review of published kindreds with familial uveal melanoma reveals that involvement over many generations, typical of autosomal dominant inheritance, is uncommon. Therefore, the possibility of two individuals in a given family developing uveal melanoma by chance alone (1 in 10 million) cannot be completely ignored.[8]

Table 35-1. Published Reports on National Incidence of Uveal Melanoma

Author	Period	Country	Definition	Number of Cases	Criteria	Incidence/Million
Mork	1953-1960	Norway	Ocular melanoma	220	Histologic	9.0
Jensen	1943-1952	Denmark	Uveal melanoma	305	Histologic	7.4
Scotto	1969-1971	United States	Eye melanoma	341	Clinical	5.6
Raivio	1953-1973	Finland	Cbd + choroid	359	Histologic	5.3
Strickland	1950-1974	United States	Eye melanoma	-	-	9.0 (Male)
						8.0 (Female)
Kaneko	1977-1979	Japan	Uveal melanoma	82	Histologic	0.3
Swerdlow	1962-1977	England (UK)	Ocular melanoma	4284	Clinical	7.2 (Male)
						5.7 (Female)
Gislason	1955-1979	Iceland	Cbd + choroid	29	Histologic	7.0 (Male)
						5.0 (Female)
Lommatzsch	1961-1980	East Germany	Eye melanoma		Clinical	10.0
Teikari	1973-1980	Finland	Cbd + choroid	382	Clinical	7.6
Iscovich	1961-1989	Israel	Cbd + choroid	502	Clinical	5.7 (Jews)
Vidal	1992	France	Uveal melanoma	412	Clinical	7.0
Bergman	1960-1998	Sweden	Uveal melanoma	2997	Clinical	9.4 (Male)
						8.8 (Female)
Singh	1973-1997	United States	Uveal melanoma	2493	Clinical	4.9 (Male)
						3.7 (Female)
Kricker	1996-1998	Australia	Choroidal melanoma	539	Clinical	11.0 (Male)
						7.8 (Female)

Uveal melanoma, iris, ciliary body (Cbd), and choroidal melanoma; Eye melanoma, uveal and conjunctival melanoma; ocular melanoma, uveal, conjunctival, and eyelid melanoma.

(Adapted from Singh AD, Topham A. Incidence of uveal melanoma in the United States: 1973-1997. *Ophthalmology.* 2003;110:956-961.)

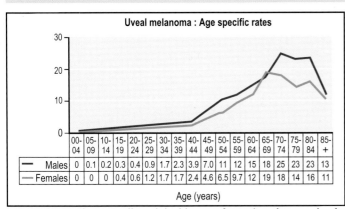

Figure 35-1. The age-adjusted incidence of uveal melanoma in the United States. (Adapted from Singh AD, Topham A. Incidence of uveal melanoma in the United States: 1973–1997. *Ophthalmology.* 2003;110:956-961.)

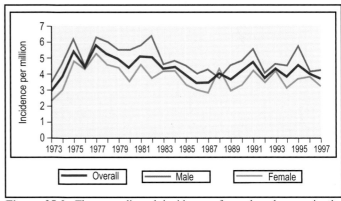

Figure 35-2. The age-adjusted incidence of uveal melanoma in the United States between 1973 and 1997. (Adapted from Singh AD, Topham A. Incidence of uveal melanoma in the United States: 1973–1997. *Ophthalmology.* 2003;110:956-961.)

Uveal Melanoma in Young Individuals

Approximately 1% of all uveal melanomas occur in patients younger than 20 years of age.[9] Young patients with uveal melanoma may display associations with oculo(dermal) melanocytosis or atypical cutaneous moles.[10]

Bilateral uveal melanoma is rare.[11] It should be distinguished from paraneoplastic melanocytic proliferations such as benign diffuse uveal melanocytic proliferation (Chapter 63).

Phenotypic Associations

Oculo(dermal) Melanocytosis

Features of ODM include a congenital hyperpigmentation of skin, episclera, uvea, orbit, and meninges (Chapter 34).

Familial Atypical Mole and Melanoma Syndrome

This denotes a specific clinicopathologic entity that is associated with an increased risk for the development of cutaneous melanoma.[12] Because cutaneous and uveal melanocytes share similar embryologic origin, it is plausible that uveal melanoma may sometimes occur within FAM-M syndrome.[7]

ENVIRONMENTAL FACTORS

Sunlight Exposure

In contrast to cutaneous melanoma, evidence for sunlight exposure in the etiopathogenesis of uveal melanoma is at best weak.[13]

Occupation

Although several case–control studies have evaluated occupation as a risk factor for uveal melanoma, there is no consistent evidence indicating occupational exposure to UV light or other agents as a risk factor.[6,13]

REFERENCES

1. Chang AE, Karnell LH, Menck HR. The National Cancer Data Base report on cutaneous and noncutaneous melanoma: a summary of 84,836 cases from the past decade. The American College of Surgeons Commission on Cancer and the American Cancer Society. *Cancer.* 1998;83:1664-1678.
2. Singh AD, Topham A. Incidence of uveal melanoma in the United States: 1973-1997. *Ophthalmology.* 2003;110:956-961.
3. Vajdic CM, Kricker A, Giblin M, et al. Incidence of ocular melanoma in Australia from 1990 to 1998. *Int J Cancer.* 2003;105:117-122.
4. Michalova K, Clemett R, Dempster A, et al. Iris melanomas: are they more frequent in New Zealand? *Br J Ophthalmol.* 2001;85:4-5.
5. Strickland D, Lee JA. Melanomas of eye: stability of rates. *Am J Epidemiol.* 1981;113:700-702.
6. Egan KM, Seddon JM, Glynn RJ, et al. Epidemiologic aspects of uveal melanoma. *Surv Ophthalmol.* 1988;32:239-251.
7. Singh AD, Damato B, Howard P, Harbour JW. Uveal melanoma: genetic aspects. *Ophthalmol Clin North Am.* 2005;18:85-97.
8. Singh AD, Demirci H, Shields CL, et al. Concurrent choroidal melanoma in son and father. *Am J Ophthalmol.* 2000;130:679-680.
9. Singh AD, Shields CL, Shields JA, Sato T. Uveal melanoma in young patients. *Arch Ophthalmol.* 2000;118:918-923.
10. Singh AD, Shields JA, Eagle RC, et al. Iris melanoma in a ten-year-old boy with familial atypical mole-melanoma (FAM-M) syndrome. *Ophthalm Genet.* 1994;15:145-149.
11. Singh AD, Shields CL, Shields JA, De Potter P. Bilateral primary uveal melanoma. Bad luck or bad genes? *Ophthalmology.* 1996;103:256-262.
12. Salopek TG. The dilemma of the dysplastic nevus. *Dermatol Clin.* 2002;20:617-628.
13. Singh AD, Rennie IG, Seregard S, et al. Sunlight exposure and pathogenesis of uveal melanoma. *Surv Ophthalmol.* 2004;49:419-428.

Uveal Malignant Melanoma: Clinical Features

Leonidas Zografos

INTRODUCTION

The presentation of uveal melanoma is mostly influenced by the site of origin (iris, ciliary body, or choroidal), size, pigmentation, extent of secondary changes, and any associated extrascleral extension, hemorrhage, or inflammation.

IRIS MELANOMA

Iris melanoma may be circumscribed or diffuse. Slit-lamp examination, gonioscopy, and ultrasound biomicroscopy (UBM) allow staging of the tumor to guide the most appropriate treatment (Box 36-1).[1]

Circumscribed iris melanoma has a nodular shape with variable pigmentation (Figure 36-1). Iris melanoma tends to arise in the inferior half of the iris. It often has an irregular or rarely a smooth surface, covered by a surface plaque. In lightly pigmented tumors, the vessels are often visible.[2,3]

Diffuse iris melanoma can develop in two ways. The first consists of primary infiltration of the iris stroma. The iris is thickened, without any obvious nodule formation. The second mechanism consists of seeding of tumor cells from a circumscribed iris or ciliary body melanoma (Figure 36-2).

CILIARY BODY MELANOMA

Ciliary body melanoma may be circumscribed or annular (ring) (Figure 36-3). Slit-lamp examination, gonioscopy, transillumination, and UBM allow staging of the tumor to guide the most appropriate treatment (see Box 36-1).[1]

CHOROIDAL MELANOMA

According to various statistical series, 80% to 90% of uveal melanomas arise in the posterior uvea. The clinical features of choroidal melanomas are varied, and multiple symptoms tend to occur sequentially (Box 36-2).

Size and Shape

Small and medium-sized tumors that are still contained by an intact Bruch's membrane are dome shaped, with a thickness equal to about half their diameter (Figure 36-4). If Bruch's membrane ruptures at the apex of the tumor, the melanoma has a mushroom or collar-button shape (Figure 36-5). Diffuse melanoma[4] constitutes a particular, infiltrative form of flat or slightly raised melanoma with predominantly horizontal growth (Figure 36-6).

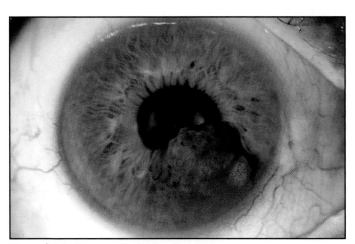

Figure 36-1. Circumscribed iris melanoma.

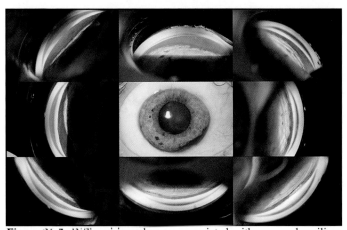

Figure 36-2. Diffuse iris melanoma associated with an annular ciliary body melanoma. Clinical and gonioscopic images.

Pigmentation

Melanoma is usually gray or greenish-brown, but the color can range from dark brown to white. Tumor pigmentation is sometimes heterogeneous. Amelanotic melanoma must be distinguished from solitary metastases.

Alterations of the Retina

Choroidal melanoma is almost always accompanied by a secondary exudative retinal detachment. In some cases, pigmented cells accumulate in the subretinal fluid, outlining the edges of the

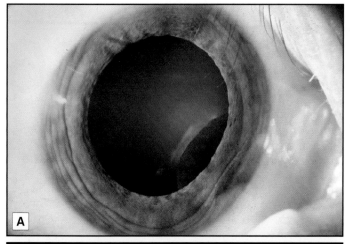

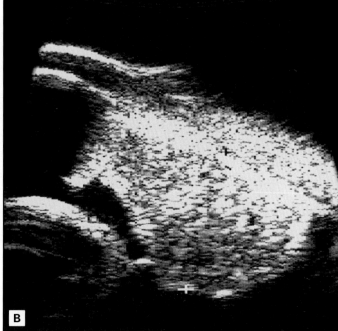

Figure 36-3. Circumscribed ciliary body melanoma. (A) Clinical appearance. (B) 20 MHz immersion ultrasonograph.

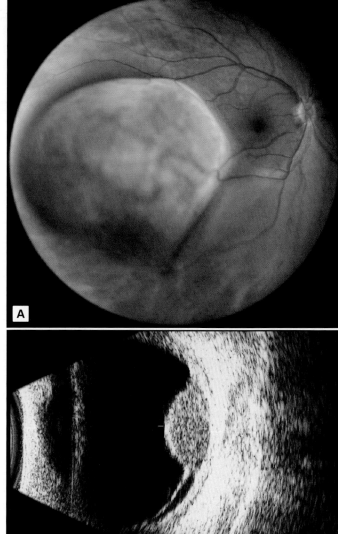

Figure 36-4. Dome-shaped melanoma. (A) Clinical appearance. (B) Ultrasonograph.

Box 36-1. Clinical Features of Iridociliary Melanomas

- Circumscribed or diffuse
- Secondary glaucoma, cataract, keratopathy, and hyphema
- Annular growth
- Seeding of cells in anterior chamber

Box 36-2. Clinical Features of Choroidal Melanomas

- Visual symptoms in most patients
- Dome, mushroom, or diffuse configuration
- Variable pigmentation
- Abnormal RPE over tumor
- Extraocular extension

retinal detachment. These cells are mainly pigment-laden macrophages, sometimes mixed with tumor cells. Disseminated pigmented cells may also be observed in the vitreous cavity when the retina is invaded or when the tumor is situated in the ciliary body.

Alterations of the Retinal Pigment Epithelium

Small melanomas frequently show confluent orange pigment (Figure 36-7). On histological examination, the orange pigment corresponds to clumps of macrophages containing lipofuscin and melanin derived from retinal pigment epithelial cells.[5]

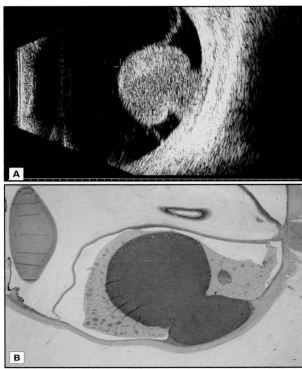

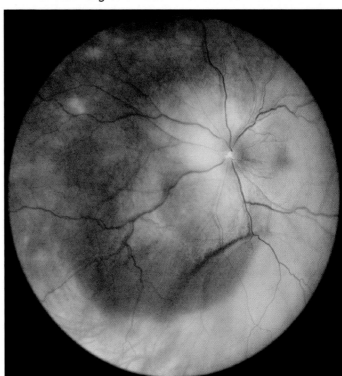

Figure 36-5. Mushroom-shaped melanoma. (A) Ultrasonograph of a mushroom-shaped melanoma with rupture of Bruch's membrane at the apex of the tumor. (B) Histopathological image of a mushroom-shaped melanoma with eccentric rupture of Bruch's membrane, inducing an irregular mushroom shape.

Figure 36-6. Diffuse choroidal melanoma.

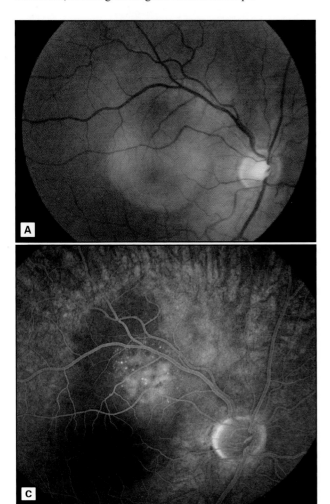

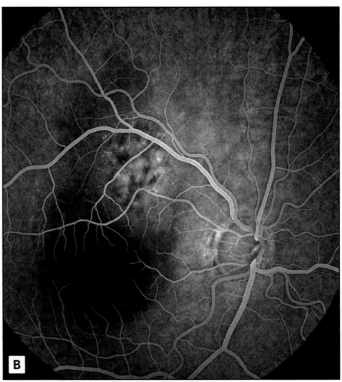

Figure 36-7. Small melanoma with orange pigment associated with serous retinal detachment in the macular region. (A) Ophthalmoscopic appearance. (B) Fluorescein angiography. The orange pigment blocks fluorescence in the early sequences. (C) Fluorescein leakage with pinpoints in late sequences.

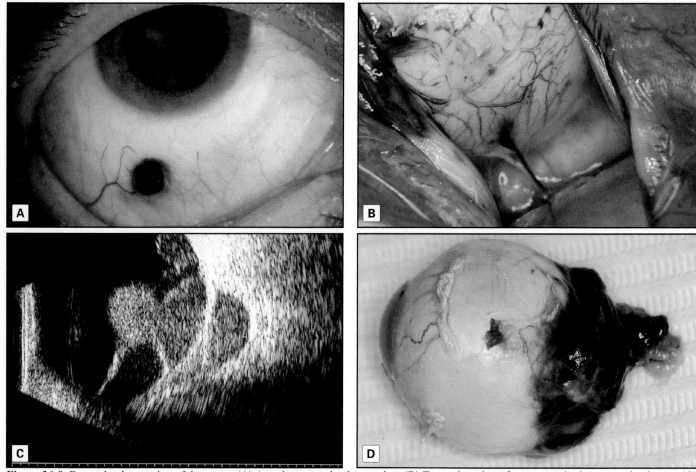

Figure 36-8. Extrascleral extension of the tumor. (A) Anterior extrascleral extension. (B) Tumor invasion of a vortex vein, intraoperative image. (C) Large posterior extrascleral extension, ultrasonograph. (D) Diffuse posterior extrascleral extension, macroscopic image.

Extrascleral Extension

The sclera presents a considerable resistance to tumor expansion. However, the sclera is traversed by many nerves and vessels, along which tumor cells tend to spread to reach the episclera and orbit (Figure 36-8).

Optic Nerve Invasion

Invasion of the optic disc and optic nerve by the tumor is rare. It is generally secondary to a large peripapillary tumor, associated with elevated intraocular pressure, a tumor of epithelioid cell type, and areas of necrosis.

REFERENCES

1. Zografos L, Uffer S. Tumeurs iriennes pigmentées. In: Zografos L, ed. *Tumeurs Intraoculaires*. Paris: Masson; 2002:281-313.
2. Arentsen JJ, Green WR. Melanoma of the iris: report of 72 cases treated surgically. *Ophthalmic Surg.* 1975;6:23-37.
3. Shields CL, Shields JA, Materin M, et al. Iris melanoma: risk factors for metastasis in 169 consecutive patients. *Ophthalmology.* 2001;108:172-178.
4. Font RL, Spaulding AG, Zimmerman LE. Diffuse malignant melanoma of the uveal tract: a clinicopathologic report of 54 cases. *Trans Am Acad Ophthalmol Otolaryngol.* 1968;72:877-895.
5. Font RL, Zimmerman LE, Armaly MF. The nature of the orange pigment over a choroidal melanoma. Histochemical and electron microscopical observations. *Arch Ophthalmol.* 1974;91:359-362.

Uveal Malignant Melanoma: Differential Diagnosis

Devron H. Char

INTRODUCTION

Making the correct diagnosis in a patient with a possible uveal tumor can be difficult. Although newer imaging techniques, including optical coherence tomography (OCT), high-resolution MR, positron emission tomography (PET) scans, and combination CT/PET scans have been very helpful in many body sites, their accuracy at differentiating uveal tumors and delineating their margins remains inferior to most purely ophthalmic diagnostic techniques.

CHOROIDAL MELANOMA

An abbreviated differential diagnosis for choroidal tumors is given in Table 37-1. Several clinical findings are suspicious for a simulating, non-malignant choroidal lesion (Box 37-1). These include patients younger than 20 (less than 2% of uveal melanomas), non-white race, and a recent history of an open intraocular procedure such as cataract extraction or glaucoma filtering (a localized subretinal hemorrhagic process [Figure 37-1]), a lesion associated with severe eye pain (scleritis), and a recent history of a visceral malignancy (metastases).

Differential Diagnosis

Choroidal Nevus

The differentiation of a small choroidal melanoma from a benign, pigmented, atypical choroidal nevus can be challenging.[1] Choroidal nevi are usually flat, less than 6 mm in diameter (<1/2 the aerial diameter of a 20 D Nikon lens), and may have overlying drusen and a surrounding hypopigmentation. Much less commonly, nevi can be amelanotic, but unlike a small choroidal metastasis, these lesions are not associated with exudative detachment. In indeterminate pigmented lesions (1.5 to 3.0 mm thick and <10.0 mm in diameter), a group we labeled with the neologism "choroidal nevoma," the differentiation between a small melanoma and a nevus can be more challenging.[2]

Choroidal hemangioma is a benign simulating lesion (Figure 37-2).[3] Clinically, on fluorescein angiography, ICG, and ultrasound, the pattern is characteristic.[4]

Choroidal metastases can present prior to the discovery of the primary neoplasm in between 10% and 90% of cases, depending on histology.[5]

Table 37-1. Lesions That Simulate Choroidal Melanoma

Choroidal neoplasms
  Choroidal nevus
  Choroidal metastasis
  Choroidal hemangioma
  Choroidal osteoma
  Choroidal neurilemmoma
  Choroidal neurofibroma
  Peripheral melanocytoma
  Benign lymphoid tumor
  Choroidal hemangiopericytoma
  Choroidal leiomyoma
Hemorrhagic processes
  Involutional macular degeneration
  Extramacular disciform lesion
  Ruptured arteriolar macroaneurysm
  Localized choroidal detachment/hemorrhage
Retinal pigment epithelial processes
  Retinal pigment epithelial hyperplasia
  Retinal pigment epithelial hypertrophy
  Retinal pigment epithelial adenocarcinoma
Inflammatory processes
  Posterior scleritis
  Posterior uveitis
Miscellaneous
  Hemorrhagic retinal detachment
  Retinoschisis with hemorrhage
  Staphyloma
  Intraocular foreign body granuloma
  Massive retinal gliosis
  Acquired retinal hemangioma
  Retinal glioma

Box 37-1. Clinical Features Not Suggestive of Choroidal Melanoma

- Age <20 years
- Recent intraocular procedure
- Black tumor
- Multiple tumors
- Vitreous hemorrhage associated with a small tumor

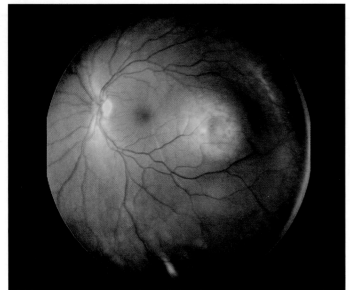

Figure 37-1. Subchoroidal hemorrhage referred as a melanoma. On fluorescein angiography, this completely blocks fluorescence.

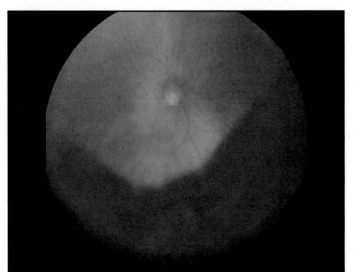

Figure 37-2. Choroidal hemangiomas have an orange–red color and typical fluorescein, ICG, and ultrasound patterns.

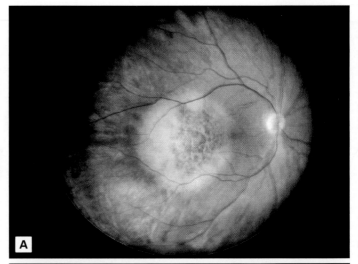

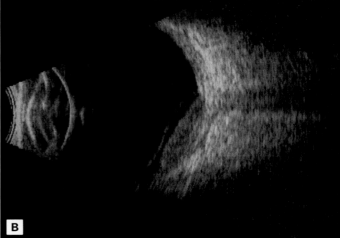

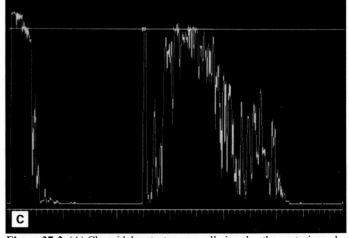

Figure 37-3. (A) Choroidal metastases usually involve the posterior pole, are amelanotic, and almost never produce a collar button-shaped mass. (B) On B-scan of the choroidal metastasis, there is no acoustic quiet zone, no choroidal excavation, and no orbital shadowing. (C) On A-scan, there is medium to high reflectivity with coarse spikes and a climbing posterior spike.

Choroidal metastases, because they are spread hematogenously, usually occur in the posterior pole (Figure 37-3). They are amelanotic and almost never produce a collar button-shaped configuration. Unlike choroidal melanoma, ultrasonography of a metastatic lesion shows no choroidal excavation, acoustic quiet zone, or orbital shadowing. On A-scan, the lesion has medium to high reflectivity with a climbing posterior spike (Chapter 32).

Melanocytoma can simulate a melanoma on clinical, fluorescein, and ultrasonographic criteria (Figure 37-4).[6]

Retinal Pigment Epithelium Tumors

Congenital hypertrophy of retinal pigment epithelium (CHRPE) in the periphery can occasionally be mistaken for a uveal melanoma (Figure 37-5). Typically, these tumors are flat, have very sharp margins that can be scalloped, and can develop lacunae. RPE hyperplastic lesions secondary to various insults have deep black pigmentation, but usually, despite having sharply

defined margins, they are somewhat jagged and less regular; lacunae do not occur.

Scleritis may or may not produce intense pain and inflammatory signs. Often with scleritis there is exudative detachment,

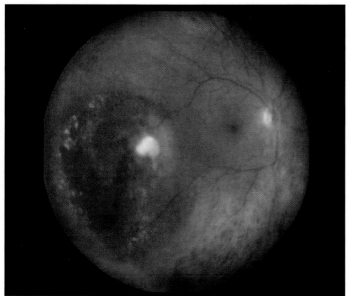

Figure 37-4. Fine needle aspiration biopsy diagnosed melanocytoma.

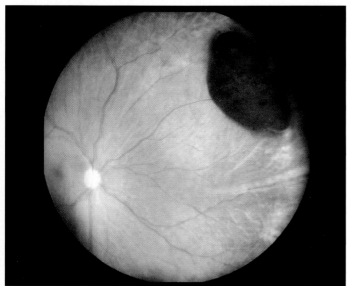

Figure 37-5. Congenital RPE hypertrophy can simulate a melanoma, but is flat.

and if the eye is red and painful, the diagnosis is usually obvious. On ultrasound, there is often fluid in sub-Tenon's space, as well as inflammatory changes in the sclera, and these findings can also be documented with either CT or MRI.

IRIS, CILIARY BODY, AND CILIOCHOROIDAL TUMORS

Diagnostic Features

Iris Nevus

This small, flat lesion usually does not distort the pupil, invade the angle, or produce tumor angiogenesis.

Table 37-2. Differential Diagnosis of Iris and Ciliary Body Tumors

Iris tumors
  Iris nevi
  Iris melanoma
  Iris metastases
  Cogan-Reese
  Essential iris atrophy
  Variant of ICE syndrome
  Central iris atrophy
  Iris stromal cyst
  Posterior pigment cyst
  Forward extension of a uveal melanoma to involve the iris
  Iris foreign body
  Amyloid
  JXG
  Sarcoid
  Leiomyoma
  Melanocytoma
  Lymphoma
Ciliary body tumors
  Staphyloma
  Leiomyoma
  Mesoectodermal leiomyoma
  Medulloepithelioma
  Melanoma
  Metastasis
  Scleritis
  Lymphoma
  Amyloid
  Plasmacytoma

Iris Pigment Epithelial Cyst

The most common simulating iris lesion we evaluate is a posterior pigment epithelial cyst (Table 37-2).[7] These do not distort the iris surface, or if they do, they mainly have a pressure effect. High-frequency ultrasound is very useful in differentiating iris melanoma from a posterior pigment epithelial cyst (Figure 37-6).

Metastases

Iris metastases are always amelanotic unless they are from a cutaneous melanoma. In atypical difficult cases, fine needle biopsy is diagnostic (Chapter 56).

REFERENCES

1. Gass JD. Problems in the differential diagnosis of choroidal nevi and malignant melanoma. XXXIII Edward Jackson Memorial Lecture. *Trans Am Acad Ophthalmol Otolaryngol.* 1977;83:19-48.
2. Butler P, Char DH, Zarbin M, Kroll S. Natural history of indeterminate pigmented choroidal tumors. *Ophthalmology.* 1994;101:710-717.
3. Bardenstein DS, Char DH, Irvine AR, Stone RD. Extramacular disciform lesions simulating uveal tumors. *Ophthalmology.* 1992;99:944-951.
4. Char DH. *Tumors of the Eye and Ocular Adnexa.* New York, NY: BC Decker; 2001.

SECTION 4 Uveal Tumors

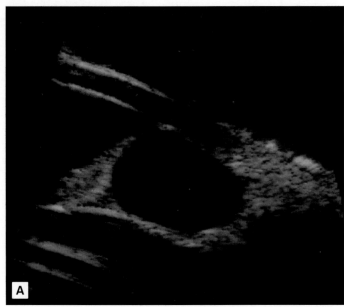

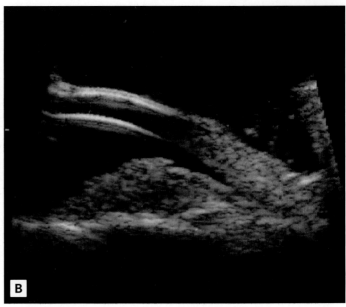

Figure 37-6. (A) A posterior pigment epithelial cyst demonstrable on high-frequency ultrasound, in contrast to (B), which shows an iris melanoma. Rarely, iris–ciliary body melanomas can have cysts or even become cavitary.

5. Char DH, Schwartz A, Miller TR, Abele JS. Ocular metastases from systemic melanoma. *Am J Ophthalmol.* 1980;90:702-707.

6. Shields JA, Font RL. Melanocytoma of the choroid clinically simulating a malignant melanoma. *Arch Ophthalmol.* 1972;87:396-400.

7. Shields JA, Kline MW, Augsburger JJ. Primary iris cysts: a review of the literature and report of 62 cases. *Br J Ophthalmol.* 1984;68:152-166.

Chapter

38

Uveal Malignant Melanoma: Histopathologic Features

Tero Kivelä

INTRODUCTION

Uveal melanomas develop from melanocytes that reside within the stroma of the choroid, ciliary body, and iris. No basement membrane needs to be breached when the tumor develops.[1]

Cell Type

Originally, six histopathologic types of uveal melanoma were described, but the categories were later simplified into three (Table 38-1).[2-4]

Spindle Cell Melanoma

Spindle cell melanoma is composed of fusiform cells oriented in bundles and whorls (Figure 38-1). Spindle cells have variable amounts of fibrillar cytoplasm, and their borders are difficult to distinguish because the cells adhere to each other. Originally, spindle cell melanomas were divided into spindle A and B types. The former have narrow, oval nuclei and inconspicuous nucleoli, and the latter contain larger, round nuclei and more conspicuous nucleoli (see Figure 38-1). Most spindle A cell tumors are currently classified as spindle cell nevi (see Table 38-1).[3]

Epithelioid Cell Melanoma

Epithelioid cell melanoma is composed of polyhedral cells, which are usually but not always large and which morphologically resemble epithelial cells (see Figure 38-1). Their abundant cytoplasm is eosinophilic, and they characteristically crack apart from their neighbors during tissue processing, resulting in a non-cohesive appearance. The nucleoli are large and prominent.

Mixed-Cell Type Melanoma

This contains variable proportions of spindle and epithelioid cells. Opinion is divided as to what proportion of epithelioid cells distinguishes spindle- from mixed- and mixed- from epithelioid-cell melanomas.[3] Increasingly, even a single well-defined epithelioid cell precludes classification as a spindle cell melanoma because the tumor is likely to harbor additional epithelioid cells.

Necrotic Melanoma

Significant necrosis is uncommon, but rarely the tumor is too necrotic to be classified by cell type. These necrotic melanomas have a prognosis comparable to that of tumors with epithelioid cells. Widespread necrosis will cause a secondary inflammatory reaction.

Pigmentation

Uveal melanomas range from heavily pigmented to amelanotic, and many show regional variations in pigmentation.

Nucleolar Size

Uveal melanoma cells typically have conspicuous nucleoli, which are visible in hematoxylin–eosin-stained sections but which can be better appreciated with special stains, especially the silver stain.[5] Melanin is first bleached with potassium permanganate and oxalic acid. Large nucleoli are associated with a high risk of metastasis.[6]

Mitotic Figures

Most uveal melanomas are slow growing, and mitotic figures are consequently usually few in number.

Extravascular Matrix Patterns

The stroma of uveal melanomas is scanty. The extravascular matrix can be highlighted with several stains, of which periodic acid–Schiff stain without counterstain is most popular (Figure 38-2).[7] Nine matrix patterns are distinguished, which often occur in combination in any given tumor (see Figure 38-2).[7] Several extravascular matrix patterns are associated with a higher-than-average chance of metastasis. The association is strongest for loops, and in particular for networks.[7,8]

Tumor-Infiltrating Macrophages

Uveal melanomas contain variable numbers of tumor-infiltrating macrophages, which can be identified by immunohistochemistry, especially using antibodies to the CD68 epitope (Figure 38-3).[9]

A high number of immunopositive cells is associated with an increased risk of metastasis.[9] A similar observation has been made with regard to infiltrating lymphocytes in uveal melanomas.[9,10]

Cell Proliferation Antigens

Cycling tumor cells can be identified with several antibodies, of which those recognizing proliferating cell nuclear antigen (PCNA) and Ki-67 antigen have been most widely used to evaluate uveal melanoma. Larger numbers of cells with immunopositive nuclei are associated with a higher risk of metastasis.[11,12]

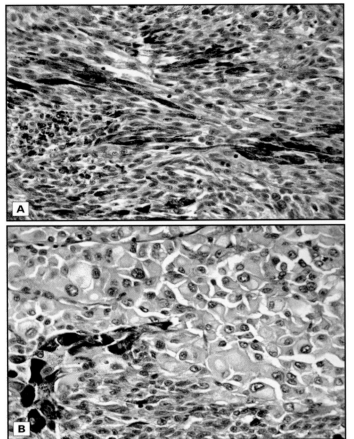

Figure 38-1. Main cell types of uveal melanoma. A spindle cell melanoma with mostly B-type cells with round nucleoli intermixed with occasional slender A-type cells with oval nuclei. Both are fusiform, with indistinct borders and arranged in bundles (A). A mixed cell melanoma with a population of polyhedral, non-cohesive, eosinophilic epithelioid cells, which have prominent nucleoli (B).

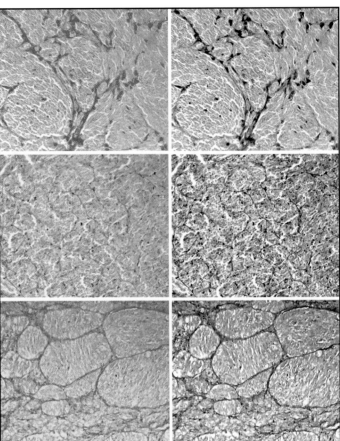

Figure 38-2. Extravascular matrix patterns are purple in specimens stained with periodic acid–Schiff stain (left column) and appear dark in red-free photographs (right column). The arcs with branching (top row), loops (middle row), and network patterns (bottom row) all belong to the family of curved patterns. Note that the thickness of the patterns varies, and some are pencil-thin (middle row).

Table 38-1. Classification of Uveal Melanoma Based on Cell Type

Original Callender	AFIP	Histopathologic Characteristics			
		Cell Shape and Appearance	Cell Borders	Nucleus	Nucleolus
Spindle A melanoma*	Spindle cell nevus*	Fusiform cohesive cells	Indistinct	Narrow, oval	Inconspicuous
Spindle B melanoma	Spindle cell melanoma*	Fusiform cohesive cells	Indistinct	Plump	Conspicuous
Mixed cell melanoma	Mixed cell melanoma	Mixed population of spindle and epithelioid cells Fusiform cohesive cells mixed with (at least single) non-cohesive epithelioid cells			
Epithelioid cell melanoma	Epithelioid cell melanoma	Large polygonal cells, abundant eosinophilic cytoplasm	Distinct	Large, round	Large, prominent
Fascicular melanoma		Spindle cells arranged in fascicles			
Necrotic melanoma		Too extensive tumor necrosis to allow classification into other groups			

*The majority of spindle A melanoma of the Callender's classification were reclassified as spindle cell nevi and a minority as spindle cell melanoma in the AFIP classification.

AFIP, Armed Forces Institute of Pathology, Washington, DC.

REFERENCES

1. Folberg R. Tumor progression in ocular melanomas. *J Invest Dermatol.* 1993;100:326S-331S.

2. Callender GR. Malignant melanocytic tumors of the eye. A study of histologic types in 111 cases. *Trans Am Acad Ophthalmol Otolaryngol.* 1931;36:131-140.

3. McLean IW, Zimmerman LE, Evans RM. Reappraisal of Callender's spindle a type of malignant melanoma of choroid and ciliary body. *Am J Ophthalmol.* 1978;86 557-564.

4. McLean IW, Foster WD, Zimmerman LE, Gamel JW. Modifications of Callender's classification of uveal melanoma at the Armed Forces Institute of Pathology. *Am J Ophthalmol.* 1983;96:502-509.

5. Moshari A, McLean IW. Uveal melanoma: mean of the longest nucleoli measured on silver-stained sections. *Invest Ophthalmol Vis Sci.* 2001;42:1160-1163.

6. McLean IW, Keefe KS, Burnier MN. Uveal melanoma: comparison of the prognostic value of fibrovascular loops, mean of the ten largest nucleoli, cell type, and tumor size. *Ophthalmology.* 1997;104:777-780.

7. Folberg R, Rummelt V, Parys-van Ginderdeuren R, et al. The prognostic value of tumor blood vessel morphology in primary uveal melanoma. *Ophthalmology.* 1993;100:1389-1398.

8. Mäkitie T, Summanen P, Tarkkanen A, Kivelä T. Microvascular loops and networks as prognostic indicators in choroidal and ciliary body melanomas. *J Natl Cancer Inst.* 1999;91:359-367.

9. Mäkitie T, Summanen P, Tarkkanen A, Kivelä T. Tumor-infiltrating macrophages (CD68+ cells) and prognosis in malignant uveal melanoma. *Invest Ophthalmol Vis Sci.* 2001;42:1414-1421.

10. de la Cruz POJ, Specht CS, McLean IW. Lymphocytic infiltration in uveal malignant melanoma. *Cancer.* 1990;65:112-115.

11. Al Jamal RT, Kivelä T. KI-67 immunopositivity in choroidal and ciliary body melanoma with respect to nucleolar diameter and other prognostic factors. *Curr Eye Res.* 2006;31:57-67.

12. Seregard S, Spångberg B, Juul C, Oskarsson M. Prognostic accuracy of the mean of the largest nucleoli, vascular patterns, and PC-10 in posterior uveal melanoma. *Ophthalmology.* 1998;105:485-491.

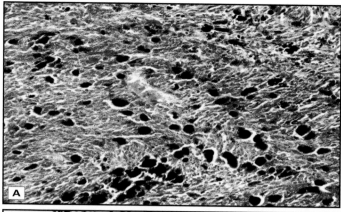

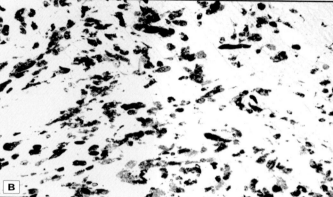

Figure 38-3. Extravascular matrix patterns are purple in specimens stained with periodic acid–Schiff stain (left column) and appear dark in red-free photographs (right column). The arcs with branching (top row), loops (middle row), and network patterns (bottom row) all belong to the family of curved patterns. Note that the thickness of the patterns varies, and some are pencil-thin (middle row).

Management of Patients With Uveal Melanoma

Bertil E. Damato

INTRODUCTION

The management of patients with uveal melanoma encompasses detection, diagnosis, prognostication, treatment, counseling, and surveillance (Box 39-1).

DETECTION

Early detection of uveal melanoma greatly improves the chance of conserving a useful eye and is perhaps vital in the prevention of metastatic spread, especially if the tumor is small.

REFERRAL PROCEDURE

The time between initial tumor detection and treatment depends greatly on the method of patient referral. The author has seen long delays with tragic consequences because the referral letter or fax was not received by the ocular oncology center. It is therefore important to give the patient a contact telephone number together with advice as to what to do if an appointment is not received within a specified time. It is also essential to inform the patient of any suspicion of malignancy, together with any caveats if the diagnosis is uncertain. Investigations such as fluorescein angiography and systemic screening can cause unnecessary delays in the referral process and could be left to ocular oncologists.

DIAGNOSIS

Diagnosis of uveal tumors requires an awareness of the wide range of conditions and of the diverse clinical manifestations of each (Chapters 33 and 37).

PROGNOSTICATION

Tumor Staging

Tumor staging is fundamental to patient care, and uveal melanoma is no exception (Chapter 33). Unfortunately, unlike other cancers, the tumor, node, metastasis (TNM) staging system has not proved acceptable for uveal melanoma.[1] A variety of alternative systems based on clinical features such as largest basal tumor diameter, tumor thickness, extraocular extension, and ciliary body involvement have been devised (Chapter 46).

Box 39-1. Aspects of Management of Patients With Uveal Melanoma

- Detection of tumor
- Referral for specialist care
- Diagnosis and differential diagnosis
- Tumor staging, according to size and extent
- Tumor grading according to histology, cytogenetics, and molecular genetics
- Counseling, to inform on condition and therapeutic options
- Ocular treatment, if possible conserving function
- Systemic investigation, detecting metastatic spread as early as possible
- Long-term surveillance, to enable timely treatment of any complications
- Psychological support for patients and relatives

Tumor Grading

As mentioned in other chapters, uveal melanoma tends to fall into two distinct categories of low and high grade. These two varieties are more accurately distinguishable using cytogenetic and molecular genetic techniques rather than traditional histopathologic evaluation.[2]

TREATMENT

There is a growing acceptance of selecting between the various methods according to tumor size and location and of a multimodality approach wherein different modes of treatment are used to improve local control while minimizing collateral damage to other parts of the eye.

Episcleral Plaque Radiotherapy

In most centers, when applicable, the first choice of treatment is episcleral plaque radiotherapy, brachytherapy, administered with a radioactive plaque containing ruthenium-106 or iodine-125 (Chapter 41). Ruthenium plaques are suitable for uveal melanomas up to 5 mm thick, because of the limited range of β radiation they emit.

Proton Beam Radiotherapy

This type of radiotherapy enables a high dose of radiation to be aimed precisely at a uveal melanoma irrespective of the tumor's size, shape, or location (Chapter 42). Facilities for this treatment are available in only a small number of centers around the world.

Stereotactic Radiotherapy

This method is generally used as an alternative to proton beam radiotherapy, in centers where a cyclotron unit is not available (Chapter 43).

Photocoagulation

Photocoagulation of choroidal melanomas is associated with a high complication rate and has been superseded by transpupillary thermotherapy.

Transpupillary Thermotherapy

With transpupillary thermotherapy, the tumor is heated by only a few degrees for about 1 minute using a 3 mm diode laser beam (Chapter 40). This treatment has been advocated for tumors up to 4-mm thick. Adjunctive brachytherapy is advocated as a means of avoiding local recurrence from intrascleral tumor ("sandwich technique").[3]

Photodynamic Therapy

Photodynamic therapy using verteporfin has recently been described but it is still too soon to assess the efficacy of this treatment, both as primary therapy and as adjunctive treatment for radiation-induced exudation.[4]

Such surgical procedures are difficult. They are therefore performed only in a few centers, where they are reserved for tumors that are considered too large for radiotherapy or as a treatment for the "toxic tumor syndrome" after radiotherapy (ie, exudation, retinal detachment, and neovascular glaucoma) (Chapter 44).

COUNSELING

Patients with uveal melanoma can have special psychological needs, which may change as they progress through their care pathway (Chapter 11).

SURVEILLANCE FOR SYSTEMIC DISEASE

There is no consensus about which patients should be screened for metastatic disease (Chapter 48). Some form of liver imaging is required, ideally every 6 months.[5] Chest radiography and liver function tests are not helpful.[5]

ORGANIZATION OF PATIENT CARE

Increasingly, patients with uveal melanoma are being managed by a multidisciplinary team comprising an ocular oncologist, general oncologist, radiation oncologist, pathologist, and psychologist. Ocular oncology services may also provide logistic assistance as well as information leaflets, Internet support, and a telephone helpline.

REFERENCES

1. Kujala E, Kivelä T. Tumor, node, metastasis classification of malignant ciliary body and choroidal melanoma: evaluation of the 6th edition and future directions. *Ophthalmology.* 2005;112:1135-1144.
2. Scholes AG, Damato BE, Nunn J, et al. Monosomy 3 in uveal melanoma: correlation with clinical and histologic predictors of survival. *Invest Ophthalmol Vis Sci.* 2003;44:1008-1011.
3. Bartlema YM, Oosterhuis JA, Journee-de Korver JG, Tjho-Heslinga RE, Keunen JE. Combined plaque radiotherapy and transpupillary thermotherapy in choroidal melanoma: 5 years' experience. *Br J Ophthalmol.* 2003;87:1370-1373.
4. Wachtlin J, Bechrakis NE, Foerster MH. [Photodynamic therapy with verteporfin for uveal melanoma]. *Ophthalmologe.* 2005;102:241-246.
5. Eskelin S, Pyrhonen S, Summanen P, Prause JU, Kivelä T. Screening for metastatic malignant melanoma of the uvea revisited. *Cancer.* 1999;85:1151-1159.

Uveal Malignant Melanoma: Management Options— Thermotherapy

Hanneke J. G. Journée-de Korver, Nicoline E. Schalij-Delfos, and Saskia M. Imhof

The heat treatment modalities for intraocular tumors include photocoagulation, hyperthermia, and thermotherapy.

PHOTOCOAGULATION

Photocoagulation involves heating of the tumor to temperatures above 65°C and provides only inadequate local tumor control and has largely been abandoned.

THERMOTHERAPY

During thermotherapy, the tumor is heated to a temperature of 60° to 65°C by means of an infrared diode laser introduced via the pupil (transpupillary thermotherapy, TTT). TTT was introduced by Oosterhuis and co-workers in 1994 (Box 40-1).[1] Histopathology after experimental TTT with a single 1-minute application shows tumor necrosis and occlusion of tumor vessels up to a maximum depth of 3.9 mm (Figure 40-1).[2]

Indications

The high rate of late recurrences has diminished enthusiasm for TTT as sole therapy, which is now reserved for small tumors less than 3-mm thick.[3,4]

To avoid insufficient treatment of the sclera, a combination of TTT and plaque radiotherapy (sandwich therapy) may be considered.[5] The two treatment modalities are complementary to each other, as TTT destroys approximately 3 mm of the superficial part of the tumor, and plaque radiotherapy adequately treats the deeper portions of the tumor as well as the underlying sclera.

In selected cases, secondary TTT may be useful when there is a lack of adequate tumor regression after radiotherapy; for local tumor recurrence after radiotherapy or local resection[6]; and for radiation-induced tumor exudation following plaque or proton beam radiotherapy.[7]

Contraindications

TTT is contraindicated in patients with media opacities that obscure the retinal image; insufficient dilatation of the pupil; peripherally located tumors; pretreatment subretinal fluid measuring more than 3 mm in elevation; and tumor basal diameter exceeding 10 mm and/or thickness more than 4 mm for TTT as sole treatment.

Technique

Prior to treatment, the pupil is dilated and parabulbar anesthesia administered.[8,9] The laser beam is directed at the tumor apex through a contact lens with infrared antireflective coating (Figure 40-2). The entire surface of the tumor is covered by overlapping applications extending at least 1.5 mm beyond its margin. Treatment starts with a central 1-minute application on the tumor apex at a relatively low laser power. In the authors' experience, the power setting is begun at 450 mW in normal pigmented tumors, at 600 mW in amelanotic tumors, and at 300 mW laser output power in heavily pigmented tumors (Figure 40-3). Tumor necrosis with vascular occlusion is obvious after a few days. Clearance of the necrotic debris takes 3 to 4 months.

Follow-Up

After TTT, patients are reviewed and examined every 2 to 3 months by ophthalmoscopy and ultrasonography. As a rule, the tumor shows gradual regression, eventually resulting in either an area of choroidal atrophy or a hypertrophic retinal pigment epithelial scar. With ultrasonography, special attention should be paid to the retrobulbar region, to exclude extraocular recurrence.[10]

RESULTS

Tumor Control

Treatment of melanomas measuring 2.2- to 4.0-mm thick is successful, with a reduction in tumor thickness to a flat scar in

---

Box 40-1. Essential Features of Transpupillary Thermotherapy

- Indicated for small, posterior tumors not involving the optic disc
- Administered with a 3 mm diode laser beam
- Heats the tumor to 60° to 65°C for about 1 minute
- Is preferably administered with adjunctive radiotherapy
- Is useful after radiotherapy for tumor recurrence or exudation
- Can be augmented using indocyanine green

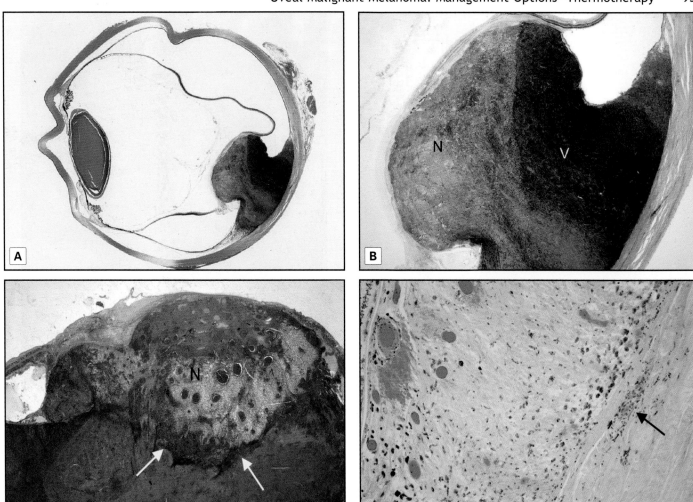

Figure 40-1. Experimental pre-enucleation single 1-minute TTT application to a choroidal melanoma (height 7.3 mm). (A) Enucleation was performed 72 hours later. On histopathology, the cornea, lens, and vitreous remain clear. (B) Higher magnification clearly shows the sharp demarcation between the necrotic (N) and viable (V) parts of the tumor. Atrophy of the retina overlying the tumor corresponds to the diameter of the laser spot. (C) Experimental pre-enucleation single 1-minute TTT application to a choroidal melanoma (height 9.1 mm). Enucleation was performed 48 hours later. Histopathology reveals tumor necrosis to a depth of 3.9 mm. All the blood vessels in the necrotic area are dilated and occluded with thrombi. Scattered small hemorrhages are present in the transitional zone (arrows) between the necrotic and viable parts of the tumor. (D) Experimental preenucleation single 1-minute TTT application to a choroidal melanoma (height 2.0 mm). Enucleation was performed 20 hours later. Histopathology demonstrates tumor necrosis bordering on the sclera and intrascleral tumor cells (arrow) appear viable. Intrascleral cells may not be adequately heated due to the low absorption of infrared light by the non-pigmented sclera.

more than 90% of cases.[3] The number of treatment sessions ranges from one to six. In patients treated with "sandwich therapy" a reduction in thickness to a flat scar in tumors originally up to 8-mm thick was found in 82% of patients after a mean follow-up of 20.5 months.[11]

Anterior Segment Complications

Occasionally, mild inflammation may be observed after TTT. Focal iris atrophy with posterior synechiae and a sectoral, non-progressive cataract may occur when the laser beam accidentally hits the pupillary margin.

Tumor Recurrence

Incidence

Kaplan–Meier estimates for recurrence in 256 consecutive cases treated only with TTT were 4% at 1 year, 12% at 2 years, and 22% at 3 years' follow-up.[3] However, the recurrence rate following sandwich therapy is much lower (3% to 4% at 5 years).[12]

Clinical Features

In general, tumor recurrences are observed at a mean interval of about 2 years following TTT, emphasizing the need for prolonged careful follow-up. Failure of local tumor control can be marginal, central, or external (Figures 40-4 and 40-5).

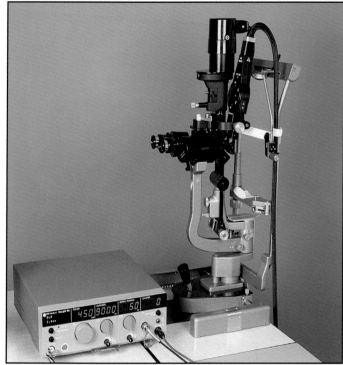

Figure 40-2. The infrared diode laser at 810 nm (Iris, Mountain View, CA), which is attached to a slit lamp (Haag-Streit, Bern, Switzerland).

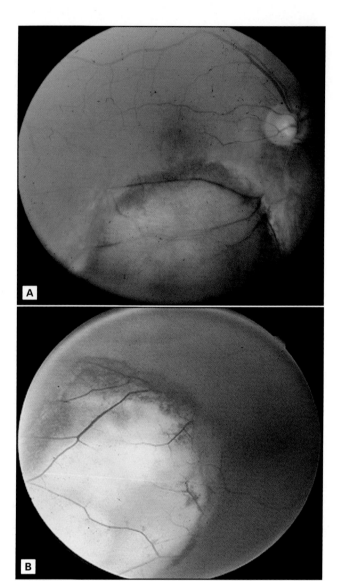

Figure 40-3. Fundus photograph showing an inferior choroidal melanoma measuring 10.7 x 10.4 x 2.8 mm that was treated with sandwich therapy. Note the grayish discoloration of tumor tissue after TTT, indicating that a subphotocoagulation-level temperature has been achieved (A). Laser power settings producing a prematurely white coagulation effect should be avoided because the increased reflection and scatter restricts the depth penetration of heat, resulting in only superficial damage to the tumor (B).

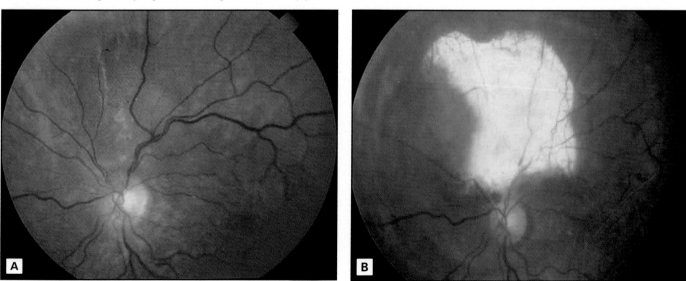

Figure 40-4. Marginal recurrence following TTT. (A) Before transpupillary thermotherapy. (B) Fifteen months after transpupillary thermotherapy, with recurrence along the posterior margin. Enucleation was performed. (Reprinted from Shields CL, Shields JA, Perez N, Singh AD, Cater J. Primary transpupillary thermotherapy for choroidal melanoma in 256 consecutive cases. Outcomes and limitations. *Ophthalmology.* 2001;23:763-767.)

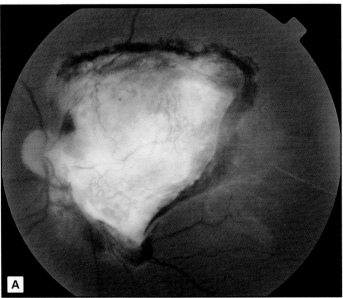
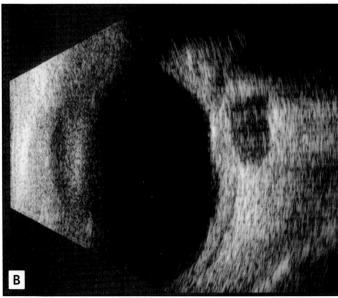

Figure 40-5. External recurrence following TTT. Fundus photograph showing fibrotic membrane with fine retinal neovascularization at the treated site of small choroidal melanoma following three sessions of TTT (A). (B) B-scan ultrasonography demonstrated a nodular extrascleral extension along the base of the original tumor. (Reproduced with permission from Singh AD, Rundle PA, Berry–Brincat A, Parsons MA, Rennie IG. Extrascleral extension of choroidal malignant melanoma following transpupillary thermotherapy. *Eye.* 2004;18:91-93.)

Visual Results

The visual outcome depends on the size and location of the original tumor.

Complications

Fine superficial hemorrhages at the tumor apex are commonly observed after TTT, as well as a transient increase in subretinal fluid that resolves within weeks. Branch retinal artery and vein occlusion can occur if excessive laser power is used. Retinal traction folds and epiretinal membranes may occur in 20% of cases.[13]

REFERENCES

1. Oosterhuis JA, Journée-de Korver JG, Kakebeeke-Kemme HM, et al. Transpupillary thermotherapy in choroidal melanoma. *Arch Ophthalmol.* 1995;113:315-321.
2. Journée-de Korver JG, Oosterhuis JA, de Wolff-Rouendaal D, et al. Histopathological findings in human choroidal melanomas after transpupillary thermotherapy. *Br J Ophthalmol.* 1997;81:234-239.
3. Shields CL, Shields JA, Perez N, et al. Primary transpupillary thermotherapy for small choroidal melanoma in 256 consecutive cases: outcomes and limitations. *Ophthalmology.* 2002;109:225-234.
4. Shields CL, Shields JA, Cater J, et al. Transpupillary thermotherapy for choroidal melanoma: tumor control and visual results in 100 consecutive cases. *Ophthalmology.* 1998;105:581-590.
5. Keunen JEE, Journée-de Korver JG, Oosterhuis JA. Transpupillary thermotherapy with or without brachytherapy: a dilemma. *Br J Ophthalmol.* 1999;83:987-988.
6. Robertson DM. TTT as rescue treatment for choroidal melanoma not controlled with iodine-125 brachytherapy. *Ocul Immunol Inflamm.* 2002;10:247-252.
7. Damato B, Patel I, Campbell IR, Mayles HM, Errington RD. Local tumor control after (106)Ru brachytherapy of choroidal melanoma. *Int J Radiat Oncol Biol Phys.* 2005;63:385-391.
8. Journée-de Korver HG, Midena E, Singh AD. Infrared thermotherapy from laboratory to clinic. *Ophthalmol Clin North Am.* 2005;18:99-110.
9. Journée-de Korver JG, Keunen JEE. Thermotherapy in the management of choroidal melanoma. *Prog Retinal Eye Res.* 2002;21:303-317.
10. Singh AD, Eagle RC Jr, Shields CL, Shields JA. Enucleation following transpupillary thermotherapy of choroidal melanoma: clinicopathologic correlations. *Arch Ophthalmol.* 2003;121:397-400.
11. Oosterhuis JA, Journée-de Korver JG, Keunen JEE. Transpupillary thermotherapy: results in 50 patients with choroidal melanoma. *Arch Ophthalmol.* 1998;116:157-162.
12. Seregard S, Landau I. Transpupillary thermotherapy as an adjunct to ruthenium plaque radiotherapy for choroidal melanoma. *Acta Ophthalmol Scand.* 2001;79:19-22.
13. Bartlema YM, Oosterhuis JA, Journée-de Korver JG, et al. Combined plaque radiotherapy and transpupillary thermotherapy in choroidal melanoma: 5 years' experience. *Br J Ophthalmol.* 2003;87:1370-1373.

Uveal Malignant Melanoma: Management Options— Brachytherapy

Stefan Seregard, Bertil E. Damato, and Peter Fleming

INTRODUCTION

Moore first used brachytherapy for uveal melanoma in 1930 by inserting radon-222 seeds into the tumor.[1] This technique was later modified by Stallard.[2] In the United States, this radionuclide was gradually replaced by plaques loaded with iodine-125 seeds, as this provided less radiation to surrounding tissues.[3] In Europe, the pioneering work of Lommatzsch in the 1970s led to the introduction of ruthenium-106 as a radioactive source for episcleral brachytherapy of uveal melanoma (Box 41-1).[4]

EPISCLERAL RADIOACTIVE PLAQUE

Plaque Design

Most episcleral plaques are bowl shaped and usually about 15 to 20 mm in diameter. The inner part contains the radioactive sources (Table 41-1), which are either integrated in the plaque or held in place by glue or a silicone mold (Figure 41-1). The outer surface is lined by a heavy metal, such as silver or gold, to prevent the radiation of tissues external to the eye. Two or more eyelets near the edge of the plaque allow the plaque to be sutured to the episcleral surface.

Dosimetry

Typically, the total dose provided and the radioactive dose per time unit of exposure (dose rate) are estimated at various distances from the radioactive source. The optimal tumoricidal dose ranges from 80 to 100 Gy.

TREATMENT

Preoperative Assessment

The basal diameter and height of the tumor are measured by funduscopy, fundus photographs, ultrasonography (standardized A- and B-scans), and transillumination, individually or in any combination. A correct estimate of the largest basal diameter is important for the selection of an appropriately sized plaque, and often a 2-mm safety margin around the tumor is added. The height measurement is usually obtained by ultrasonography and is critical for calculation of the appropriate delivery time and hence the radiation dose. Most centers deliver an apex dose of 80 to 100 Gy, so that the sclera receives a much higher dose of radiation.

Box 41-1. Brachytherapy of Uveal Melanoma

- Administered with plaques containing iodine-125 ruthenium-106
- Delivers a minimum apex dose of 80–100 Gy
- May be combined with TTT
- Can cause damage to ocular tissue, especially with large tumors
- The most common complications include optic neuropathy, maculopathy, cataract, and neovascular glaucoma
- Survival is not significantly worse than after enucleation

Table 41-1. Characteristics of Radionuclides Used for Brachytherapy of Uveal Melanoma

Element	Nuclide	Energy (MeV)	Half-Life
Cobalt	Co-60	1.25	5.26 years
Iodine	I-125	2.392	59.4 days
Ruthenium	Ru-106	6.547	373.6 days
Iridium	Ir-192	1.460	73.8 days
Palladium	Pd-103	2.660	17.0 days
Gold	Au-198	1.372	2.7 days
Strontium	Sr-90	6.697	28.8 years

(Data from chemlab.pcmaricopa.edu)

Plaque Positioning

The tumor margins are localized by transillumination, indentation, or both, and marked on the sclera with a pen. If necessary, any overlying extraocular muscles are disinserted. A template is sutured to the sclera, and once it is well placed in relation to the tumor, it is replaced with the radioactive plaque. The position of the template or plaque in relation to the tumor is checked by intraoperative ultrasonography. Another approach is to perform indirect ophthalmoscopy while indenting the eye with the edge of

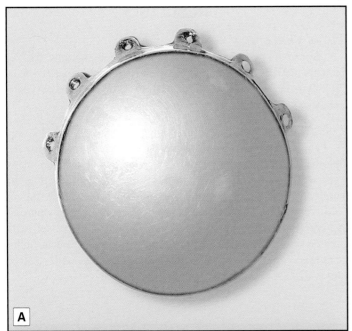

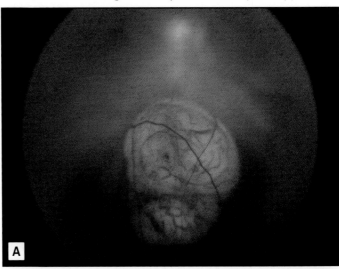

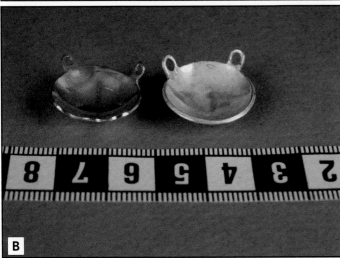

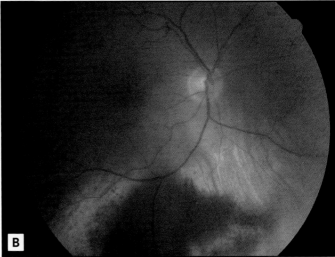

Figure 41-2. Fundus with a large uveal melanoma before (A) and 12 months after (B) ruthenium brachytherapy. Significant tumor regression is evident. The patient succumbed to metastatic disease 2 years after brachytherapy.

Figure 41-1. Episcleral plaques loaded with iodine-125 seeds (A) and containing ruthenium-106 integrated in the applicator (B).

the plaque or with a right-angled fiberoptic transilluminator, the tip of this instrument inserted in a hole in the template.[5] Once the plaque is in place, any rectus muscles are repositioned, and the conjunctiva is closed. When the prescribed dose of radiotherapy has been delivered, usually after 2 to 7 days, the plaque is removed by a second procedure.

Follow-Up

As with other forms of conservative therapy, lifelong surveillance is indicated, with assessment initially every 3 to 6 months, then every 6 months for about 5 years, and eventually once every year. Comparison of ophthalmoscopic appearances with a baseline color photograph or serial fundus photography should reveal any marginal recurrence at an early stage. Ultrasonography is especially useful for measuring changes in tumor thickness. Tumor regression is usually not apparent for the first 3 to 6 months after brachytherapy. The rate of regression varies significantly between tumors, being more rapid and complete in patients who subsequently develop metastatic disease (Figure 41-2). Recur-

rence should be suspected only if any apparent growth exceeds 0.5 mm and if a trend is confirmed by repeated examination.

Radiation Safety

Once the plaque is inserted, visitors and healthcare personnel working by the bedside should receive minimal doses of radiation. Each hospital has its own safety rules, which must be strictly enforced.

COLLATERAL DAMAGE TO OCULAR TISSUES

Using simulation software programs, the risk of radiation-related side effects can usually be estimated before brachytherapy.[6] At least 50% of patients with a large uveal melanoma experience significant ocular morbidity.[7] With small tumors, ocular adverse effects are less common and less severe, especially with a low-energy b-emitting source such as ruthenium-106.[8] Most radiation-related ocular side effects occur in the early postoperative years (Figures 41-3 and 41-4), but adverse effects may present after a prolonged period (Chapter 9).

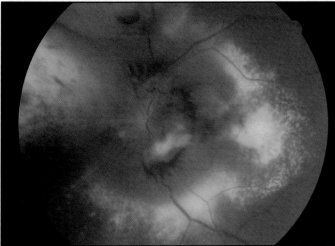

Figure 41-3. Fundus featuring radiation retinopathy and papillopathy 3 years after iodine brachytherapy for a large choroidal melanoma.

RESULTS

Visual Outcome

Approximately 3 to 5 years after brachytherapy, half of patients (49% to 55%) maintain a best corrected visual acuity of 20/200 or better, and one third (31% to 33%) have 20/50 visual acuity or better in the affected eye.[9,10]

Local Tumor Recurrence

This is the main reason for secondary enucleation following episcleral brachytherapy for uveal melanoma. However, many eyes with local recurrence can be retained after repeating the brachytherapy, or performing transpupillary thermotherapy or local resection. The overall tumor recurrence rate is approximately 10% at 5 years, and treatment failure is associated with greater size and posterior extension of the tumor.[11] Local tumor recurrence after plaque radiotherapy is associated with reduced survival.[11]

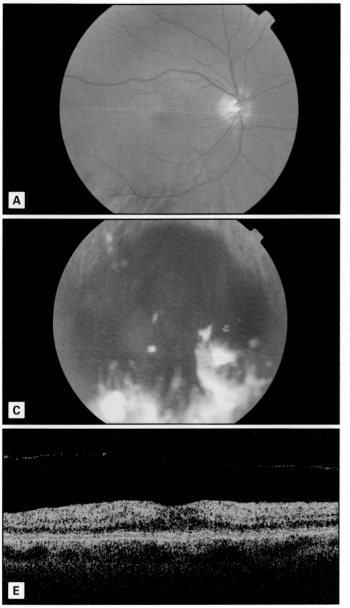

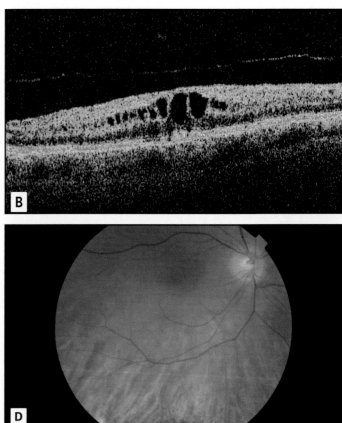

Figure 41-4. Clinical features (A) and imaging by optical coherence tomography (OCT) (B) of macular edema 9 months after ruthenium brachytherapy for a medium-sized uveal melanoma. Visual acuity was reduced from 20/20 before radiotherapy to 20/50. Intravitreal injection of triamcinolone (C) induced prompt resolution of edema, both clinically (D) and by OCT (E). Visual acuity improved to 20/30 within 2 weeks.

Ocular Conservation

Generally, eyes are enucleated following episcleral brachytherapy in 12% to 17% of patients at 3 to 5 years follow-up.[10,11] The reasons for enucleation vary from one study to another and include local tumor recurrence, recurrent vitreous hemorrhage, and painful neovascular glaucoma.

SURVIVAL

The COMS trials suggest that patient survival following brachytherapy is not significantly different from that after enucleation.[12] Patients randomized to either enucleation or iodine brachytherapy had unadjusted 5-year survival rates of 81% and 82%, respectively, and histopathologically confirmed melanoma metastases occurred in 11% and 9%, respectively.[12] Patients treated with ruthenium brachytherapy had similar 5- and 10-year survival rates of 84% and 72%, respectively.[10]

REFERENCES

1. Moore RF. Choroidal sarcoma treated by the intraocular insertion of radon seeds. *Br J Ophthalmol.* 1930;14:145-152.
2. Stallard HB. Radiotherapy of malignant intraocular neoplasm. *Br J Ophthalmol.* 1948;32:618-639.
3. Packer S, Rotman M. Radiotherapy of choroidal melanoma with iodine-125. *Ophthalmology.* 1974;87:582-590.
4. Lommatzsch PK. Treatment of choroidal melanomas with 106Ru/106Rh beta-ray applicators. *Surv Ophthalmol.* 1974;19:85-100.
5. Damato BE, Patel I, Campbell IR, et al. Local tumor control after (106)Ru brachytherapy of choroidal melanoma. *Int J Radiat Oncol Biol Phys.* 2005;63:385-391.
6. Puusaari I, Heikkonen J, Kivela T. Effect of radiation dose on ocular complications after iodine brachytherapy for large uveal melanoma: empirical data and simulation of collimated plaques. *Invest Ophthalmol Vis Sci.* 2004;45:3425-3434.
7. Puusaari I, Heikkonen J, Kivela T. Ocular complications after iodine brachytherapy for large uveal melanomas. *Ophthalmology.* 2004;111:1768-1777.
8. Damato B, Patel I, Campbell IR, et al. Visual acuity after ruthenium (106) brachytherapy of choridal melanomas. *Int J Radiat Oncol Biolol Phys.* 2005;63:392-400.
9. The Collaborative Ocular Melanoma Study Group. Collaborative Ocular Melanoma Study (COMS) randomized trial of I-125 brachytherapy for medium choroidal melanoma. 1. Visual acuity after 3 years. COMS report no. 16. *Ophthalmology.* 2001;108:348-366.
10. Bergman L, Nilsson B, Lundell G, et al. Ruthenium brachytherapy for uveal melanoma, 1979-2003. Survival and functional outcomes in the Swedish population. *Ophthalmology.* 2005;112:834-840.
11. Jampol LM, Moy CS, Murray TG, et al. The COMS randomized trial of iodine 125 brachytherapy for choroidal melanoma: IV. Local treatment failure and enucleation in the first 5 years after brachytherapy. COMS report no. 19. *Ophthalmology.* 2002;109:2197-2206.
12. The Collaborative Ocular Melanoma Study Group. The COMS Randomized trial of iodine 125 brachytherapy for choroidal melanoma, III: Initial mortality findings. COMS report no. 18. *Arch Ophthalmol.* 2001;119:969-982.

Uveal Malignant Melanoma: Management Options— Proton Beam Radiotherapy

Anne Marie Lane and Evangelos S. Gragoudas

RADIOTHERAPY

The properties of protons, specifically the manner in which they lose energy in tissue, with minimal scatter due to their mass, low LET (linear energy transfer), and the deposition of most energy at the end of their range (Bragg peak), permit the design of a beam that covers the target volume with a uniform dose and reduces or eliminates the dose proximal and distal to the target. By varying or modulating the beam energy, the Bragg peak can be broadened to conform to any tumor (Box 42-1).[1]

PROTON BEAM IRRADIATION

Patient Evaluation

Proton irradiation is not recommended for patients with very large melanomas that occupy more than 30% of the ocular volume, large extrascleral extensions, or extensive neovascularization in a painful eye. Such cases are unlikely to benefit from conservative treatment, and, therefore, enucleation is recommended.

Pre-Radiation Surgery

Most patients with uveal melanomas have surgery to localize the tumor prior to receiving proton therapy. This is done by trans-illumination and/or indirect ophthalmoscopy followed by suturing of four 2.5-mm radio-opaque tantalum rings on the sclera around the borders of the tumor, which serve as reference points for placement of the proton beam at the time of treatment.

Proton Treatment Planning

Proton treatment planning is used to design an aperture that approximates the shape of the tumor and gives a 3-mm margin laterally (1.5 mm at the 90% dose level), to calculate the maximum and minimum depths of the target, and the beam range and modulation width, which includes a 2.5- to 4-mm margin both distally and proximally. The dose distribution is calculated, and dose volume histograms for the globe, lens, ciliary body, retina, macula, and disc are generated.

Irradiation Procedure

The patient is treated in the sitting position, with the head immobilized by using a facemask and bite block, which are attached to a headholder (Figure 42-1). During treatment, the eyelids are retracted by the ophthalmologist using an eye speculum to reduce radiation exposure to the eyelid, and the patient is asked to fixate. A fluoroscopic system is used to monitor eye position. A total dose of 70 CGE (63.6 proton Gy times 1.1 relative biologic effectiveness) in five equal fractions is delivered at the MEEI.[2]

Follow-Up Protocol

Ophthalmological examinations are performed 6 weeks, 6 months, and 12 months after treatment, biannually thereafter up to 5 years after treatment, and then annually, to monitor the status of both tumor and patient.

PATIENT CHARACTERISTICS

Two large series of uveal melanoma patients (more than 2000 patients each) have been treated at the Massachusetts Eye and Ear Infirmary/Harvard Cyclotron/Francis H. Burr Proton Therapy Center and the Hôpital Ophthalmique Jules Gonin/Paul Scherrer Institute.

OPHTHALMIC OUTCOMES

Local Control

Disappearance of the tumor or the formation of a flat scar occurs infrequently, and the vast majority of lesions continue to regress years after therapy (Figure 42-2). The 10-year cumulative rate of regrowth (confirmed and suspected cases) is 4%.[3]

Eye Loss

Neovascular glaucoma and tumor recurrence are the main reasons for enucleation.[2] The probability of retaining the eye is 91% at 5 years, 88% at 10 years, and 84% at 15 years after irradiation.[4]

Vision Loss

The overall 5-year rate of vision loss is 52% (20/200 or worse). This rate rises to 68% in patients with tumors located near the optic nerve or macula.[5] Tumor location within two disc diameters of these structures is the strongest predictor of poor visual outcome.[2]

Complications

The most serious anterior segment complications are rubeosis iridis and neovascular glaucoma. Five-year cumulative rates of maculopathy and papillopathy, two common posterior complications, are 40% and 24%, respectively.[4]

Box 42-1. Proton Beam Radiotherapy of Uveal Melanoma

- Deposits most energy at end of beam (Bragg peak)
- Allows good control of radiation
- Is administered with safety margins, 3 mm laterally and up to 4 mm longitudinally
- Achieves a high rate of local tumor control
- The main complications are neovascular glaucoma, maculopathy, optic neuropathy, and cataract
- Survival rates are not significantly different from those after enucleation

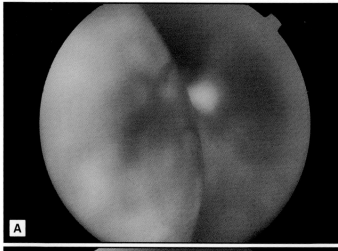

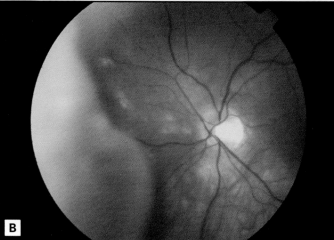

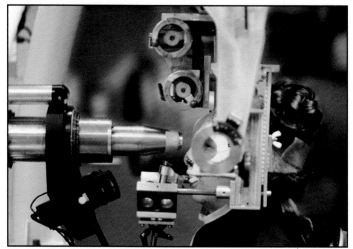

Figure 42-1. Patient immobilized for treatment with use of headholder, facemask and bite block. (This figure was published in Gragoudas ES. Charged particle irradiation of uveal melanoma. In: Ryan SJ, ed. *Retina.* 4th ed. © Elsevier 2006.)

Figure 42-2. Large ciliochoroidal melanoma extending up to the optic nerve and associated with serous retinal detachment. (A) Before proton irradiation. (B) Approximately 1 year post-treatment, a significant reduction of the tumor is seen.

METASTASIS AND SURVIVAL

Annual melanoma-related death rates are highest between 3 and 6 years after proton therapy, varying between 3.5% and 4.4%.[4] Five-, 10-, and 15-year tumor-specific survival rates are 86%, 77%, and 73%, respectively.[2] Patient and tumor characteristics associated with metastatic death include largest tumor diameter, patient age, tumor pigmentation, presence or absence of symptoms, tumor origin, and iris color.[2]

The most common site of metastasis is the liver.[6] Prognosis after diagnosis of metastasis is poor, with few patients surviving more than 1 year.[6]

REFERENCES

1. Suit HD, Gotein M, Tepper J, et al. Exploratory study of proton radiation therapy using large field techniques and fractionated dose schedules. *Cancer.* 1975;35:1646-1657.
2. Gragoudas E, Li W, Goitein M, Lane AM, Munzenrider JE, Egan KM. Evidence-based estimates of outcome in patients irradiated for intraocular melanoma. *Arch Ophthalmol.* 2002;120:1665-1671.
3. Gragoudas ES, Lane AM, Munzenrider J, Egan KM, Li W. Long-term risk of local failure after proton therapy for choroidal/ciliary body melanoma. *Trans Am Ophthalmol Soc.* 2002;100:43-48.
4. Gragoudas ES, Lane AM. Uveal melanoma: proton beam irradiation. *Ophthalmol Clin North Am.* 2005;18:111-118.
5. Gragoudas ES, Li W, Lane AM, Munzenrider J, Egan KM. Risk factors for radiation maculopathy and papillopathy after intraocular irradiation. *Ophthalmology.* 1999;106:1571-1578.
6. Gragoudas E, Egan K, Seddon J, et al. Survival of patients with metastases from uveal melanoma. *Ophthalmology.* 1991;98:383-390.

Uveal Malignant Melanoma: Management Options— Stereotactic Radiotherapy

Karin Dieckmann, Gerald Langmann, Roy Ma, Mona Schmutzer, Richard Poetter, Werner Wackernagel, and Martin Zehetmayer

INTRODUCTION

Stereotactic radiotherapy involves precise positioning of the tumor in three-dimensional space by appropriate scanning and the delivery of ionizing radiation to the tumor from multiple directions.[1] A high dose of radiation is therefore focused on the target tissue, with relatively little irradiation of surrounding healthy tissues.

INDICATIONS

Stereotactic radiotherapy is considered for cases that are unsuitable for brachytherapy, either because of posterior location or large size.

TYPES OF STEREOTACTIC RADIOTHERAPY

There are two techniques for delivering stereotactic radiation to the eye: stereotactic radiosurgery and fractionated stereotactic radiotherapy (Box 43-1).

Stereotactic Radiosurgery

Stereotactic radiosurgery involves multiple radiation beams focused on the tumor simultaneously from different directions, the treatment usually being completed in a single session, or occasionally fractionated over several days. Radiosurgery is delivered using the Leksell Gamma Knife (LGK). This device comprises 201 cobalt sources localized in a hemisphere around the patient's head so that all beams of gamma radiation converge on the tumor (Figure 43-1).

Fractionated Stereotactic Radiotherapy

A single beam of radiation is aimed at the tumor from successively different directions, the entire treatment being delivered either in a single session or, more usually, in a fractionated manner over several sessions.

STEREOTACTIC RADIOSURGERY

Treatment planning is based on MRI scans.

Critical structures such as the optic nerve, retina, macula, lens, and ciliary body are identified. A dose of 30 Gy is administered. A safety margin of 1 to 2 mm around the tumor is treated (planned treatment volume) (Figure 43-2). Dose-volume histo-

Box 43-1. Stereotactic Radiotherapy

- Ionizing radiation is delivered to the tumor from multiple directions, either concurrently (stereotactic radiosurgery) or sequentially (stereotactic radiotherapy)
- The tumor is positioned precisely in three-dimensional space by appropriate scanning
- The patient's head and eye are immobilized using a variety of methods
- Stereotactic radiotherapy delivers a high dose of radiation to the tumor with small doses to surrounding tissues
- Early results are encouraging, indicating that this modality has a place in the treatment of uveal melanoma
- These methods are used mostly for posterior tumors that are difficult to treat with a plaque and for large tumors

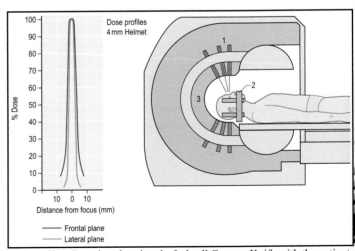

Figure 43-1. Drawing showing the Leksell Gamma Knife with the patient lying in the supine position. The beams of the 201 sources (1) converge in the eye (crossfiring); the patient's head is fixed with the stereotactic frame (2) to the inner collimator helmet (3).

gram analysis is also performed to determine the likelihood of complications.[2]

Results

Tumor regression is achieved in 93% of patients. Neovascular glaucoma develops in patients with larger tumors and in proximity to the ciliary body.[3]

FRACTIONATED STEREOTACTIC RADIOTHERAPY

Treatment Planning

A computerized three-dimensional model of the eye and tumor is generated. The CT and MRI images are fused so that they can be viewed in axial, sagittal, or coronal planes. A total dose of 50 to 60 Gy is usually delivered in five fractions over a period of up to 10 days.[4,5] The tumor is treated with a safety margin of 2.0 to 2.5 mm in all directions. Additionally, critical structures (lens, optic nerve, anterior eye segment, lacrimal gland) are contoured for treatment plan optimization, which includes dose-volume histograms.

Results

Tumor Control and Complications

Between 1997 and 2004, 158 patients were treated with LINAC SRT in Vienna. This therapy was selected for tumors with a thickness exceeding 7.0 mm or extending to within 3 mm of the optic disc or macula. Interim results have been published and more recent data are in press. With a median follow-up time of 33 months, local control is achieved in 98% of patients. Long-term side effects included retinopathy (n=70; 44%); cataract (n=30; 23%); optic neuropathy (n=65; 41%); and secondary neovascular glaucoma (n=23; 13.8%).[6]

REFERENCES

1. McKenzie MR, Ma R, Clark B, et al. Stereotactic radiosurgery and radiation therapy in British Columbia. *Br Columbia Med J.* 2001;43:567-572.

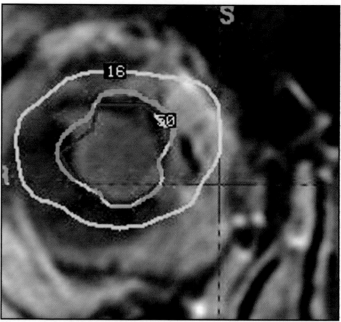

Figure 43-2. MRI scans showing juxtapapillary choroidal melanoma (red line). The 50% and 16% isodoses (coronal) view are represented by the green and yellow lines, respectively.

2. Langmann G, Wackernagel W, Stucklschweiger G, et al. [Dose-volume histogram regression analysis of uveal melanomas after single fraction gamma knife radiosurgery]. *Ophthalmologe.* 2004;101:1111-1119.

3. Langmann G, Pendl G, Klaus M, et al. Gamma knife radiosurgery for uveal melanomas: an 8-year experience. *J Neurosurg.* 2000;93(Suppl 3):184-188.

4. Zehetmayer M, Dieckmann K, Kren G, et al. Fractionated stereotactic radiotherapy with linear accelerator for uveal melanoma—preliminary Vienna results. *Strahlenther Onkol.* 1999;175(Suppl 2):74-75.

5. Muller K, Nowak PJ, de Pan C, et al. Effectiveness of fractionated stereotactic radiotherapy for uveal melanoma. *Int J Radiat Oncol Biol Phys.* 2005;63:116-122.

6. Dieckmann D, Georg D, Zehetmayer M, et al. Stereotactic photon beam irradiation of uveal melanoma: indications and experience at the University of Vienna since 1997. *Strahlenther Onkol.* 2007;183:11-13.

Uveal Malignant Melanoma: Management Options— Resection Techniques

Bertil E. Damato and Carl Groenewald

INTRODUCTION

Local resection of uveal melanoma was for many years restricted to small iris and ciliary body melanomas, mostly because of the technical difficulties associated with the excision of larger and more posterior tumors. There are now several tumor resection techniques reported by a number of authors.[1-9]

IRIDECTOMY

Indications and Contraindications

Iridectomy is indicated if the iris tumor is considered to be a malignant melanoma. Contraindications include the involvement of more than four clock hours of the iris and diffuse spread or seeding.

Surgical Technique (Figure 44-1)

The pupil is dilated if a broad iridectomy is planned and constricted if conservation of the iris sphincter is intended. The tumor is removed with a safety margin of approximately 1 to 2 mm. If possible, the iris sphincter is preserved or sutured with 10-0 Prolene to reform the pupil. The corneoscleral wound is closed with 10-0 nylon.

Results and Complications

Local recurrence can occur if the tumor is incompletely excised. The iris coloboma tends to cause a cosmetic deficit and photophobia, which may require treatment with a painted contact lens or an artificial iris implant. Lens touch can result in cataract.

IRIDOCYCLECTOMY

Indications and Contraindications

Iridocyclectomy is indicated for an iris melanoma involving the angle and for ciliary body melanomas or adenocarcinomas. This procedure is contraindicated if the tumor involves more than 4 clock hours of the ciliary body or angle, or if there is diffuse spread. Extraocular spread is a relative contraindication, depending on whether or not it is small and encapsulated.

Surgical Technique (Figure 44-1)

A fornix-based conjunctival flap is prepared, and two traction sutures are placed in the sclera. The tumor extent is defined by transpupillary transillumination and marked on the sclera with a pen. Using a Desmarres scarifier, a limbus-based lamellar scleral flap is prepared, extending into cornea if the tumor involves the iris. A deep scleral incision is made, approximately 1 mm within the superficial incision, so as to create a stepped wound edge. This is done first posteriorly, then laterally, and finally anterior to the tumor. The tumor is excised with safety margins of about 1 to 2 mm. An incision is made in the peripheral iris to prevent iris prolapse and is extended either along the anterior margin of the tumor or along the lateral and posterior margins. Alternatively, if the tumor is mostly ciliary, the uvea is perforated in the region of the pars plana and resected either posteroanteriorly or in a circumferential (transverse) direction so as to preserve as much of the iris as possible. The tumor is lifted from the eye using the deep scleral lamella as a handle. Care is taken to avoid damage to the lens. It may be possible to conserve some of the zonules and ciliary epithelium. The vitreous base can usually be left intact, either repositioning prolapsed vitreous as the sclera is closed or performing a limited vitrectomy, either using the open-sky technique or through a separate sclerotomy. The sclera is closed with interrupted sutures. An alternative technique is to perform full-thickness corneoscleral excision with grafting, using a corneal trephine.[9]

Results and Complications

The results and complications of iridocyclectomy are similar to those of iridectomy. In addition, ocular hypotony can occur as a result of excessive cyclectomy (more than four clock hours), wound leakage, or cyclodialysis (which is more likely to occur if adjunctive radiotherapy is administered at the same time as the resection, instead of being delayed by a few weeks). If more than four clock hours of the ciliary body is excised, the lens can subluxate, causing keratopathy if it comes into contact with the corneal endothelium.

TRANS-SCLERAL CHOROIDECTOMY

Indications and Contraindications

Trans-scleral local resection is difficult and requires hypotensive anesthesia.

Surgical Technique (Figure 44-1)

A fornix-based conjunctival flap is prepared. Extraocular muscles in the operative field are disinserted after placing sutures

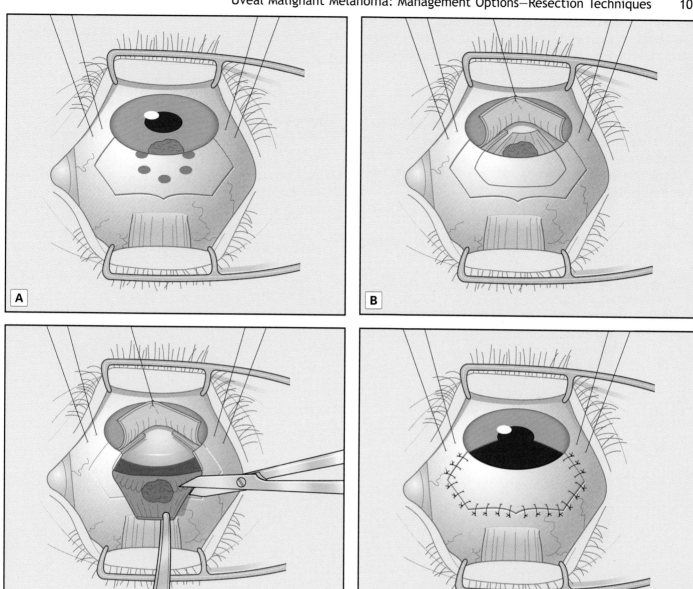

Figure 44-1. Iridectomy (A). Iridocyclectomy. Preparation of lamellar scleral flap hinged at the limbus (B). Starting anteriorly if broad iridectomy is performed (as shown) or posteriorly if only peripheral iridectomy is done (C). Suturing of scleral flap (D). (This figure was published in Damato B. *Ocular Tumours: Diagnosis and Treatment.* © Elsevier 1999.)

and measuring the knot-to-limbus distances. The tumor is localized by transpupillary transillumination. A lamellar scleral flap is dissected, hinged posteriorly. Any vortex veins or long posterior ciliary arteries entering the flap are cauterized and divided. The eye is partially collapsed by performing a limited pars plana vitrectomy, thereby preventing retinal prolapse through the scleral window. The deep sclera is incised with scissors around the tumor, first laterally, then posteriorly, and finally anteriorly. The deep scleral incision is made about 1 to 2 mm within the superficial incisions so as to create a stepped wound edge. The choroid is opened by gently holding it with two pairs of notched microforceps, which are slowly pulled apart. The uveal incision is made with blunt-tipped spring scissors, first anterior to the tumor, then along each side, and finally posteriorly. With ciliochoroidal tumors,

it is usually possible to conserve most of the ciliary epithelium if the uveal incision is started posterior to the ora serrata. As the uveal incision is made, the tumor is slowly lifted out of the eye using the deep lamellar handle. The retina usually separates spontaneously from the tumor, but if not, it may be necessary to separate these two structures. As soon as the tumor has been removed, the traction sutures are pulled gently until the retina starts to bulge through the scleral window. Two sponge cells are placed posterior to the scleral flap to indent the eye, thereby avoiding subretinal hematoma. Using a fresh set of instruments, the eye is closed with interrupted nylon sutures. A balanced salt solution is injected through the pars plana sclerotomy. If adjunctive brachytherapy is to be administered, a 25-mm ruthenium plaque is inserted, reattaching any disinserted extraocular muscles with slings, so that they are in approximately their correct anatomical locations. The conjunctiva is closed in the usual fashion. If adjunctive brachytherapy is administered, the plaque is removed after delivering a dose of 100 Gy to a depth of approximately 1 to 2 mm.

ENDORESECTION

Primary transretinal local resection of choroidal melanoma is controversial because of concerns regarding intraocular, extraocular, and systemic tumor dissemination.[10] Secondary endoresection after radiotherapy can be effective treatment for exudation, when less invasive methods have failed.

REFERENCES

1. Stallard HB. Partial choroidectomy. *Br J Ophthalmol.* 1966;50:660-662.
2. Damato BE, Foulds WS. Surgical resection of choroidal melanoma. In: Schachat AP, Ryan SJ, eds. *Retina.* 4th ed. St Louis, MO: Mosby; 2006:769-778.
3. Peyman GA, Gremillion CM. Eye wall resection in the management of uveal neoplasms. *Jpn J Ophthalmol.* 1989;33:458-471.
4. Shields JA, Shields CL. Surgical approach to lamellar sclerouvectomy for posterior uveal melanomas: the 1986 Schoenberg lecture. *Ophthalmic Surg.* 1988;19:774-780.
5. Garcia-Arumi J, Sararols L, Martinez V, Corcostegui B. Vitreoretinal surgery and endoresection in high posterior choroidal melanomas. *Retina.* 2001;21:445-452.
6. Bornfeld N, Talies S, Anastassiou G, Schilling H, Schuler A, Horstmann GA. Endoscopic resection of malignant melanomas of the uvea after preoperative stereotactic single dose convergence irradiation with the Leksell gamma knife. *Ophthalmologe.* 2002;99:338-344.
7. Char DH, Miller T, Crawford JB. Uveal tumour resection. *Br J Ophthalmol.* 2001;85:1213-1219.
8. Kertes PJ, Johnson JC, Peyman GA. Internal resection of posterior uveal melanomas. *Br J Ophthalmol.* 1998;82:1147-1153.
9. Naumann GO, Rummelt V. Block excision of tumors of the anterior uvea. Report on 68 consecutive patients. *Ophthalmology.* 1996;103:2017-2027.
10. Robertson DM. Melanoma endoresection: a perspective. *Retina.* 2001;21:403-407.

Uveal Malignant Melanoma: COMS Results

Arun D. Singh and Tero Kivelä

INTRODUCTION

Until the 1980s, most studies on the treatment of uveal melanoma were retrospective and included only small numbers of patients treated at a given center. The optimal management for uveal melanomas was debatable. Therefore, in 1984, at the request of Dr Kupfer, Director of the National Eye Institute (Bethesda, MD), the Collaborative Ocular Melanoma Study (COMS) trials were designed.[1]

The COMS is a multicenter study with 43 participating clinical centers in North America with centralized units dealing with echography, photography, pathology, radiation physics, and general coordination. The details of the entire protocol and procedures of the study are available elsewhere.[2]

ELIGIBILITY AND EXCLUSION CRITERIA

The general eligibility criteria and exclusion criteria are listed in Box 45-1 and Box 45-2, respectively.

COMS CLASSIFICATION OF CHOROIDAL MELANOMA

The COMS divided choroidal melanomas into small, medium, or large tumors according to largest basal diameter (LBD) and height (Figure 45-1).[2] In December 1990, the lower boundary of height for medium-sized tumors was redefined from 3.0 to 2.5 mm so as to increase patient recruitment in this group.

MAIN OUTCOME MEASURES

Although the main outcome measure in COMS was all-cause mortality,[2] the cause of death was graded by the Mortality Coding Committee as follows: confirmed melanoma metastasis; suspected melanoma metastasis; other malignant tumor; no evidence of malignancy; and insufficient evidence to establish melanoma metastasis.[3]

COMS TRIALS AND OBSERVATIONAL STUDIES

The COMS includes two randomized trials, for medium[4] and large tumors respectively,[5] and two observational studies (Figure 45-2).[6,7] In addition, several adjunct papers have been published.[8,9]

Box 45-1. Eligibility Criteria for Collaborative Ocular Melanoma Study

- Primary choroidal melanoma in one eye
- Age 21 years or older
- Ability to give informed consent
- Ability to return for scheduled follow-up
- No contraindication for surgery or radiation

Box 45-2. Exclusion Criteria for Collaborative Ocular Melanoma Study

- Previous biopsy of choroidal melanoma
- Previous treatment of choroidal melanoma
- 50% or more of tumor involving the ciliary body
- Gross extrascleral extension
- Use of immunosuppressive therapy
- Any other primary or metastatic malignancy except nonmelanotic skin cancer and carcinoma in situ of uterine cervix

Small Choroidal Melanoma Observational Study

A total of 204 patients with a small melanoma (ie, 93% of those eligible) were enrolled in an observational study aimed at determining the proportion of small melanomas that grew and their impact on survival.[6]

Growth of Small Choroidal Melanoma

This prospective study identified clinical features associated with time to tumor growth, using a standard set of fundus photographs. Growth was defined as increase from small to either medium or large. Initial observation was chosen for 188 tumors. The Kaplan–Meier estimates of the probability of growth were 11%, 21%, and 31% at 1, 2, and 5 years of enrollment, respectively (Figure 45-3). Interestingly, 63% of small tumors classified as melanoma did not grow during 5 years.

By multivariate analysis, small melanomas with prominent orange pigment were 6.4 times more likely to grow than tumors lacking this feature, and tumor thickness of at least 2 mm and largest basal diameter of 12 mm or more were respectively 4.4

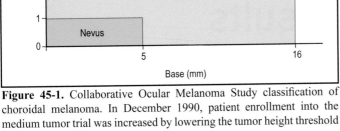

Figure 45-1. Collaborative Ocular Melanoma Study classification of choroidal melanoma. In December 1990, patient enrollment into the medium tumor trial was increased by lowering the tumor height threshold from 3 mm to 2.5 mm.

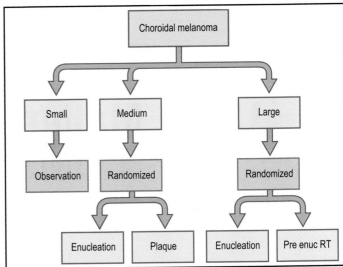

Figure 45-2. Component trials of Collaborative Ocular Melanoma Study.

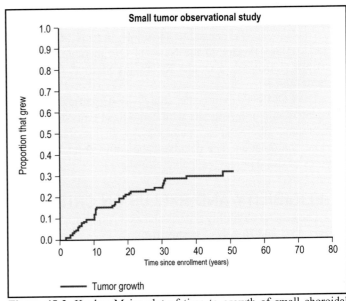

Figure 45-3. Kaplan–Meier plot of time to growth of small choroidal melanoma. (From COMS Group. Factors predictive of growth and treatment of small choroidal melanoma: COMS report no. 5. *Arch Ophthalmol.* 1997;115:1537-1544. Copyright © 1997 American Medical Association. All rights reserved.)

and 5.2 times more likely to grow than smaller tumors. Additionally, the absence of drusen on the tumor surface and the absence of retinal pigment epithelial (RPE) changes adjacent to the tumor were associated with a higher likelihood of growth (Table 45-1).

Mortality With Small Choroidal Melanoma

The Kaplan–Meier estimate of all-cause mortality was 6% (95% CI 3–9) and of melanoma-related mortality was 1% (95% CI 0–3) at 5 years (Figure 45-4).[6] This study indicated a low risk of death from a small melanoma within 5 years, even though the majority of these patients were not treated.

Medium Choroidal Melanoma: Randomized Trial of Enucleation Versus Brachytherapy

Patients with medium-sized choroidal melanomas were randomized to receive enucleation or iodine-125 brachytherapy.[4] The rationale was a concern that any treatment other than enucleation might increase mortality. Of the 5046 patients with medium choroidal melanoma, 2882 were eligible, and 1317 (46% of eligible patients) were enrolled.

Visual Outcome Following Brachytherapy

Visual loss due to radiation-induced complications following brachytherapy was associated with greater tumor thickness, proximity to the foveal avascular zone, a history of diabetes, and the presence of exudative retinal detachment. Three years after brachytherapy, the median visual acuity was 20/125, and 31% and 41% of eyes had 20/40 or better and 20/200 or worse vision, respectively.[10] When counseling the patient, it is useful to know that about 43% (95% CI 38–48) will have a final visual acuity of <20/200 at 3 years, and the majority will depend on their fellow eye for visual function, which is expected to remain good.[11]

Mortality With Medium Choroidal Melanoma

The Kaplan–Meier estimates of 5-year all-cause mortality were comparable for both treatment arms: 19% for enucleation and 18% for brachytherapy (P=0.48; Figure 45-5). The Kaplan–Meier estimate of 5-year melanoma-related mortality based on histopathologically confirmed metastasis was also comparable for both treatment arms: 11% for enucleation and 9% for brachytherapy (P=0.56).

Large Choroidal Melanoma: Randomized Trial of Enucleation Alone Versus Pre-Enucleation Irradiation

Patients with a large choroidal melanoma were randomly assigned to enucleation with and without prior radiation (20 Gy was delivered in five daily fractions).[5,12]

Local Complications of Enucleation

In all patients undergoing enucleation, pain (2%) and hemorrhage (1%) were the main complications.

Minor complications such as eyelid swelling were slightly more common among those treated with pre-enucleation radiation, but the risk of wound dehiscence and infection was equal between the treatment arms. Long-term complications, in both groups, were mainly cosmetic and related to motility of the prosthesis, alignment of the prosthesis, and ptosis.

Table 45-1. Features Associated With Growth of Small Choroidal Melanoma

Feature	Dimensions	Risk Ratio	95% Confidence Interval
Height (mm)	1.0-1.9	1.0	Reference category
	2.0-2.4	4.41	(0.56-34.9)
	2.5-3.0	17.74	(2.36-133)
Basal diameter (mm)	4.0-8.0	1	Reference category
	8.1-12.0	0.77	(0.29-2.03)
	12.1-16.0	5.16	(1.86-14.3)
Drusen	Absent	1.0	Reference category
	Present	0.24	(0.10-0.59)
Area of RPE changes	Absent	1.0	Reference category
	Present	0.23	(0.09-0.57)
Orange pigment	Absent	1.0	Reference category
	Minimal	1.56	(0.70-3.45)
	Prominent	6.38	(2.80-14.5)

(From Group COMS. Factors predictive of growth and treatment of small choroidal melanoma. COMS report No. 5. *Arch Ophthalmol.* 1997;115:1537-1544. Copyright © 1997 American Medical Association. All rights reserved.)

Mortality With Large Choroidal Melanoma

The Kaplan–Meier estimates of 5-year all-cause mortality were comparable for both treatment arms: 57% for enucleation alone and 62% for pre-enucleation radiation (P=0.32; Figure 45-6). The 10-year death rates from histopathologically confirmed metastases were 45% for the pre-enucleation radiation group and 40% for enucleation alone (risk ratio 1.02 [95% CI 0.93–1.42]).[13]

Natural History Observational Study: Medium and Large Choroidal Melanoma

Of the 77 patients with medium and large choroidal melanoma who refused treatment, 45 (42 medium and three large tumors) were enrolled to the natural history study. The unadjusted risk of death in patients who deferred treatment was about twice the risk of patients who were treated promptly (RR 1.8), but after adjusting for differences in age at enrollment and LBD, which differed significantly between the observational study and the randomized trial, the hazard ratio was smaller (RR 1.5; 95% CI 0.9–2.6).

Given the small number of patients, the study did not rule out that prompt treatment of medium-sized melanoma, by either enucleation or brachytherapy, prolongs survival.

Adjunct Studies

The quality of life cross-sectional study of medium choroidal melanoma was designed to measure the impact of disease and its treatment on quality of life.[14] Appearance scores were significantly associated with appearance-altering complications, recurrence scores with secondary enucleation following brachytherapy, and stereopsis–binocularity scores were higher in patients with good visual acuity in both eyes. Quality-of-life comparisons between treatment arms are pending.

Local Treatment Failure and Secondary Enucleation

The Kaplan–Meier estimate of the probability of treatment failure was 10% at 5 years. Risk factors for treatment failure were older age, greater tumor thickness, and proximity of the tumor to the foveal avascular zone. Most of these cases were managed by enucleation. Ocular pain from radiation-related complications was the second leading cause of enucleation.

Histopathologic Features of Choroidal Melanoma

Of the 1527 eyes enucleated in the medium-sized and large tumor trials, the participating investigators were more than 99% accurate in clinically diagnosing melanoma.[8] Mixed cell type choroidal melanoma (<50% of cells epithelioid in type) was the most commonly observed type both among medium (85%) and large (82%) melanomas.

Screening for Metastasis

Patients enrolled in the medium and large choroidal melanoma trials were screened annually for metastasis using liver function tests ([LFTs] alkaline phosphatase, AST, ALT, or bilirubin). In addition, chest radiographs were routinely taken. Abnormal findings prompted a diagnostic or imaging test to confirm or rule out cancer recurrence.[15] The sensitivity, specificity, positive predictive value, and negative predictive values associated with abnormal LFTs before the diagnosis of metastasis were 15%, 92%, 46%, and 71%, respectively. Because the LFTs had low sensitivity, liver imaging is recommended to identify earlier metastatic disease.[16] The benefit of annual chest X-ray as a screening method for metastasis is questionable.

REFERENCES

1. Schachat AP. Management of uveal melanoma: a continuing dilemma. Collaborative Ocular Melanoma Study Group. *Cancer.* 1994;74:3073-3075.

2. Group COMS. *COMS Manual of Procedures: accession no. PBS 179693.* Springfield, VA: National Technical Information Service; 1995.

3. Moy CS, Albert DM, Diener-West M, et al. Cause-specific mortality coding. Methods in the Collaborative Ocular Melanoma Study. COMS report no. 14. *Control Clin Trials.* 2001;22:248-262.

4. Diener-West M, Earle JD, Fine SL, et al. The COMS randomized trial of iodine 125 brachytherapy for choroidal melanoma, III: initial mortality findings. COMS report no. 18. *Arch Ophthalmol.* 2001;119:969-982.

5. Group COMS. The Collaborative Ocular Melanoma Study (COMS) randomized trial of pre-enucleation radiation of large choroidal melanoma II: initial mortality findings. COMS report no. 10. *Am J Ophthalmol,* 1998;125:779-796.

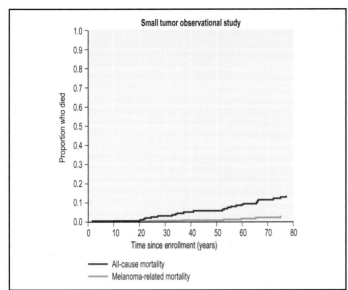

Figure 45-4. Kaplan–Meier plot of all-cause (red line) and melanoma-related (green line) mortality from small choroidal melanoma. (From COMS Group. Mortality in patients with small choroidal melanoma. COMS report no. 4. *Arch Ophthalmol.* 1997;115:886-893. Copyright © 1997 American Medical Association. All rights reserved.)

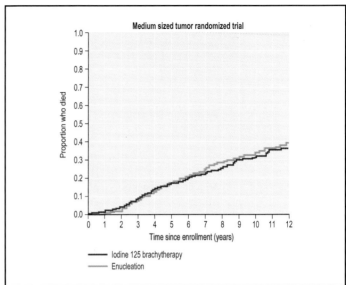

Figure 45-5. Kaplan–Meier plot of all-cause mortality after iodine-125 brachytherapy (red line) and enucleation (green line) for medium-sized choroidal melanoma. Note similar outcome in both study arms. (From Diener-West M, Earle JD, Fine SL, et al. The COMS randomized trial of iodine 125 brachytherapy for choroidal melanoma, III: initial mortality findings. COMS report no. 18. *Arch Ophthalmol.* 2001;119:969-982. Copyright © 2001 American Medical Association. All rights reserved.)

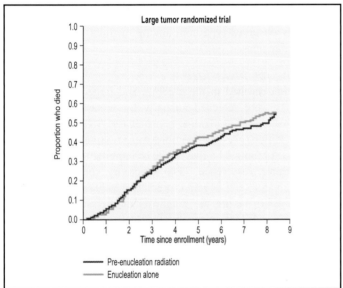

Figure 45-6. Kaplan–Meier plot of all-cause mortality after pre-enucleation radiation (red line) and enucleation alone (green line) for large choroidal melanoma. Note similar outcome in both study arms. (From *Am J Ophthalmol,* 125, OMS Group, The Collaborative Ocular Melanoma Study (COMS) randomized trial of pre-enucleation radiation of large choroidal melanoma II: initial mortality findings. COMS report no. 10, 779-796 © Elsevier 1998.)

6.   Group COMS. Mortality in patients with small choroidal melanoma. COMS report no. 4. The Collaborative Ocular Melanoma Study Group. *Arch Ophthalmol,* 1997;115:886-893.

7.   Straatsma BR, Diener-West M, Caldwell R, Engstrom RE. Mortality after deferral of treatment or no treatment for choroidal melanoma. *Am J Ophthalmol.* 2003;136:47-54.

8.   Group COMS. Histopathologic characteristics of uveal melanomas in eyes enucleated from the Collaborative Ocular Melanoma Study. COMS report no. 6. *Am J Ophthalmol.* 1998;125:745-766.

9.   Group COMS. Trends in size and treatment of recently diagnosed choroidal melanoma, 1987-1997: findings from patients examined at collaborative ocular melanoma study (COMS) centers: COMS report no. 20. *Arch Ophthalmol.* 2003;121:1156-1162.

10. Melia BM, Abramson DH, Albert DM, et al. Collaborative ocular melanoma study (COMS) randomized trial of I-125 brachytherapy for medium choroidal melanoma. I. Visual acuity after 3 years. COMS report no. 16. *Ophthalmology.* 2001;108:348-366.

11. Group COMS. Ten-year follow-up of fellow eyes of patients enrolled in Collaborative Ocular Melanoma Study randomized trials: COMS report no. 22. *Ophthalmology.* 2004;111:966-976.

12. Group COMS. The Collaborative Ocular Melanoma Study (COMS) randomized trial of pre-enucleation radiation of large choroidal melanoma III: local complications and observations following enucleation COMS report no. 11. *Am J Ophthalmol.* 1998;126:362-372.

13. Group COMS. The Collaborative Ocular Melanoma Study (COMS) randomized trial of pre-enucleation radiation of large choroidal melanoma: IV. Ten-year mortality findings and prognostic factors. COMS report number 24. *Am J Ophthalmol.* 2004;138:936-951.

14. Group COMS. Quality of life assessment in the collaborative ocular melanoma study: design and methods. COMS-QOLS Report No. 1. COMS Quality of Life Study Group. *Ophthalm Epidemiol.* 1999;6:5-17.

15. Diener-West M, Reynolds SM, Agugliaro DJ, et al. Screening for metastasis from choroidal melanoma: the Collaborative Ocular Melanoma Study Group Report 23. *J Clin Oncol.* 2004;22:2438-2444.

16. Eskelin S, Pyrhonen S, Summanen P, et al. Screening for metastatic malignant melanoma of the uvea revisited. *Cancer.* 1999;85:1151-1159.

Chapter

46

Uveal Malignant Melanoma: Prognostic Factors

Robert Folberg and Jacob Pe'er

TUMOR CHARACTERISTICS DETECTABLE BY CONVENTIONAL CLINICAL EXAMINATION

The most consistent clinical (and pathological) feature that correlates with mortality is the largest basal tumor diameter (Box 46-1).[1] This can be estimated by indirect ophthalmoscopy and by echography. The recent development of wide-angle digital cameras has also made it possible to measure tumor diameter photographically, with great accuracy (Figure 46-1).

Other clinical features of prognostic significance are advanced age of the patient at the time of treatment, extrascleral tumor extension, male gender, and rare growth patterns such as diffuse type of melanoma and ring melanomas.[2] Anterior extension beyond the equator, and especially ciliary body involvement, have been shown to indicate a poor prognosis for survival.[3]

PATHOLOGICAL FEATURES DERIVED FROM THE EXAMINATION OF RESECTED TUMORS

Histologic prognostic factors are described in Box 46-2 and Figure 46-2. Most iris melanocytic lesions follow a benign course unless they involve the ciliary body.

Assignment of cell type to the tumor by the Callender classification[4] or its modification[5] has been shown to be independently associated with outcome. The classification is based on assessments of cell shape and nuclear characteristics. Elongated cells with a longitudinally folded nucleus and without conspicuous nucleoli are designated spindle A cells. Spindle B cells have a more "open" nucleus and more prominent nucleoli. Round cells with abundant cytoplasm and prominent nucleoli are designated epithelioid. Tumors composed exclusively of spindle A cells may be classified as nevi. Tumors containing only spindle A and B cells are now classified as "spindle cell melanomas." Melanomas composed of a mixture of spindle and epithelioid cells are classified as being of the "mixed cell type." Tumors composed largely of epithelioid cells are classified as "epithelioid" melanomas. There is no consensus among pathologists as to the number of epithelioid cells required to change a tumor from mixed to epithelioid. Many pathologists have therefore adapted a two-tiered classification system by simply reporting whether epithelioid cells are present or absent.[6]

Box 46-1. Clinical Prognostic Factors

- Largest basal tumor diameter
- Tumor thickness/height
- Anterior tumor location/ciliary body involvement
- Extrascleral extension
- Diffuse melanoma
- Older age
- Male gender
- Faster-growing tumor
- Initial tumor regression rate after radiotherapy

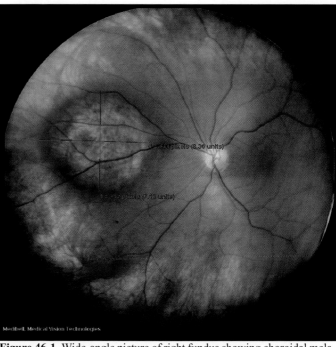

Medibell, Medical Vision Technologies

Figure 46-1. Wide-angle picture of right fundus showing choroidal melanoma nasal to the disc, permitting accurate measurements of the basal tumor diameter.

Nucleolar diameter also is of prognostic significance.[7] Other factors include looping patterns that are positive on periodic acid–

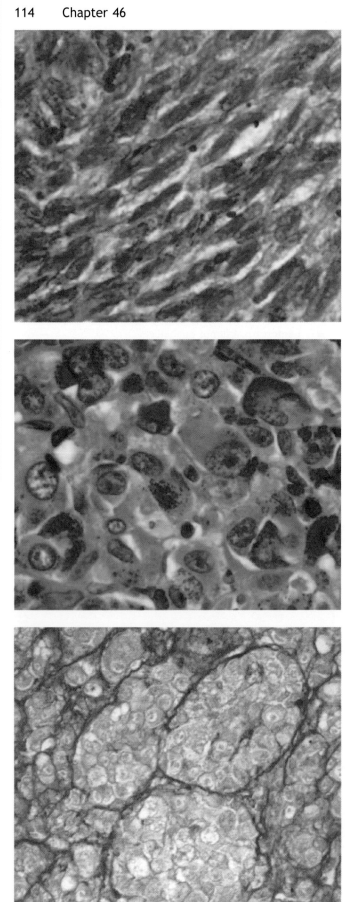

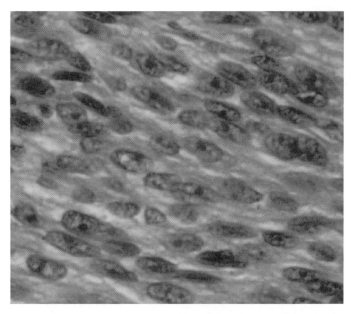

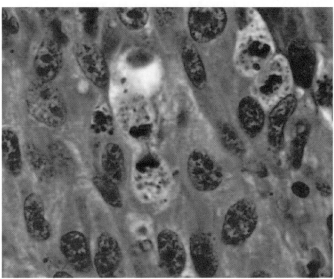

Figure 46-2. Histological prognostic markers in uveal melanoma. Upper left: Spindle A melanoma cells. Note the absence of prominent nucleoli and the longitudinal fold in the nucleus. Upper right: Spindle B melanoma cells. The nucleoli are more "open" than in spindle A cells, and prominent nucleoli are identified. Middle left: Epithelioid cells. The cytoplasm is abundant, and the nucleus is round and "open," with large nucleoli. Middle right: Mitotic figures in choroidal melanoma. Bottom: Vasculogenic mimicry patterns in uveal melanoma. This tissue was stained with the periodic acid–Schiff (PAS) reagent without hematoxylin counterstaining.

Box 46-2. Histological Prognostic Factors

- Location (iris, ciliary body, choroid)
- Extraocular extension (yes, no)
- Growth pattern (focal, diffuse, ring)
- Dimension of largest diameter in contact with the sclera (mm)
- Cell type (Callender classification: spindle, mixed, epithelioid, necrotic)
- Number of mitotic figures per 40 high-power fields or proliferation index
- Presence of >100 tumor infiltrating lymphocytes per 20 high-power fields
- Vasculogenic mimicry patterns (networks or loops, present or absent)

(Adapted from Folberg R, Salomão D, Grossniklaus HE, et al. Recommendations for reporting of tissues removed as part of the surgical treatment of common malignancies of the eye and adnexa. *Am J Surg Pathol.* 2003;27:999-1004.)

Schiff (PAS) staining.[6] A high number of mitotic figures[8] and a high proliferation index has been associated with an adverse outcome in uveal melanoma.[9] Microvascular density (MVD) is measured by counting discrete points of staining using endothelial cell markers. Several studies indicate that MVD is associated with adverse outcome.[10]

ANALYSIS OF CELLS EXTRACTED BY FINE NEEDLE ASPIRATION BIOPSY

There is now considerable interest in determining the karyotype of uveal melanomas. Non-random chromosomal abnormalities such as monosomy 3 and extra copies of chromosome 8 are associated with an adverse outcome.[11] It has recently been demonstrated that it is possible to identify monosomy 3 from FNAB specimens.[11]

PROGNOSTIC FACTORS BY NON-INVASIVE TESTING

Serum melanoma inhibitory activity has been associated with the development of metastatic melanoma in one series,[12] but this result was not duplicated by others. Recently, raised serum osteopontin has been shown to correlate with hepatic metastases with high levels of sensitivity and specificity.[13]

REFERENCES

1. Shammas HF, Blodi FC. Prognostic factors in choroidal and ciliary body melanomas. *Arch Ophthalmol.* 1977;95:63-69.
2. Kaiserman I, Anteby I, Chowers I, et al. Post-brachytherapy initial tumour regression rate correlates with metastatic spread in posterior uveal melanoma. *Br J Ophthalmol.* 2004;88:892-895.
3. Augsburger JJ, Gamel JW. Clinical prognostic factors in patients with posterior uveal malignant melanoma. *Cancer.* 1990;66:1596-1600.
4. Callender GR. Malignant melanotic tumors of the eye: a study of histologic types in 111 cases. *Trans Am Acad Ophthalmol Otolaryngol.* 1931;36:131-142.
5. McLean IW, Zimmerman LE, Evans RM. Reappraisal of Callender's spindle A type of malignant melanoma of choroid and ciliary body. *Am J Ophthalmol.* 1978;86:557-564.
6. Folberg R, Rummelt V, Parys-Van Ginderdeuren R, et al. The prognostic value of tumor blood vessel morphology in primary uveal melanoma. *Ophthalmology.* 1993;100:1389-1398.
7. McLean IW, Sibug ME, Becker RL, et al. Uveal melanoma: the importance of large nucleoli in predicting patient outcome—an automated image analysis study. *Cancer.* 1997;79:982-988.
8. McLean IW, Foster WD, Zimmerman LE. Prognostic factors in small malignant melanomas of choroid and ciliary body. *Arch Ophthalmol.* 1977;95:48-58.
9. Pe'er J, Gnessin H, Shargal Y, et al. PC-10 immunostaining of proliferating cell nuclear antigen (PCNA) in posterior uveal melanoma. Enucleation versus enucleation postirradiation groups. *Ophthalmology.* 1994;101:56-62.
10. Foss AJ, Alexander RA, Jefferies LW, et al. Microvessel count predicts survival in uveal melanoma. *Cancer Res.* 1996;56:2900-2903.
11. Sisley K, Nichols C, Parsons MA, et al. Clinical applications of chromosome analysis, from fine needle aspiration biopsies, of posterior uveal melanomas. *Eye.* 1998;12:203-207.
12. Schaller UC, Bosserhoff AK, Neubauer AS, et al. Melanoma inhibitory activity: a novel serum marker for uveal melanoma. *Melanoma Res.* 2002;12:593-599.
13. Kadkol SS, Lin AY, Barak V, et al. Osteopontin expression and serum levels in metastatic uveal melanoma—a pilot study. *Invest Ophthalmol Vis Sci.* 2006;47:802-806.

Uveal Malignant Melanoma: Mortality

Bertil E. Damato and Azzam Taktak

INTRODUCTION

Many patients with uveal melanoma die as a result of systemic spread, despite successful treatment of the primary tumor. This raises important and unsettling questions about how and in whom ocular treatment influences survival.

UVEAL MELANOMA MORTALITY

Survival Probability According to Tumor Size

The cumulative melanoma-related mortality rates 25 years after treatment of the primary tumor are approximately 18%, 52%, and 59% for small, medium, and large tumors, respectively (Figure 47-1).[1]

Competing Risks

In the Finnish study, the rates of melanoma-related mortality were lower than generally reported because the authors performed cumulative incidence analysis, which takes account of competing risk events (ie, deaths unrelated to uveal melanoma).[1]

Lead-Time Bias

The increased mortality observed after treatment of large tumors may simply reflect the fact that these tumors and any metastases have been present for a relatively long time.

Loss to Follow-Up

This can cause bias in different ways. Melanoma-related mortality rates would be exaggerated if patients lost to follow-up subsequently contacted the oncology center for advice when they developed metastatic disease. Conversely, melanoma-related mortality might be underestimated if patients lost to follow-up stopped attending the center because of ill health, and if such disease was usually caused by metastasis.

Erroneous Death Certification

In a study by Kujala and associates,[1] about 10% of all autopsies discovered metastatic melanoma in patients who were thought to have died of unrelated disease.[1]

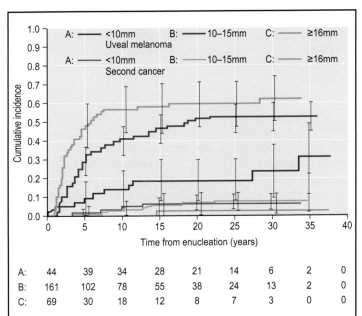

Figure 47-1. Cumulative incidence of death from uveal melanoma (thick lines) and from second malignancy (thin lines) according to largest basal tumor diameter at the time of treatment. (Reproduced with permission from Kujala E, Mäkitie T, Kivelä T. Very long-term prognosis of patients with malignant uveal melanoma. *Invest Ophthalmol Vis Sci.* 2003;44:4651-4659.)

ONSET OF METASTASIS

Late-Onset Hypothesis

The strong correlation between large tumor size at treatment and high mortality is the logical basis for the hypothesis that most metastatic spread commences after tumors grow large (Figure 47-2).

Early-Onset Hypothesis

A rival hypothesis is that metastatic spread occurs before tumor growth, years before treatment (Figure 47-3).[2-4] This model would suggest that large tumor size at the time of treatment merely reflects faster tumor growth and increased malignancy. There is growing evidence that uveal melanomas differentiate into low- and high-grade varieties at an early stage.[5] It is therefore

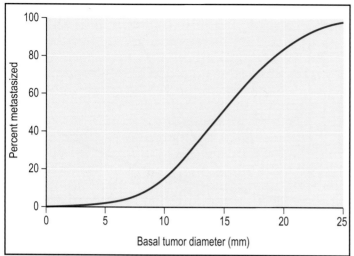

Figure 47-2. Schematic graph showing how the percentage of tumors that have metastasized before treatment might increase with basal tumor diameter. This model implies that all uveal melanomas tend to become more malignant and to metastasize, given time.

possible that low-grade tumors remain small or grow large over many years, rarely or never metastasizing; high-grade tumors metastasize early and then rapidly grow large (Figure 47-4).

IMPACT OF THERAPY ON MORTALITY

The impact of ocular treatment on mortality from uveal melanoma is still speculative because there have been no randomized, prospective studies comparing treatment with no treatment.

Enucleation

In 1978, Zimmerman and colleagues[6] hypothesized that two thirds of all fatalities occurring after enucleation could be attributed to the dissemination of tumor emboli at the time of surgery. This impression was based on the correct observation that the mortality rate rises abruptly following enucleation, reaching a peak of about 8% during the second postoperative year (Figure 47-5). The "Zimmerman hypothesis," as it came to be known, was challenged by Manschot[2] and others.[7]

Local Resection

Predictive factors for survival are similar to those of enucleation (ie, large basal tumor diameter and tumor cell type).[8] There is no evidence that survival is worse after local resection than after enucleation. According to the "early-metastasis hypothesis," this is because metastatic spread has already occurred by the time the patient first presents.

Transpupillary Thermotherapy

Transpupillary thermotherapy (TTT) is associated with a significant rate of local tumour recurrence. However, it is in this group of patients that recurrence is most life threatening.

Radiotherapy

The Collaborative Ocular Melanoma Study (COMS) did not show that survival was worse after plaque radiotherapy than after enucleation (Chapter 45); however, the results are essentially inconclusive because of insufficient patient numbers and follow-up.

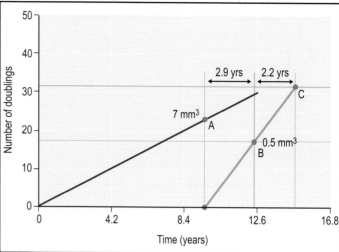

Figure 47-3. Estimated growth of primary tumor (red line) and metastasis (green line). Points A, B, and C represent the times of initial metastasis, ocular treatment, and detectable metastatic disease, respectively. Tumor doubling times suggest that the onset of metastatic spread is around 5 years before clinic metastases appear and 3.9 years before primary ocular treatment, when the uveal melanoma still has a volume of only 7 mm[3]. (This figure was published in *Ophthalmology*, 108, Eskelin S, Kivelä T, Reply: tumor doubling times in metastatic malignant melanoma of the uvea: tumor progression before and after treatment, 830-831, © Elsevier 2001.)

Systemic Therapy

Advances in the ocular treatment of uveal melanoma have not improved survival.[9] This realization is stimulating interest in systemic adjuvant therapy for the treatment of micrometastases.

IRIS MELANOMA

The actuarial rate of metastasis is 5% at 10 years.[10] Risk factors for increased mortality were identified as age at primary treatment, angle involvement, secondary glaucoma, extraocular extension, and prior surgical treatment before referral. The method of treatment (ie, radiotherapy, enucleation, or local resection) was considered not to influence survival.

CONCLUSION

It is with small tumors that treatment deferral, pre-enucleation radiotherapy, and local tumor recurrence are most likely to influence survival. Studies undertaken with medium-sized and large tumors are probably of no relevance to small melanomas. Randomized studies of treatment versus no treatment of small uveal melanomas would seem to be indicated, but are prevented by logistical difficulties. From this review, it is obvious that studies on uveal melanoma are fraught with difficulties. Weighing risks against benefits in the face of uncertainty, while considering the patient's own utilities or priorities, is a challenge. With recent advances in statistics and molecular biology, one can expect new insights into the pathogenesis of metastatic disease from uveal melanoma and the impact of any treatment on survival.

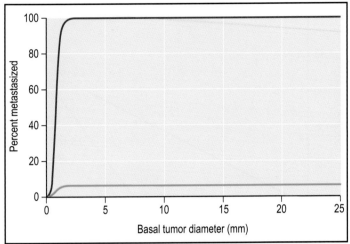

Figure 47-4. Schematic graph showing how high-grade uveal melanomas all metastasize early (red line) and how few, if any, low-grade tumors do (green line). According to this model, size essentially indicates only the duration of ocular tumor and any metastases. If the tumor has metastasized, size is inversely proportional to the time to metastatic death.

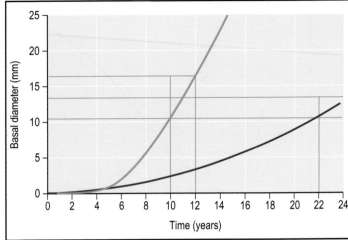

Figure 47-5. Peak in mortality after treatment of uveal melanoma. (Reproduced with permission from Zimmerman LE, McLean IW, Foster WD. Does enucleation of the eye containing a malignant melanoma prevent or accelerate the dissemination of tumour cells? *Br J Ophthalmol.* 1978;62:420-425.)

REFERENCES

1. Kujala E, Makitie T, Kivela T. Very long-term prognosis of patients with malignant uveal melanoma. *Invest Ophthalmol Vis Sci.* 2003;44:4651-4659.
2. Manschot WA, Lee WR, van Strik R. Uveal melanoma: updated considerations on current management modalities. *Int Ophthalmol.* 1995;19:203-209.
3. Eskelin S, Pyrhonen S, Summanen P, et al. Tumor doubling times in metastatic malignant melanoma of the uvea: tumor progression before and after treatment. *Ophthalmology.* 2000;107:1443-1449.
4. Singh AD. Uveal melanoma: implications of tumor doubling time. *Ophthalmology.* 2001;108:829-831.
5. Tschentscher F, Husing J, Holter T, et al. Tumor classification based on gene expression profiling shows that uveal melanomas with and without monosomy 3 represent two distinct entities. *Cancer Res.* 2003;63:2578-2584.
6. Zimmerman LE, McLean IW, Foster WD. Does enucleation of the eye containing a malignant melanoma prevent or accelerate the dissemination of tumour cells? *Br J Ophthalmol.* 1978;62:420-425.
7. Singh AD, Rennie IG, Kivela T, et al. The Zimmerman-McLean-Foster hypothesis: 25 years later. *Br J Ophthalmol.* 2004;88:962-967.
8. Damato BE, Paul J, Foulds WS. Risk factors for metastatic uveal melanoma after trans-scleral local resection. *Br J Ophthalmol.* 1996;80:109-116.
9. Singh AD, Borden EC. Metastatic uveal melanoma. *Ophthalmol Clin North Am.* 2005;18:143-150, ix.
10. Shields CL, Shields JA, Materin M, et al. Iris melanoma: risk factors for metastasis in 169 consecutive patients. *Ophthalmology.* 2001;108:172-178.

Uveal Malignant Melanoma: Metastasis

Arun D. Singh, Julie Bray, and Ernest C. Borden

INTRODUCTION

In general, the survival of patients with metastatic uveal melanoma is poor, with a median survival of less than 6 months.[1] Despite recent advances in management, the relative survival rate of uveal melanoma appears to have remained unchanged over the past 25 years.[2]

CLINICAL FEATURES

Frequency of Metastasis

Clinically evident metastatic disease at the time of initial presentation is detected in less than 1% of all patients.[1] Nevertheless, long-term follow-up of treated patients reveals metastases in 31% of cases in 5 years, 45% in 15 years, and almost 50% in 25 years (Figure 48-1).[3] These findings suggest that subclinical metastasis is present in such cases at the time of primary treatment. The correlation of primary and metastatic uveal melanoma growth data suggests that metastasis commences when the primary tumor is still small.[4] At the time of diagnosis of the primary uveal melanoma, any metastases are too small to be clinically detected by currently available techniques.[4,5]

Sites of Metastasis

The liver is the predominant organ, being involved in 70% to 90% of cases with metastatic uveal melanoma.[6] Liver involvement also tends to be the first manifestation of metastatic disease.[7] Lymph nodes and brain are uncommonly involved (Box 48-1).[6]

Determinants of Metastasis

Several clinical, histopathological, cytogenetic, and molecular genetic factors influence the frequency of metastasis (Chapter 46).

Signs and Symptoms

Patients with metastases can present with a variety of symptoms based on organ involvement. About 60% are asymptomatic at the time of detection of their metastases.[8] Hepatomegaly, abnormal liver function tests, and abnormal appearance of the liver on imaging studies are highly suspicious of metastasis. However, liver function tests can be normal in about one third of cases in the presence of liver metastases.[8] Needle biopsy is usually performed to confirm the diagnosis (Figure 48-2).

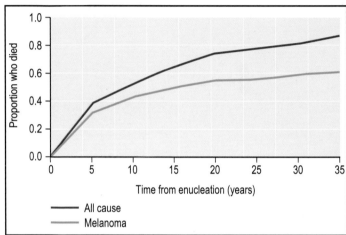

Figure 48-1. Kaplan–Meier estimate of all-cause and melanoma-specific mortality. (Data with permission from Kujala E, Mäkitie T, Kivelä T. Very long-term prognosis of patients with malignant uveal melanoma. *Invest Ophthalmol Vis Sci.* 2003;44:4651-4659.)

Box 48-1. Sites for Metastatic Uveal Melanoma

- Liver 93%
- Lungs 24%
- Bone 16%
- Skin 11%
- Lymph nodes 10%
- Brain 5%
- Fellow eye 0%

Multiple sites involved in about half the cases. In an atypical case, consider a second primary tumor.

TREATMENT OPTIONS

Several treatments have been tried for patients with metastatic uveal melanoma, and these include chemotherapy, intra-arterial hepatic chemotherapy, chemoembolization, immunotherapy, surgery, and a combined approach (Box 48-2). Most published results are based on non-randomized, non-comparative case series of a small number of patients or phase I trials.[9]

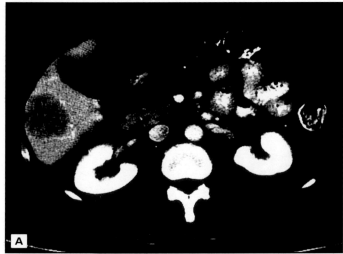

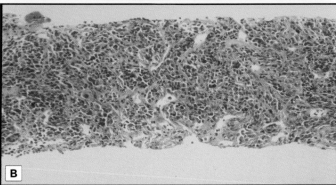

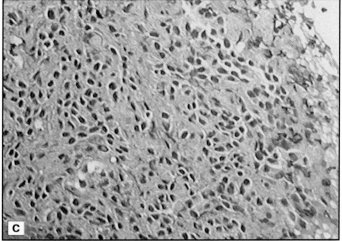

Figure 48-2. Computerized tomograph of the liver shows a focal area of metastasis in the right lobe of the liver (A). Fine needle aspiration biopsy of the liver (B). Metastatic uveal melanoma (C). (Hematoxylin and eosin ×400.)

Box 48-2. Metastatic Uveal Melanoma

- Median survival is less than 6 months
- Dacarbazine-based chemotherapy is ineffective
- Total resection of the solitary metastasis offers a survival advantage
- Total resection of the hepatic metastasis followed by intra-arterial hepatic chemotherapy (where feasible) may prolong the median survival (22 months)
- Screening protocols, although generally recommended, are of questionable benefit
- Gene profiling and proteomics may offer new therapeutic targets

PROGNOSIS

Survival with metastatic uveal melanoma is poor, with a median of less than 6 months.[1] Dacarbazine-based chemotherapy used for the treatment of metastatic cutaneous melanoma is ineffective in the treatment of metastatic uveal melanoma.[9] Total resection of the solitary metastasis in the liver or at other sites offers a distinct survival advantage.[9] However, the longest median survival is observed when it is possible to perform complete surgical excision of the hepatic metastasis, followed by intra-arterial hepatic fotemustine and/or dacarbazine + cisplatin.[10]

REFERENCES

1. Diener-West M, Reynolds SM, Agugliaro DJ, et al. Screening for metastasis from choroidal melanoma: the Collaborative Ocular Melanoma Study Group report no. 23. *J Clin Oncol.* 2004;22:2438-2444.
2. Singh AD, Topham A. Survival rate with uveal melanoma in the United States: 1973-1997. *Ophthalmology.* 2003;110:962-965.
3. Kujala E, Makitie T, Kivelä T. Very long-term prognosis of patients with malignant uveal melanoma. *Invest Ophthalmol Vis Sci.* 2003;44:4651-4659.
4. Singh AD. Uveal melanoma: implications of tumor doubling time. *Ophthalmology.* 2001;108:829-830.
5. Eskelin S, Kivelä T. Reply: Tumor doubling times in metastatic malignant melanoma of the uvea: tumor progression before and after treatment. *Ophthalmology.* 2001;108:830-831.
7. Rajpal S, Moore R, Karakousis CP. Survival in metastatic ocular melanoma. *Cancer.* 1983;52:334-336.
6. Group TCOMS. Assessment of metastatic disease status at death in 435 patients with large choroidal melanoma in the Collaborative Ocular Melanoma Study (COMS): COMS report no. 15. *Arch Ophthalmol.* 2001;119:670-676.
8. Eskelin S, Kivelä T. Imaging to detect metastases from malignant uveal melanoma. *Arch Ophthalmol.* 2002;120:676.
9. Singh AD, Borden EC. Metastatic uveal melanoma. *Ophthalmol Clin North Am.* 2005;18:143-150, ix.
10. Salmon RJ, Levy C, Plancher C, et al. Treatment of liver metastases from uveal melanoma by combined surgery—chemotherapy. *Eur J Surg Oncol.* 1998;24:127-130.

Uveal Vascular Tumors

Arun D. Singh and Peter K. Kaiser

INTRODUCTION

Uveal vascular tumors represent benign, hamartomatous disorders and are classified as hemangiomas. Although the iris and ciliary body can be involved, hemangiomas most frequently affect the choroid. Choroidal hemangioma can either be circumscribed or diffuse.[1] In general, uveal hemangioma may be confined to the globe or may be a manifestation of a widespread hemangiomatous disorder.

IRIS HEMANGIOMA

Iris hemangioma is a rare benign vascular tumor of the iris stroma. Some have even questioned its existence.[2,3] However, there are few well-documented cases with histopathologic and immunohistochemical findings that are confirmatory of the diagnosis (Figure 49-1).[4]

CILIARY BODY HEMANGIOMA

Only a few cases of well-documented ciliary body hemangioma have been published.[2,5] These tumors are mistaken for ciliary body melanomas, and a definitive diagnosis is made on histopathologic evaluation following iridocyclectomy.[5]

CIRCUMSCRIBED CHOROIDAL HEMANGIOMA

A circumscribed choroidal hemangioma is usually diagnosed between the second and fourth decades of life when it causes visual disturbances owing to the development of an exudative retinal detachment.[6] Circumscribed tumors occur sporadically, without any associated local or systemic anomalies. In contrast, a diffuse choroidal hemangioma is usually evident at birth and generally occurs as a part of neuro-oculocutaneous hemangiomatosis (Sturge–Weber syndrome).

Clinical Features

Although they are usually asymptomatic, the common symptoms are visual disturbances, such as reduced vision, metamorphopsia, and photopsia. Ophthalmoscopically, a circumscribed choroidal hemangioma appears as an orange choroidal mass with margins that blend with the surrounding choroid (Figures 49-2 and 49-3). Circumscribed choroidal hemangiomas are usually

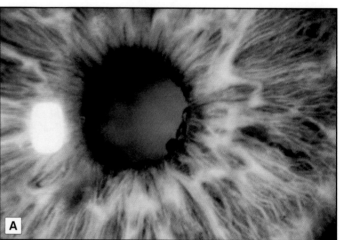

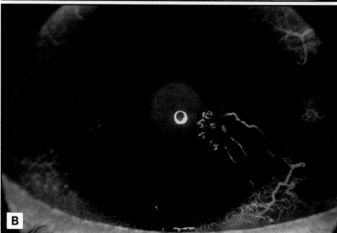

Figure 49-1. Abnormal collection of iris vessels at the pupillary margin with prominent feeder vessel (A). Iris angiography confirms the vascular nature of the tumor (B). (Reproduced with permission from Giessler S, Tost F, Duncker GI. Vascular convolute of the iris. Cavernous iris hemangioma. *Der Ophthalmologe.* 1999;96[11]:752-753. © Springer-Verlag 1999.)

located in the posterior pole and are no thicker than 6 mm.[1] Although they are vascular tumors, prominent intrinsic tumor vessels or feeder vessels are not seen ophthalmoscopically. Exudative retinal detachment is generally present in symptomatic cases.

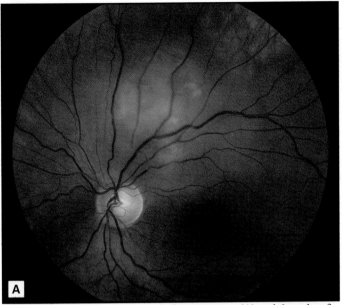
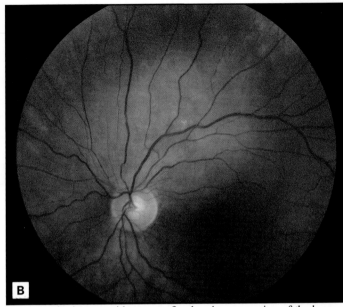

Figure 49-2. Fundus appearance before treatment (A) and 6 weeks after photodynamic therapy with verteporfin showing regression of the hemangioma (B).

Table 49-1. Differential Diagnosis of a Circumscribed Choroidal Hemangioma

Feature		Choroidal Melanoma	Choroidal Metastasis	Choroidal Granuloma	Posterior Scleritis	Choroidal Hemangioma
Pain		-	-	-	+	-
Color		Brown Yellow (amelanotic)	Yellow	Yellow	Orange	Orange
Location		Anywhere	Anywhere	Anywhere	Posterior pole	Posterior pole
Number		Single	Multiple	Single or multiple	Single	Single
Intrinsic vessels		Visible	-	-	-	-
Subretinal fluid		+	+	+	+	+
Hard exudates		-	-	-	-	-
Vitreous cells		-	-	+	+/-	-
Fluorescein angiography	Early	Hypo	Hypo	Hypo	Hypo	Hyper
	Late	Hyper	Hyper	Hyper	Hyper	Hyper
ICG fluorescence		Late hyper	Late hyper	Late hyper	Late hyper	Early hyper
Ultrasonographic internal reflectivity		Low	Medium	High	High, Tenons lucency	High

Hypo, hypofluorescent; Hyper, hyperfluorescent; -, absent; +, present.

Differential diagnosis can be easily misdiagnosed (Table 49-1).

Treatment

The aim of treatment is to induce tumor atrophy with resolution of subretinal fluid and foveal distortion without destroying overlying retina. Some asymptomatic cases can be observed. Laser photocoagulation,[6] cryotherapy, radiotherapy, transpupillary thermotherapy,[7] and more recently photodynamic therapy with verteporfin[8] have been reported to be efficacious (see Figure 49-2).

Prognosis

The long-term visual prognosis is poor even in adequately treated patients.[9] With the increasing use of photodynamic therapy, it may be possible to achieve better long-term visual results.[10]

DIFFUSE CHOROIDAL HEMANGIOMA

About half of patients with Sturge–Weber syndrome have a diffuse choroidal hemangioma (Chapter 63).[11] It is usually unilateral and ipsilateral to the nevus flammeus (Figure 49-4A, B).[12,13]

Treatment

In asymptomatic cases, especially in the absence of an exudative retinal detachment, observation is recommended. Tumor regression and resolution of subretinal fluid can be induced with low-dose lens-sparing radiation (20 Gy, 10 fractions) or proton beam irradiation.[14,15]

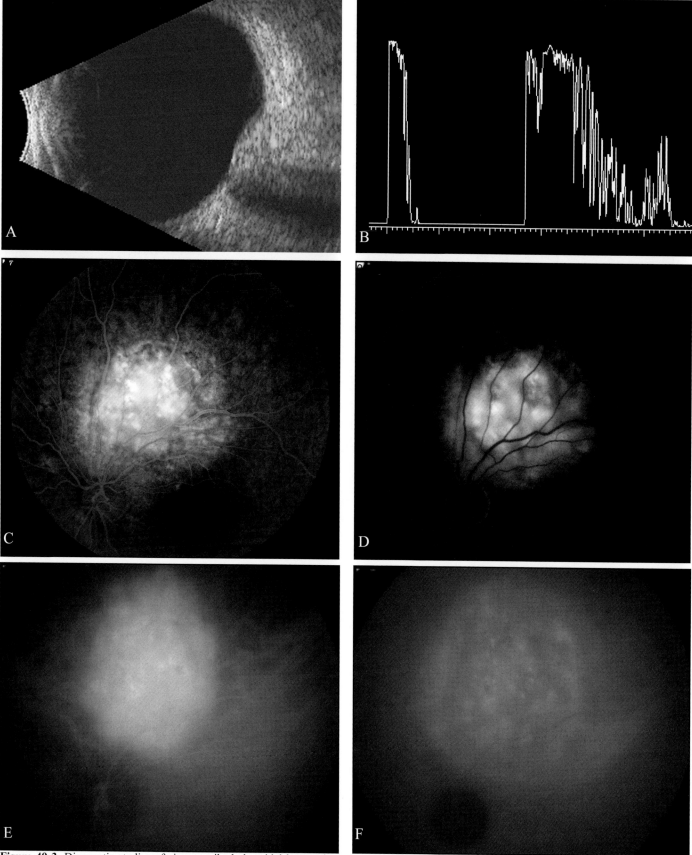

Figure 49-3. Diagnostic studies of circumscribed choroidal hemangioma. On B-scan ultrasonography there is a smooth, contoured, dome-shaped choroidal mass (A) that demonstrates high internal reflectivity on A-scan (B). Fluorescein angiography shows early hyperfluorescence (53 s) (C). The hyperfluorescence increases through most of the phases of the angiogram, with variable amounts of late leakage (10 min) (D). Indocyanine green angiogram showing early hyperfluorescence (within 30 seconds) (E). In the late phase, a "washout" effect with reduction of the initial hyperfluorescence due to egress of dye from the hemangioma is observed (20 minutes) (F).

SECTION 4 Uveal Tumors

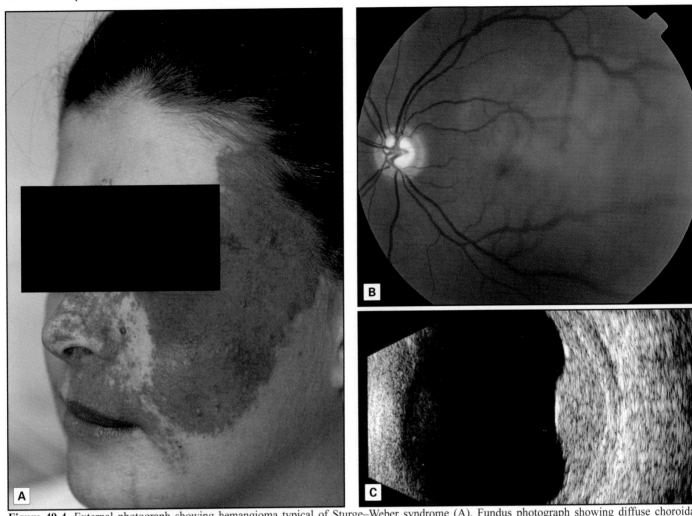

Figure 49-4. External photograph showing hemangioma typical of Sturge–Weber syndrome (A). Fundus photograph showing diffuse choroidal thickening with shallow subretinal fluid (B). Note glaucomatous cupping of the optic disc. B-scan ultrasonograph demonstrating a dome-shaped choroidal mass that blends with diffusely thickened choroid (C).

REFERENCES

1. Witschel H, Font RL. Hemangioma of the choroid. A clinicopathologic study of 71 cases and a review of the literature. *Surv Ophthalmol.* 1976;20:415-431.

2. Ferry AP. Hemangiomas of the iris and ciliary body. Do they exist? A search for a histologically proved case. *Int Ophthalmol Clin.* 1972;12:177-194.

3. Naidoff MA, Kenyon KR, Green WR. Iris hemangioma and abnormal retinal vasculature in a case of diffuse congenital hemangiomatosis. *Am J Ophthalmol.* 1971;72:633-644.

4. Woo SJ, Kim CJ, Yu YS. Cavernous hemangioma of the iris in an infant. *J Aapos.* 2004;8:499-501.

5. Isola VM. Hemangioma of the ciliary body: a case report and review of the literature. *Ophthalmologica.* 1996;210:239-243.

6. Anand R, Augsburger JJ, Shields JA. Circumscribed choroidal hemangiomas. *Arch Ophthalmol.* 1989;107:1338-1342.

7. Gunduz K. Transpupillary thermotherapy in the management of circumscribed choroidal hemangioma. *Surv Ophthalmol.* 2004;49:316-327.

8. Singh AD, Kaiser PK, Sears JE, et al. Photodynamic therapy of circumscribed choroidal haemangioma. *Br J Ophthalmol.* 2004;88:1414-1418.

9. Shields CL, Honavar SG, Shields JA, et al. Circumscribed choroidal hemangioma: clinical manifestations and factors predictive of visual outcome in 200 consecutive cases. *Ophthalmology.* 2001;108:2237-2248.

10. Michels S, Michels R, Beckendorf A, Schmidt-Erfurth U. Photodynamic therapy for choroidal hemangioma. Long-term results. *Ophthalmologe.* 2004;101:569-575.

11. Sullivan TJ, Clarke MP, Morin JD. The ocular manifestations of the Sturge-Weber syndrome. *J Pediatr Ophthalmol Strab.* 1992;29:349-356.

12. Amirikia A, Scott IU, Murray TG. Bilateral diffuse choroidal hemangiomas with unilateral facial nevus flammeus in Sturge-Weber syndrome. *Am J Ophthalmol.* 2000;130:362-364.

13. Scott IU, Alexandrakis G, Cordahi GJ, Murray TG. Diffuse and circumscribed choroidal hemangiomas in a patient with Sturge-Weber syndrome. *Arch Ophthalmol.* 1999;117:406-407.

14. Schilling H, Sauerwein W, Lommatzsch A. Long term results after low dose ocular irradiation for choroidal hemangioma. *Br J Ophthalmol.* 1997;81:267-273.

15. Zografos L, Bercher L, Chamot L, et al. Cobalt-60 treatment of choroidal hemangiomas. *Am J Ophthalmol.* 1996;121:190-199.

Uveal Neural Tumors

Arun D. Singh and Jonathan E. Sears

INTRODUCTION

Neurofibroma and schwannoma (neurilemmoma) are two types of neural tumor having distinct clinical and histopathologic features.

UVEAL NEUROFIBROMA

Neurofibromatosis type 1 can affect the uvea in several ways. Almost all patients develop Lisch nodules, which are melanocytic hamartomas of the iris, albeit not strictly neural in origin. Another abnormality that is almost universal is the presence of choroidal bright spots, which are believed to correspond to histologically observed ovoid bodies.[1] Choroidal neurofibromas (solitary or diffuse)[2] and ganglioneuromas[3] are extremely unusual ophthalmic manifestations of NF1.

Clinical Features

A solitary uveal neurofibroma appears as a circumscribed amelanotic choroidal tumor.[4] Diffuse uveal neurofibroma can be associated with congenital glaucoma presenting as a classic triad of unilateral buphthalmos, homolateral eyelid plexiform neurofibroma, and homolateral facial hypertrophy (François syndrome) (Figure 50-1).[2]

Treatment

There is no effective treatment for uveal neurofibroma.

UVEAL SCHWANNOMA

A review of the clinical findings of a uveal schwannoma, based on features of about 20 published cases, reveals that they can arise in the ciliary body, the choroid, or diffusely in the whole uvea.[5,6] Typically, uveal schwannoma presents as a solitary amelanotic tumor,[5] but multifocal uveal involvement due to plexiform schwannoma has rarely been described (Figure 50-2).[6]

Treatment

For smaller tumors located anteriorly, resection may be feasible.[7] However, most cases are enucleated because they are mistaken for melanoma.

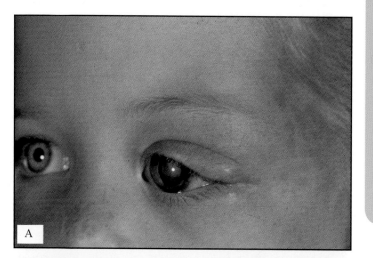

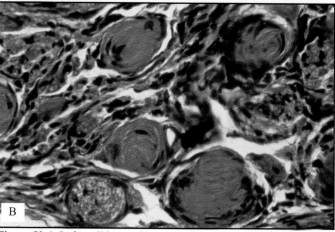

Figure 50-1. Left eyelid neurofibroma, café au lait spot, and buphthalmic globe (A). The choroid is thickened by diffuse neurofibroma. Ovoid bodies in choroidal neurofibroma (B). (Hematoxylin and eosin x400.) (This figure was published in *Ophthalmology,* 90, Brownstein S, Little JM, Ocular neurofibromatosis, 1595-1599, © Elsevier 1983.)

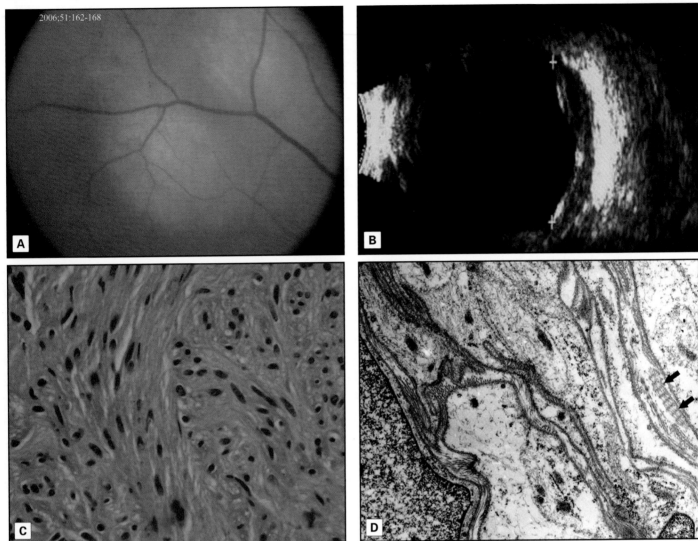

Figure 50-2. A 9-year-old white girl with iris and choroidal masses in her left eye. There was hyperpigmentation of the nasal iris and irregularity of the pupillary margin, with nasal pupillary margin cysts. Fundus photograph showing two raised amelanotic choroidal nodules in the superonasal quadrant (A). There is multifocal thickening of the choroid in the corresponding areas on B-scan ultrasonography (B). Photomicrograph of the iridectomy specimen reveals spindle-shaped cells with abundant eosinophilic cytoplasm and bland nuclei tending to palisade (C). (Hematoxylin and eosin x250.) Electron photomicrograph microscopy shows spindle cells with long-spaced collagen (Luse bodies, arrows) (D). (Reprinted from Saavedra E, Singh AD, Sears JE, Ratliff NB. Plexiform pigmented schwannoma of the uvea. *Surv Ophthalmol.* 2006;51:162-168.)

REFERENCES

1. Yasunari T, Shiraki K, Hattori H, Miki T. Frequency of choroidal abnormalities in neurofibromatosis type 1. *Lancet.* 2000;356:988-992.
2. Brownstein S, Little JM. Ocular neurofibromatosis. *Ophthalmology.* 1983;90:1595-1599.
3. Woog JJ, Albert DM, Craft J, et al. Choroidal ganglioneuroma in neurofibromatosis. *Graefes Arch Clin Exp Ophthalmol.* 1983;220:25-31.
4. Shields JA, Sanborn GE, Kurz GH, Augsburger JJ. Benign peripheral nerve tumor of the choroid: a clinicopathologic correlation and review of the literature. *Ophthalmology.* 1981;88:1322-1329.
5. Fan JT, Campbell RJ, Robertson DM. A survey of intraocular schwannoma with a case report. *Can J Ophthalmol.* 1995;30:37-41.
6. Saavedra E, Singh AD, Sears JE, Ratliff NB. Plexiform pigmented schwannoma of the uvea. *Surv Ophthalmol.* 2006;51:162-168.
7. Kuchle M, Holbach L, Schlotzer-Schrehardt U, Naumann GO. Schwannoma of the ciliary body treated by block excision. *Br J Ophthalmol.* 1994;78:397-400.

Uveal Osseous Tumors

Arun D. Singh

INTRODUCTION

Choroidal osteoma consists of cancellous bone and must be differentiated from calcium deposition (ie, calcification), which can be dystrophic or metastatic.[1] Dystrophic calcification occurs in dead or degenerated tissues despite normal calcium metabolism. An example of this condition is sclerochoroidal calcification. In contrast, metastatic calcification involves normal tissues and is secondary to hypercalcemia (Table 51-1).

CHOROIDAL OSTEOMA

Clinical Features

About 90% of cases are observed in females, presenting at a mean age of 21 years.[2] About 75% of cases are unilateral.[2] Most patients are asymptomatic.[3]

The lesion is yellow-white in color, with varying degrees of overlying retinal pigment epithelium (RPE) changes (Figure 51-1A).[4] The typical location is juxtapapillary or peripapillary, with some extension into the macular region. The tumor is round or oval in shape, with well-defined wavy margins. Fine vascular tufts are visible on its surface and are distinct from secondary choroidal neovascularization, which manifests as exudation, hemorrhage, or subretinal fluid in the vicinity of the tumor.[5]

Diagnostic Evaluation (Box 51-1)

Treatment

Choroidal osteoma by itself is untreatable. However, its main complication of choroidal neovascularization may respond to photocoagulation, photodynamic therapy, and anti-angiogenic agents in a similar fashion to age-related disease.

SCLEROCHOROIDAL CALCIFICATION

In most patients, sclerochoroidal calcification is apparently unrelated to any metabolic disease. Some cases occurred in patients with calcium metabolic disorders, which include hyperparathyroidism, hypervitaminosis D, and hypokalemic metabolic alkalosis (see Table 51-1).[6]

Clinical Features

Sclerochoroidal calcification is a disease of the elderly, detected at a mean age of 76 years.[7] Bilateral involvement occurs in about 85% of cases.[6] As a rule, patients are asymptomatic, and the condition is detected on a routine examination.

Typically, nodular conglomerations of round, yellow-white lesions in the supero- and infero-temporal mid-periphery, beneath the major retinal vascular arcades, are observed (Figure 51-2A).[6,7] The lesions vary in basal diameter from 3 to 8 mm, and may either be elevated (up to 6 mm) or flat with overlying RPE atrophy. Calcific deposits along the insertion of the medial or lateral rectus muscles (Cogan plaque) may be evident on external examination.

Diagnostic Evaluation (Box 51-2)

Differential Diagnosis

Some might confuse sclerochoroidal calcification with other amelanotic lesions, such as choroidal metastasis and subpigment epithelial infiltrates of primary central nervous system–ocular lymphoma, and choroidal osteoma (Table 51-2).

Treatment

Treatment may be necessary for secondary choroidal neovascularization or for any underlying metabolic disorder.

REFERENCES

1. Cotran RS, Kumar V, Collins T. *Robbins' Pathologic Basis of Disease.* 6th ed. Philadelphia, PA: WB Saunders; 1999:43-45.
2. Aylward GW, Chang TS, Pautler SE, Gass JD. A long-term follow-up of choroidal osteoma. *Arch Ophthalmol.* 1998;116:1337-1341.
3. Kadrmas EF, Weiter JJ. Choroidal osteoma. *Int Ophthalmol Clin.* 1997;37:171-182.
4. Gass JD, Guerry RK, Jack RL, Harris G. Choroidal osteoma. *Arch Ophthalmol.* 1978;96:428-435.
5. Shields CL, Shields JA, Augsburger JJ. Choroidal osteoma. *Surv Ophthalmol.* 1988;33:17-27.
6. Honavar SG, Shields CL, Demirci H, Shields JA. Sclerochoroidal calcification: clinical manifestations and systemic associations. *Arch Ophthalmol.* 2001;119:833-840.
7. Schachat AP, Robertson DM, Mieler WF, et al. Sclerochoroidal calcification. *Arch Ophthalmol.* 1992;110:196-199.

Table 51-1. Causes of Retinal, Choroidal, and Scleral Calcification

	Category		Example
Dystrophic	Degenerative		Sclerochoroidal calcification
	Metaplastic		Phthisis bulbi
	Neoplastic	Benign Hamartoma	Astrocytoma, retinocytoma
		Choristoma	Osteoma*
		Malignant	Retinoblastoma
Metabolic	Hypercalcemia	Hyperparathyroidism	Sclerochoroidal calcification
		Bone destruction	
		Vitamin D-related disorders	
		Renal failure	
	Hypokalemic metabolic alkalosis	Bartter syndrome	
		Gitelman syndrome	

*Choroidal osteoma represents bone formation and not a mere deposition of calcium salts.

Box 51-1. Features of Choroidal Osteoma

- Young healthy females with unilateral involvement
- Ophthalmoscopic appearance of a yellow-white choroidal mass, minimal elevation with a well-defined scalloped margin, located in the juxtapapillary region
- Early patchy hyperfluorescence and late staining on fluorescein angiography
- Early hypofluorescence and late staining on indocyanine angiography
- Highly reflective choroidal plaque-like lesion with orbital shadowing on ultrasonography (B-scan)
- A dense plaque-like bony opacity at the level of the choroid is noted on CT scan

Box 51-2. Features of Sclerochoroidal Calcification

- Elderly patients with bilateral involvement
- Ophthalmoscopic appearance of a yellow-white choroidal mass, minimal elevation with ill-defined margins, and in the midperipheral location
- Early hypofluorescence, progressive hyperfluorescence, and late staining on fluorescein angiography
- Highly reflective sclerochoroidal plaque-like lesion with orbital shadowing on ultrasonography (B-scan)
- A dense plaque-like bony opacity at the sclerochoroidal level on CT scan
- Systemic association with disorders of calcium, vitamin D, and magnesium

Table 51-2. Differentiating Features of Choroidal Osteoma and Sclerochoroidal Calcification

	Feature	Choroidal Osteoma	Sclerochoroidal Calcification
Clinical	Age (mean)	21 years	76 years
	Gender	Female >> male	Male = female
	Bilaterality	75% Unilateral	85% Bilateral
	Progression	Frequent	Stable
Ophthalmoscopic	Location	Juxtapapillary	Mid-periphery
	Shape	Oval with scalloped margins	Round with ill-defined margins
	Size (diameter)	2-22 mm	3-8 mm
	Elevation	<2.5 mm	<6 mm
	Focality	Unifocal	Multifocal
	Neovascularization	Frequent	Rare
Diagnostic	Fluorescein angiography	Early patchy hyperfluorescence; late staining	Early hypofluorescence; late staining
	Ultrasonography	Calcification	Calcification
Pathology		Osseous choristoma	Degenerative/metastatic calcification
Systemic association		Absent	May be present

(Adapted from Schachat AP, Robertson DM, Mieler WF, et al. Sclerochoroidal calcification. *Arch Ophthalmol.* 1992;110:196-199.)

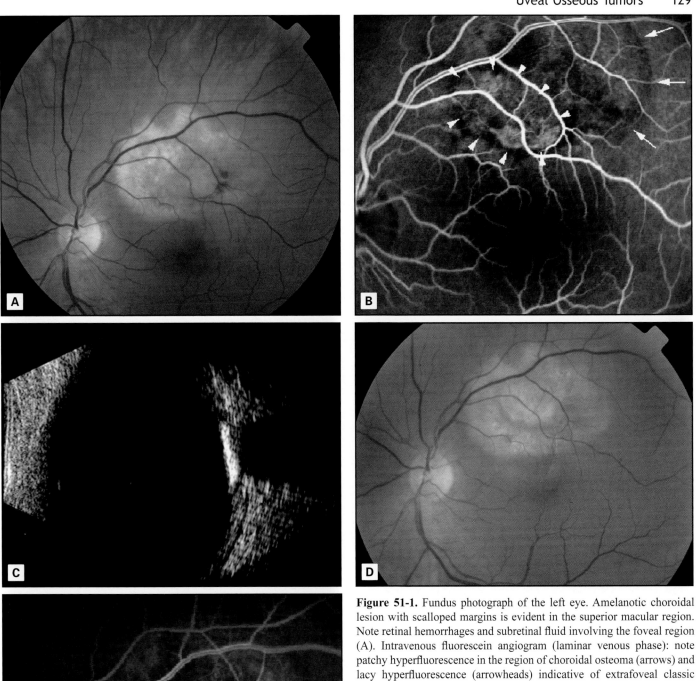

Figure 51-1. Fundus photograph of the left eye. Amelanotic choroidal lesion with scalloped margins is evident in the superior macular region. Note retinal hemorrhages and subretinal fluid involving the foveal region (A). Intravenous fluorescein angiogram (laminar venous phase): note patchy hyperfluorescence in the region of choroidal osteoma (arrows) and lacy hyperfluorescence (arrowheads) indicative of extrafoveal classic choroidal neovascularization (B). B-scan ultrasonography demonstrates high reflectivity at the level of the choroid suggestive of calcium deposition (C). Following photodynamic therapy, a grayish subretinal fibrotic membrane is present in the treated area, and there is resolution of retinal hemorrhages and subretinal fluid (D). Note the absence of lacy hyperfluorescence on the fluorescein angiogram (E). (Reproduced with permission from Singh AD, Talbot JF, Rundle PA, Rennie IG. Choroidal neovascularization secondary to choroidal osteoma: successful treatment with photodynamic therapy. *Eye*. 2005;19:482-483.)

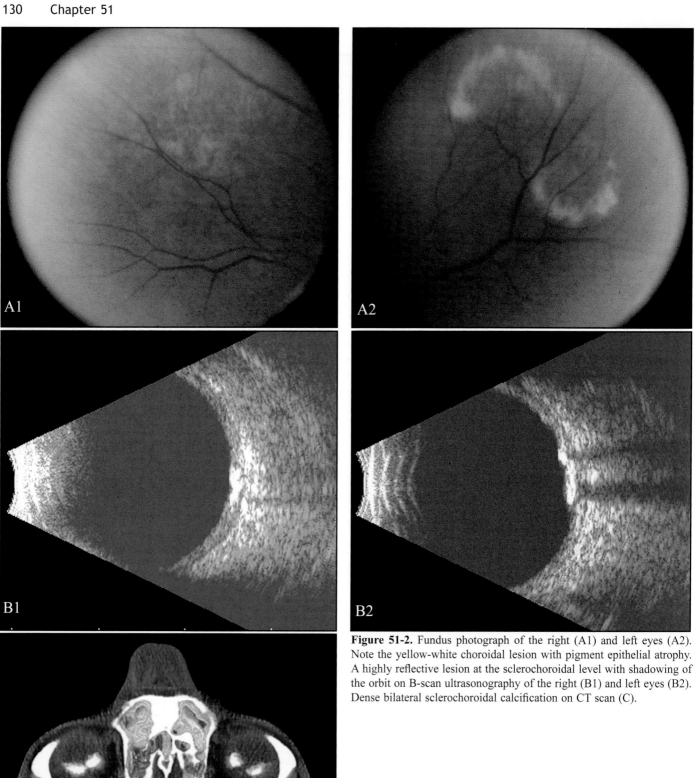

Figure 51-2. Fundus photograph of the right (A1) and left eyes (A2). Note the yellow-white choroidal lesion with pigment epithelial atrophy. A highly reflective lesion at the sclerochoroidal level with shadowing of the orbit on B-scan ultrasonography of the right (B1) and left eyes (B2). Dense bilateral sclerochoroidal calcification on CT scan (C).

Uveal Myogenic, Fibrous, and Histiocytic Tumors

Paul Rundle, Hardeep Singh Mudhar, M. Andrew Parsons, and Ian G. Rennie

LEIOMYOMA

These are rare benign tumors arising from smooth muscle components of the uveal tract.[1] Their rarity and the fact that leiomyomas often strongly resemble malignancies such as uveal melanoma makes diagnosis difficult prior to treatment.

Pathogenesis

Overall, leiomyomas occur in a younger age group (third to fifth decades) than uveal melanomas, which have a mean age at presentation of 55 years.[2] Interestingly, as with leiomyomas elsewhere in the body, uveal lesions are more common in females.[2]

Clinical Features

Leiomyomas are solitary, usually well-circumscribed lesions affecting only one eye (Figure 52-1). Leiomyomas are usually amelanotic in appearance and may show prominent intrinsic vessels, making them indistinguishable in some cases from collar-stud melanomas. One characteristic feature of leiomyomas is that they frequently transilluminate, in contrast to melanomas, which generally cast a shadow on transillumination of the globe.[2]

Diagnostic Evaluation

Making a firm diagnosis of uveal leiomyoma may be impossible without histology, although the presence of an amelanotic mass that transilluminates in a young (female) patient should certainly raise the possibility of this diagnosis. Unfortunately, there are no features that are pathognomonic of leiomyoma (Figure 52-2).

Treatment

As leiomyomas of the uveal tract are benign in the histological sense, then in theory treatment could be conservative. They do, however, have a propensity to grow, and so require treatment to prevent local damage. Unfortunately, the diagnosis may only become apparent after the lesion—or indeed the eye—has been removed.

JUVENILE XANTHOGRANULOMA

In general, juvenile xanthogranuloma (JXG) is a benign, self-limiting skin condition affecting young children.[3] Ocular involvement most commonly presents as a unilateral infiltration of the iris.[3] Ciliary body, choroidal, optic nerve, and orbital involvement

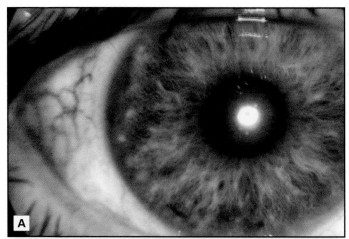
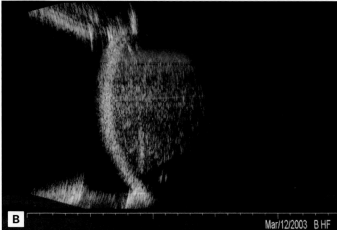

Figure 52-1. Pigmented ciliary body leiomyoma eroding through the iris root. Note the dilated episcleral vessels overlying the tumor (A). High-frequency ultrasound scan demonstrating the lesion (B).

are rare. Iris lesions are yellow in color and may be localized or diffuse.[4] Recurrent hyphema, uveitis, secondary glaucoma or heterochromia are common presenting features.[4]

The diagnosis is easily confirmed by means of a skin biopsy, paracentesis, or iris biopsy (Figure 52-3).

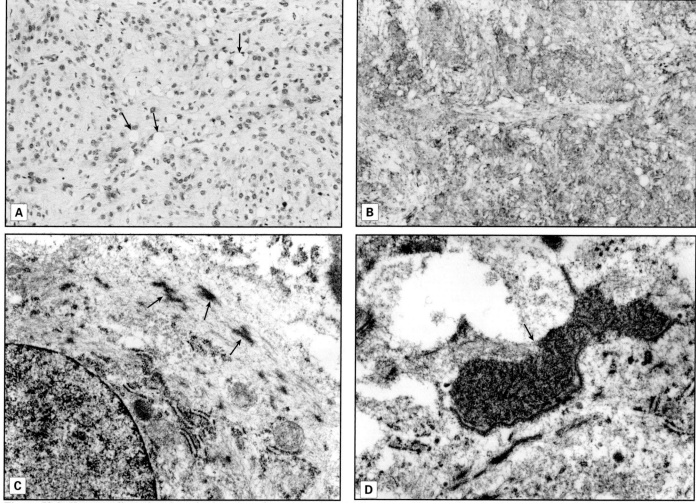

Figure 52-2. Hematoxylin and eosin-stained section of a mesectodermal leiomyoma. Note oval to circular nuclei in spindle-shaped eosinophilic cytoplasm, with some paranuclear vacuolation (arrows) (A). Diffuse, strong cytoplasmic immunoreactivity with anti-smooth muscle actin (brown reaction product) (B). Transmission electron micrograph. The arrows point to smooth muscle actin fusiform, focal densities (C). Transmission electron micrograph. The arrow points to a skenoid fiber (D).

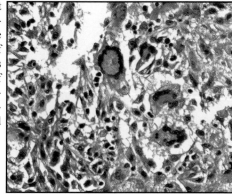

Figure 52-3. Light microscopic appearance of JXG. Note the foamy cytoplasm of the histiocytic cells and the giant cells of Touton type (peripheral wreath of circumferentially disposed nuclei).

REFERENCES

1. Blodi FC. Leiomyoma of the ciliary body. *Am J Ophthamol.* 1950;33:939-942.
2. Shields JA, Shields CL, Eagle RC, De Potter P. Observations on seven cases of intraocular leiomyoma. The 1993 Byron Demorest Lecture. *Arch Ophthalmol.* 1994;112:521-528.
3. Lyons C, Rootman J. Histiocytic, haematopoietic and lymphoproliferative disorders. In: Taylor D, Hoyt C, eds. *Paediatric Ophthalmology and Strabismus.* 3rd ed. Philadelphia, PA: Elsevier Saunders; 2006:344-353.
4. Zimmerman LE. Ocular lesions of juvenile xanthogranuloma. Nevoxanthoedothelioma. *Am J Ophthalmol.* 1965;60:1011-1035.
5. Gass JD. Management of juvenile xanthogranuloma of the iris. *Arch Ophthalmol.* 1964;71:344-347.
6. Harley RD, Romayananda N, Chan GH. Juvenile xanthogranuloma. *J Pediatr Ophthalmol Strabismus.* 1982;19:33-39.

Treatment and Prognosis

JXG is a self-limiting condition. Symptomatic cases requiring treatment usually respond to topical, periocular, or systemic steroids.[5] In cases unresponsive to steroids, low-dose radiotherapy (less than 500cGy) may be used.[6]

Uveal Lymphoproliferative Tumors

Sarah E. Coupland

INTRODUCTION

Lymphoid proliferations of the uvea can be divided into primary uveal tumors and secondary intraocular manifestations of systemic lymphoma. Approximately 75 cases of primary lymphoproliferations of the choroid have been reported in the literature.

PRIMARY CHOROIDAL LYMPHOMA

Clinical features of primary choroidal lymphoma include creamy choroidal infiltrates on fundus examination and low echogenicity on ophthalmic ultrasound (Figure 53-1).[1,2] Ultimately, a diffuse thickening of the uveal tract and, in some cases, subconjunctival or episcleral extension can occur (Box 53-1).

Diagnostic Evaluation

In most reported cases of primary choroidal lymphoma, the eyes were ultimately enucleated. Biopsies of the episcleral tumor nodules and either aspirates or biopsies of the choroidal swelling may establish the diagnosis. The morphological, immunohistochemical, and molecular biological characteristics of primary choroidal lymphomas are similar to those of extranodal marginal zone B-cell lymphomas of MALT type in other locations (Figure 53-2).[3] The neoplastic nature of the B cells in choroidal MALT lymphomas can be supported through clonality analysis, which demonstrates a monoclonal B-cell population using IgH-PCR and GeneScan (Figure 53-3).

Differential Diagnosis

Differential diagnosis of primary choroidal lymphoma includes diffuse uveal melanoma, uveal effusion syndrome, posterior scleritis, and amelanotic choroidal tumors such as choroidal metastasis, choroidal hemangioma, and choroidal osteoma (Table 53-1).

Treatment

It is essential to perform a complete staging investigation, including a complete blood count, serum protein electrophoresis, and abdominal and chest CT scanning[4] to exclude the possibility of concurrent systemic disease (eg, pulmonary MALT lymphoma) with secondary infiltration of the uvea. If no systemic disease is found, local treatment is appropriate. This includes excisional biopsy of any epibulbar mass, cryotherapy, and low-dose irradiation in divided doses.[4]

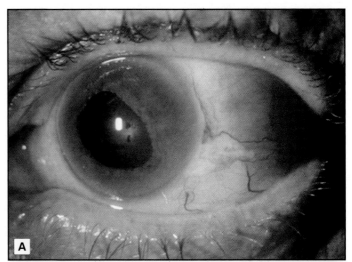

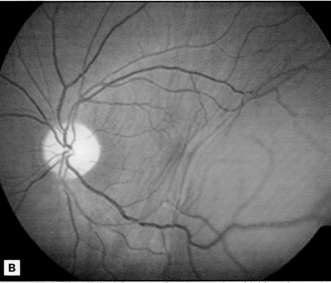

Figure 53-1. The clinical features of a primary choroidal lymphoma. (A) Yellow-orange episcleral and anterior choroidal mass. (Courtesy of Professor B. Damato.) (B) Fundus appearance of a choroidal mass and accompanying exudative retinal detachment. (Courtesy of Professor N. Bornfeld.)

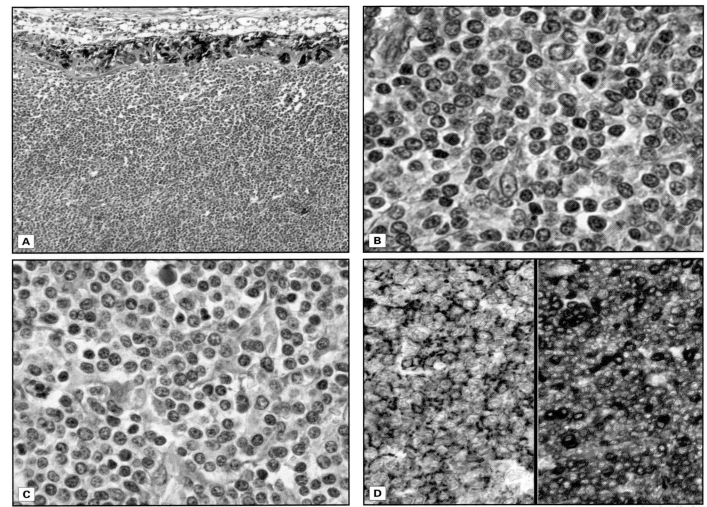

Figure 53-2. (A) Primary choroidal lymphoma with infiltration and disruption of Bruch's membrane and the RPE; the overlying retina is gliotic. (Hematoxylin and eosin, original magnification x200.) (B) Small centrocyte-like and plasmacytoid cells with occasional blasts are evident. (Hematoxylin and eosin, original magnification x400.) The tumor cells exhibit plasmacellular differentiation with Dutcher bodies (C). (PAS stain, original magnification x400.) (D) In addition, the tumor cells are positive for B-cell antigen, CD20 (left panel; APAAP x400 original magnification) and monotypic IgM (right panel; APAAP x400 original magnification).

Table 53-1. The Differential Diagnosis of Primary Choroidal Lymphoma

Features		Diffuse Melanoma	Uveal Effusion	Posterior Scleritis	Choroidal Metastasis	Choroidal Lymphoma
Symptoms	Pain	Absent	Absent	Present	Absent	Absent
External examination	Sentinel vessels	Present	Absent	Absent	Usually absent	Usually absent
	Other	Extrascleral extension	Normal	Scleritis	Trans-scleral metastasis	Salmon patch
Ophthalmoscopy	Mass	Choroidal	Absent	Scleral	Choroidal	Choroidal
	Shape	Diffuse	Dome	Dome	Variable	Variable
	Color	Usually pigmented	Normal choroid	Normal choroid	Yellow	Normal choroid or yellow
	RPE	Mottled	Mottled	Normal	Mottled	Normal
	Retina	Exudative detachment	Exudative detachment	Exudative detachment	Exudative detachment	Exudative detachment
Ultrasonography	Internal reflectivity	Low	Absent	Medium-high	Medium-high	Low
	Associated findings	Extrascleral extension	Exudative detachment	Retrobulbar edema	Trans-scleral metastasis or Exudative detachment	Exudative detachment
IVFA	Late leakage	Present	Absent	Present	Present	Present
Systemic association		Absent	Absent	Autoimmune disease	Carcinoma elsewhere	Absent

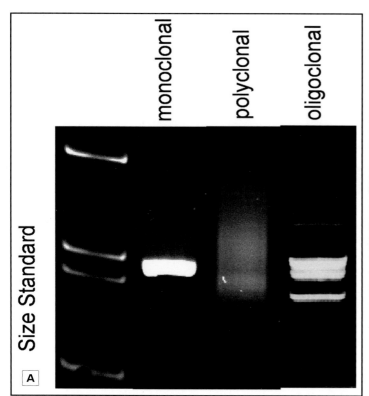

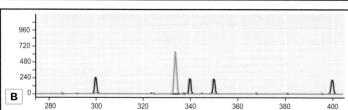

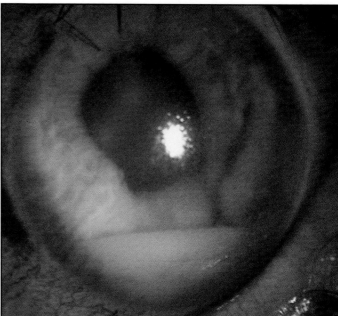

Figure 53-4. Pseudohypopyon in a 34-year-old woman with primary iridal lymphoma. Anterior chamber aspirate consisted of medium-sized atypical lymphocytes expressing the B-cell antigen CD79a. (Courtesy of Professor N. Bornfeld.)

Figure 53-3. Electophoresis gel demonstrating monoclonal, polyclonal, and oligoclonal bands (left to right) obtained by using polymerase chain reaction for immunoglobulin gene heavy chain rearrangements (A). The monoclonal band displays a monoclonal peak of 335 base pairs using the primer FR1 (B). (GeneScan). The red signals represent the internal size standard.

PRIMARY IRIDAL LYMPHOMA

Primary iridal lymphomas are exceptionally rare.[5] The typical clinical fetaures include a painful eye, photophobia, and sometimes decreased vision. The clinical signs include uveitis of uncertain origin, nodular or diffuse iridal precipitates, iris discoloration, iridal swelling, and hyphema or pseudohypopyon (Figure 53-4). An anterior chamber tap or iris biopsy may be necessary for diagnosis.

Box 53-1. Primary Choroidal Lymphoma

- Prolonged benign course
- Thickened uveal tract with confluent or nonconfluent one disc diameter creamy yellow lesions
- Depigmentation of the retinal pigment epithelium with loss of normal choroidal markings
- Anterior segment involvement in the form of fixed salmon-colored epibulbar masses with fine intrinsic vascularity
- Fluorescein angiography: early mottled or pinpoint areas of hyperfluorescence of the lesions and late staining at the level of the retinal pigment epithelium
- Ultrasonography: choroidal thickening with decreased echogenicity and extrascleral extension with an intact intervening scleral layer. Absence of scleral thickening or retrobulbar edema
- Computed tomography: thickening in the region of the mass without calcification, with a corresponding reduction in size of the vitreous cavity
- Magnetic resonance imaging: thickening in the region of the mass with a decrease in size of the vitreous cavity

REFERENCES

1. Jakobiec FA, Sacks E, Kronish JW, et al. Multifocal static creamy choroidal infiltrates. An early sign of lymphoid neoplasia. *Ophthalmology.* 1987;94:397-406.
2. Ciulla TA, Bains RA, Jakobiec FA, et al. Uveal lymphoid neoplasia: a clinical-pathologic correlation and review of the early form. *Surv Ophthalmol.* 1997;41:467-476.
3. Coupland SE, Foss H-D, Hidayat AA, Cockerham GC, et al. Extranodal marginal zone B-cell lymphomas of the uvea: an analysis of 13 cases. *J Pathology.* 2002;197(3):333-340.
4. Augsburger JJ, Greatrex KV. Intraocular lymphoma: clinical presentations, differential diagnosis and treatment. *Trans Am Acad Ophthalmol Otolaryngol.* 1989;41:796-808.
5. Velez G, de Smet MD, Whitcup SM, et al. Iris involvement in primary intraocular lymphoma: report of two cases and review of the literature. *Surv Ophthalmol.* 2000;44:518-526.

Uveal Metastatic Tumors

Norbert Bornfeld

INTRODUCTION

Numerous studies have shown that cancer metastasis to the uvea is by far the most frequent intraocular tumor and that often the ophthalmologist is the first physician to detect disseminating cancer because uveal metastasis is the first presenting symptom.

Clinical Features

Metastatic tumors may occur anywhere in the uvea, including the iris, ciliary body, and choroid. The vast majority of metastatic tumors, however, develop in the choroid, whereas metastases to the iris are relatively rare. Metastasizing breast cancer accounts for more than half of all patients with a clinical diagnosis of uveal metastasis[1] and can even occur in men (Table 54-1).[2] In a quarter of all patients with choroidal metastases, cancer of the lung is the underlying primary tumor. Other primary tumors, such as carcinoid tumor, cancer of the gastrointestinal tract, thyroid, prostate, cutaneous melanoma, and renal cell carcinoma, rarely metastasize to the uvea. Sarcomas only very exceptionally lead to uveal metastasis. Choroidal metastases usually occur in a setting of a pre-existing primary tumor (eg, in breast cancer).[1] It may also occur as the initial manifestation of a metastasizing primary tumor.[3] Choroidal metastases from an unknown or undetectable primary tumor is uncommon.

Frequently, choroidal metastases are bilateral and multifocal (Box 54-1). At presentation, up to one quarter of all patients have metastatic tumors in both eyes.[4] Choroidal metastases are located preferentially at the posterior pole. The macula is involved in 42% of eyes.[5] Choroidal metastatic tumors may appear in three different forms:

- Flat, amelanotic tumor with indistinct margins (Figure 54-1)
- Flat, pigmented tumor with indistinct margins (Figure 54-2)
- Amelanotic dome-shaped tumor (Figure 54-3).

Melanotic dome-shaped tumor as a result of uveal metastasis from cutaneous melanoma is clinically indistinguishable from primary choroidal melanoma (Figure 54-4). The presence of widespread metastasis from cutaneous melanoma and rapid growth of intraocular tumor is usually evident.

Typical signs of metastatic tumors to the iris include uni- or multifocal, non-pigmented, sometimes vascularized tumors with associated anterior chamber inflammation, hyphema, and pseudo-hypopyon (ie, layering of tumor cells).[6] The tumor, which may be located in the chamber angle or on the surface of the iris, usually undergoes rapid growth (Figure 54-5).

DIAGNOSTIC EVALUATION

Fluorescein and indocyanine angiography may be helpful in distinguishing choroidal metastases from uveal melanoma. Typical angiographic characteristics are lack of early blockage, mottling of pigment on the surface of the tumor, lack of intrinsic tumor vessels, and late pooling of the dye (Figure 54-6). In contrast, choroidal melanoma demonstrates early blockage, intrinsic tumor vessels, and late pooling of dye.

Ultrasonography is helpful in detecting the intraocular mass, particularly in cases where an extensive exudative retinal detachment is present. Metastatic lesions may have extremely variable reflectivity. Therefore, ultrasonography may not be diagnostic.

Intraocular biopsy of a suspected lesion is indicated when the diagnosis cannot be ascertained by other, less invasive procedures. Additionally, intraocular biopsy may be required when the primary tumor is undetectable on systemic evaluation. In such cases, histopathological characterization of the intraocular metastasis can facilitate identification of the primary tumor (Chapter 56).[7]

TREATMENT

The decision to treat metastasis is made in consultation with the oncologist and radiation oncologist. At the outset, systemic evaluation is performed to determine the extent of metastasis, particularly involvement of the brain, by appropriate imaging techniques, serum markers, and bone marrow biopsy (if indicated). The extent of metastatic disease may be classified as diffuse (ie, widespread to several organs in addition to uvea), focal (ie, confined to uvea), or local (ie, a solitary focus in the uvea) (Figure 54-7). If the metastatic disease is diffuse, then the treatment options include chemotherapy, hormonal therapy (for hormone-dependent tumors), immune modulation, angiogenic inhibitors, and hospice care for the terminally ill (Figure 54-8). Radiotherapy is usually recommended for focal disease (confined to the uvea). The localized disease may be treated by plaque radiotherapy. Surgical treatment may be necessary for painful eyes with secondary glaucoma.

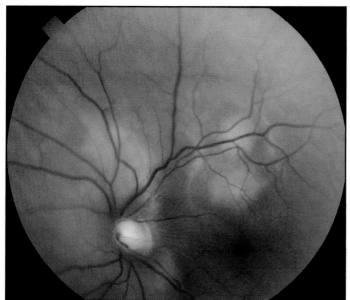

Figure 54-1. Multifocal choroidal metastases in a patient with disseminated breast cancer.

Table 54-1. Primary Tumors That Metastasize to the Uvea

Primary Site	Frequency (%)
Breast carcinoma	47
Lung carcinoma	21
Gastrointestinal tract carcinoma	4
Renal cell carcinoma	2
Cutaneous melanoma	2
Prostate carcinoma	2
Other tumors	4
Unknown	18

Note that sarcoma only very exceptionally metastasizes to the uvea.

(Adapted from Shields CL, Shields JA, Gross NE, et al. Survey of 520 eyes with uveal metastases. *Ophthalmology.* 1997;104:1265-1276.)

Box 54-1. Features of Choroidal Metastasis

- Uni- or multifocal yellow white tumors, mostly at the posterior pole
- Exudative retinal detachment
- No tumor vessels on fluorescein angiography
- Rapid growth if untreated

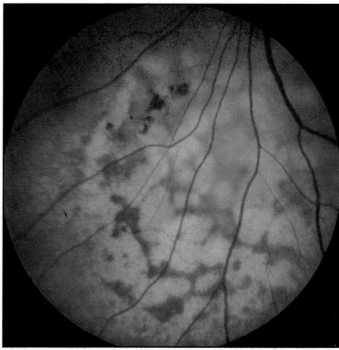

Figure 54-2. Flat, pigmented metastatic tumor in the choroid with typical pigmentary pattern on the tumor surface.

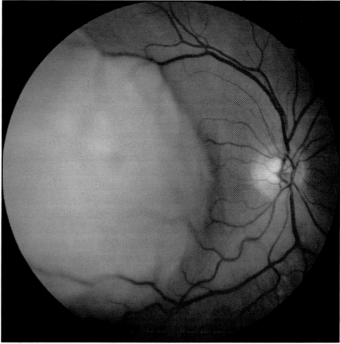

Figure 54-3. Amelanotic, dome-shaped metastatic tumor in the choroid in a patient with metastasizing cancer of the lung.

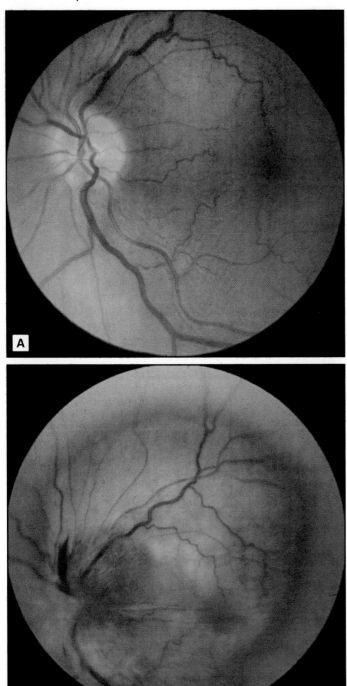

Figure 54-4. Melanotic, dome-shaped metastatic choroidal tumor from a primary cutaneous melanoma, which is ophthalmoscopically indistinguishable from a primary choroidal melanoma (A). Massive tumor growth 3 months later (B).

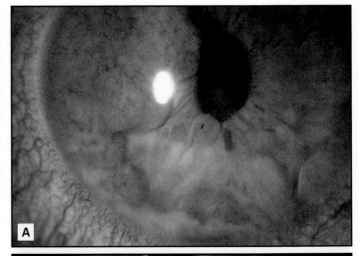

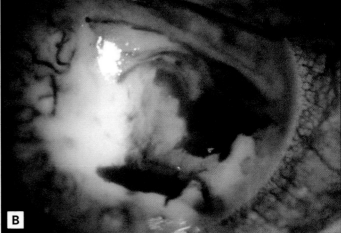

Figure 54-5. Iris metastases from a bronchial carcinoma (A). Three months later, massive tumor growth nearly fills the anterior chamber (B).

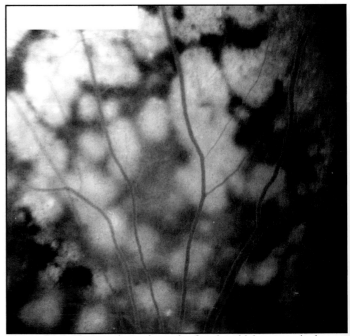

Figure 54-6. Fluorescein angiograph of a choroidal metastasis demonstrating characteristic early blockage and a mottled appearance.

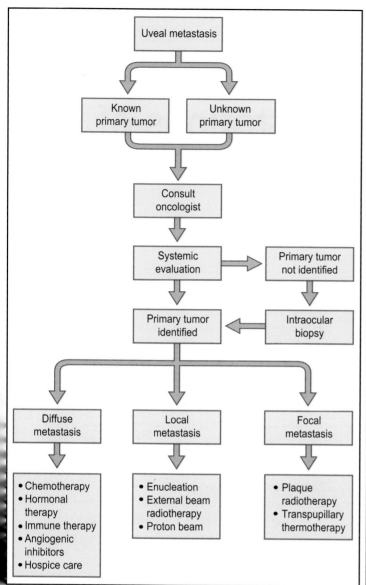

Figure 54-7. Steps in management of uveal metastasis.

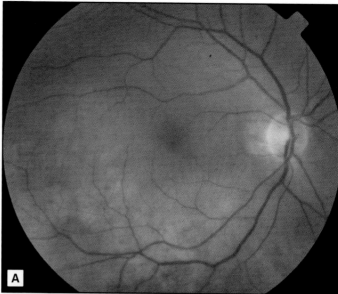

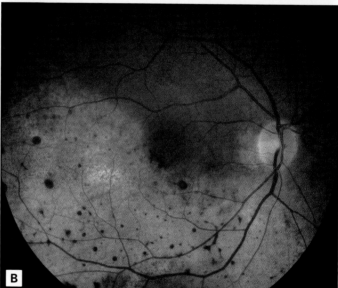

Figure 54-8. A 62-year-old woman presented with superior visual field defect OD. She gave a history of mastectomy and radiotherapy for stage IIA breast infiltrating ductal carcinoma diagnosed 3 years before. All 17 lymph nodes were negative, and the tumor was estrogen and progesterone receptor positive. FISH analysis revealed HER2 gene amplification. She was currently on tamoxifen 20 mg daily. Fundus examination revealed diffuse choroidal thickening (18 x 2.0 mm) extending into the fovea (A). Exudative retinal detachment involved the lower half of the retina. Systemic evaluation indicated metastatic disease in the lungs. In consultation with her oncologist, she was started on paclitaxel (antimicrotubular antineoplastic agent, Taxol) and trastuzumab (monoclonal antibody that binds to extracellular domain of the human epidermal growth factor receptor 2 protein—HER2, Herceptin). For more than 12 months, she has been maintained on letrozole (aromatase inhibitor, Femara) and Herceptin, with complete regression of the choroidal tumor (B).

REFERENCES

1. Demirci H, Shields CL, Chao AN, Shields JA. Uveal metastasis from breast cancer in 264 patients. *Am J Ophthalmol.* 2003;136:264-271.

2. Kreusel KM, Heimann H, Wiegel T, et al. Choroidal metastasis in men with metastatic breast cancer. *Am J Ophthalmol.* 1999;128:253-255.

3. Williams NJ, Leris AC, Kouriefs C, et al. Choroidal metastasis—the initial presentation of breast carcinoma. *Eur J Surg Oncol.* 2000;26:817-818.

4. Shields CL, Shields JA, Gross NE, et al. Survey of 520 eyes with uveal metastases. *Ophthalmology.* 1997;104:1265-1276.

5. Kreusel KM, Bechrakis N, Wiegel T, et al. Klinische Charakteristika der Aderhautmetastasierung. *Ophthalmologe.* 2003;100:618-622.

6. Shields JA, Shields CL, Kiratli H, de Potter P. Metastatic tumors to the iris in 40 patients. *Am J Ophthalmol.* 1995;119:422-430.

7. Augsburger JJ. Diagnostic biopsy of selected intraocular tumors. *Am J Ophthalmol.* 2005;140:1094-1095.

Intraocular Manifestations of Proliferative Hematopoietic Disorders

Hayyam Kiratli

INTRODUCTION

Hematopoietic disorders encompass a wide variety of neoplastic and non-neoplastic diseases of erythrocytes, leukocytes, and platelets, and their precursors.

LEUKEMIAS

The leukemias are malignancies of myelogenous and lymphocytic leukocyte precursors, which develop in the bone marrow and are characterized by the spread of leukemic blast cells to the circulation, liver, spleen, and lymph nodes.[1] The early clinical manifestations of the disease are pallor, fatigue, easy bruising, and mucosal bleeding, appearing when the malignant cell number is enough to suppress normal hematopoiesis.

Ophthalmic Features

Ocular involvement is reported in 32% to 92% of patients with leukemia (Box 55-1).[2] Nearly 50% of patients with ocular leukemia have concomitant central nervous system involvement. Isolated ocular leukemic infiltrations may also be the first clinical evidence of an extramedullary relapse in 30% of cases.[3]

IRIS AND ANTERIOR CHAMBER

The infiltrated heterochromic iris may show diffuse or nodular thickening, which is often associated with a gray-yellow pseudo-hypopyon with hemorrhage (Figure 55-1).[4]

VITREOUS

Direct involvement of the vitreous by the leukemic process is exceedingly rare.[5] The differential diagnosis includes infectious endophthalmitis, especially in immunocompromised patients.

RETINA

Clinically, the retina is the most commonly affected intraocular structure (Figure 55-2).[6] In most cases, this is in the form of leukemic retinopathy caused by anemia, hyperviscosity, and thrombocytopenia. Leukemic retinopathy is more often associated with adult acute leukemias and relapses.[5]

Box 55-1. Ocular Features of Leukemia

- Leukemic infiltrates can develop in the iris and choroid
- Anemia, increased blood viscosity, thrombocytopenia, and immunosuppression can all cause ocular abnormalities
- Anterior chamber abnormalities include hyphema and glaucoma
- Retinal disease includes white-centered hemorrhages, cotton-wool spots, microaneurysms, neovascularization, vascular sheathing, and serous retinal detachment
- Choroidal abnormalities include tumor formation and a leopard-skin appearance
- The optic nerve can be infiltrated or there may be swelling due to raised intracranial pressure

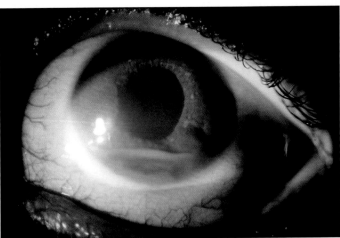

Figure 55-1. Iris and anterior chamber involvement in a 5-year-old boy with ALL L2. There is diffuse irregular thickening of the iris and a pseudohypopyon mixed with hemorrhage.

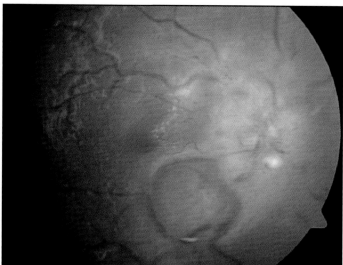

Figure 55-2. Serous retinal detachment with a subretinal "hypopyon" in a 7-year-old girl with AML M4. There is also infiltration of the optic nerve head.

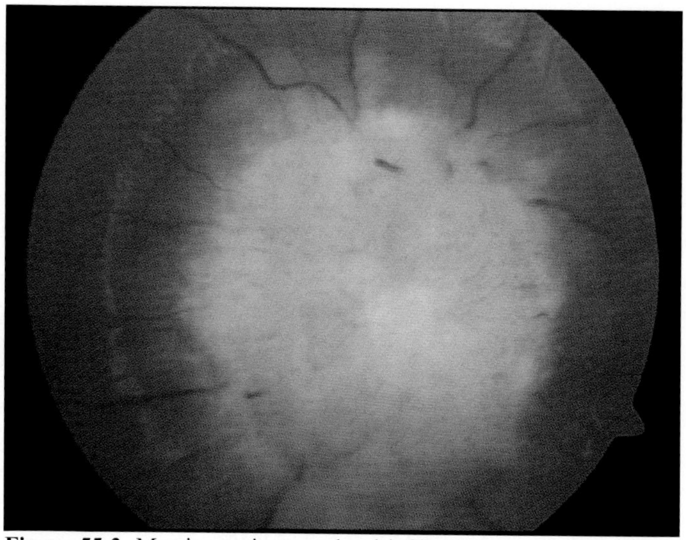

Figure 55-3. Massive optic nerve head infiltration in a 4-year-old boy with ALL L2. The patient also had central nervous system involvement.

CHOROID

Choroidal infiltration is the most frequent finding on histopathological examination, although it is rarely recognized clinically.[7]

OPTIC NERVE

Optic nerve involvement is an ominous sign because of a strong correlation with central nervous system (CNS) leukemia. It is found more commonly in children with ALL (Figure 55-3).[8]

Treatment for any type of leukemia aims to restore normal hematopoiesis, prevent the emergence of resistant leukemic clones, eradicate minimal residual disease, and provide effective prophylactic therapy to prevent recurrence from "sanctuary sites," most importantly in the CNS.

POLYCYTHEMIA VERA RUBRA

Polycythemia vera (PV) is a chronic myeloproliferative disorder that originates in a clonal hematopoietic stem cell. Ocular effects include transient visual obscurations, cyanotic fundus, dilatation and tortuosity of retinal vessels, intraretinal and vitreous hemorrhages, juxtafoveolar retinal telangiectasis, and optic disc swelling and atrophy. Retinal arterial and venous occlusions are common.[9]

GRAFT-VERSUS-HOST DISEASE

This is a particularly serious complication of hematopoietic stem cell transplantation that occurs when competent donor-derived T cells react with recipient tissue antigens. The skin, liver, and gastrointestinal tract are most severely affected. Serious ocular complications can also occur and include cicatricial lag-ophthalmos, keratoconjunctivitis sicca, pseudomembranous conjunctivitis, pathognomonic fibrotic tarsal conjunctival Arlt lines, corneal ulceration, and corneal melting.[8] Intraocular manifestations include cataract, bilateral optic disc edema, vitreous hemorrhage, retinal detachment, and cotton wool spots.[5] The treatment of graft-versus-host disease involves immunosuppression by the use of cyclosporine, tacrolimus, or prednisolone.

REFERENCES

1. Jaffe ES, Harris NL, Stein H, Vardiman JW, eds. *World Health Organization Classification of Tumors. Pathology and Genetics of Tumors of Haematopoietic and Lymphoid Tissues.* Lyon: IARC Press; 2001:76-117.
2. Kinkaid MC, Green WR. Ocular and orbital involvement in leukemia. *Surv Ophthalmol.* 1983;27:211-232.
3. Curto ML, Zingone A, Acquaviva A, et al. Leukemic infiltration of the eye: results of therapy in a retrospective multicentric study. *Med Pediatr Oncol.* 1989;17:134-137.
4. Zakka KA, Yee RD, Shorr N, et al. Leukemic iris infiltration. *Am J Ophthalmol.* 1980;89:204-209.
5. Gordon KB, Rugo HS, Duncan JL, et al. Ocular manifestations of leukemia. Leukemic infiltration versus infectious process. *Ophthalmology.* 2001;108:2293-2300.
6. Rosenthal AR. Ocular manifestations of leukemia. A review. *Ophthalmology.* 1983;90:899-905.
7. Leonardy NJ, Rupani M, Dent G, Klintworth GK. Analysis of 135 autopsy eyes for ocular involvement in leukcmia. *Am J Ophthalmol.* 1990;109:436-444.
8. Sharma T, Grewal J, Gupta S, Murray PI. Ophthalmic manifestations of acute leukaemias: the ophthalmologist's role. *Eye.* 2004;18:663-672.
9. Rothstein T. Bilateral central retinal vein closure as the initial manifestation of polycythemia. *Am J Ophthalmol.* 1972;74:256-260.

Intraocular Biopsy

Devron H. Char

INTRODUCTION

The major indication for intraocular tumor biopsy is failure to establish a diagnosis non-invasively in a patient who requires therapy. A confusing clinical pattern, such as an amelanotic uveal tumor with a history of a prior carcinoma, media opacities with ultrasound demonstration of a choroidal mass, question of a uveitis versus intraocular lymphoma, or a patient unwilling to have a surgical procedure without cytopathologic confirmation of the diagnosis, are potential indications. Newer highly accurate molecular prognostic data currently available on fine needle aspiration biopsy (FNAB) have expanded its indications.

TECHNIQUES

There are several techniques; these include vitrectomy, fine needle aspiration biopsy (trans-scleral or transvitreal), external scleral-based choroidal resection, and endoretinal biopsy (Box 56-1).

Vitrectomy is usually performed to rule out an intraocular lymphoma, although occasionally it is also used to detect metastatic tumors to the vitreous. We and others have previously reported on techniques to optimize the quality of vitreous cellular cytopathology.[1] If a patient has moderate or severe vitreous cellularity, a standard three-port vitrectomy is set up, but before using the vitrector, a sample is obtained with a 20-gauge needle and immediately transported to the laboratory. Saving these specimens in RPMI or newer preservation media can reduce cell degradation (Figure 56-1).

Fine Needle Aspiration Biopsy

Transvitreal and trans-scleral FNAB has been used mainly to diagnose adult choroidal tumors. No evidence of tumor spread has been documented in eye or orbital fine needle biopsies.[2] We prefer the use of a 25-gauge needle, which may be obtained with or without the application of negative pressure. The optimal preparation is that of direct smears on glass slides. If the material is alcohol fixed, a Papanicolaou stain is used. Air-dried samples are stained with the May–Grünwald–Giemsa method.

In addition to making the diagnosis of a uveal melanoma, cell type can also be ascertained (Figures 56-2 and 56-3).[3] We have recently documented that accurate molecular prognostic data can be obtained by FNAB in uveal melanoma.[4] FNAB is also used to

Box 56-1. Techniques of Intraocular Biopsy

- Vitrectomy
- Fine needle aspiration biopsy (trans-scleral or transretinal)
- Trans-scleral incisional tumor biopsy
- Endoretinal biopsy

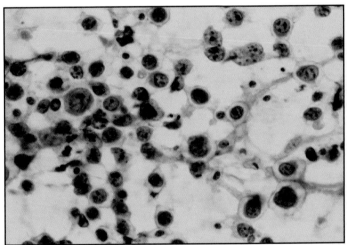

Figure 56-1. B-cell lymphoma demonstrating large single cells with irregular nuclear shapes. (Papanicolaou stain x60.)

confirm the diagnosis of lymphoma and metastatic carcinoma (see Figure 56-3).

External (Scleral-Based Choroidal Resection) Biopsy

Rarely have we required an external approach to make the diagnosis of an intraocular tumor. We prefer a scleral flap and chorioretinal biopsy if the tumor involves the choroid or deep retinal layers.[5] Under hypotensive anesthesia, we raise a 90% scleral flap around the area to be biopsied (Figure 56-4). If it is a deep lesion, we do not incise the full thickness of the retina. Figure 56-5 shows a post eye-wall biopsy patient in whom intraocular lymphoma was diagnosed after negative vitreous biopsy.

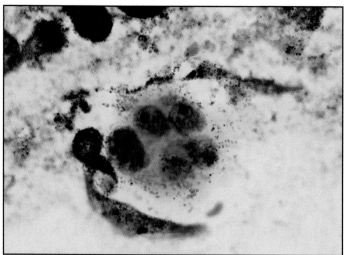

Figure 56-2. Epithelioid melanoma, note large nucleoli. (Papanicolaou stain x60.)

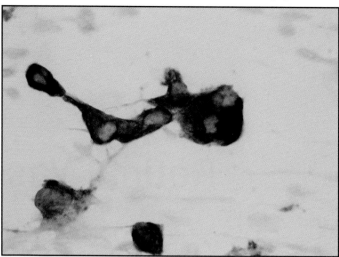

Figure 56-3. Metastatic breast carcinoma showing cohesive cell groups. (Immunohistochemical stain for keratin. AE 1/3 x60.)

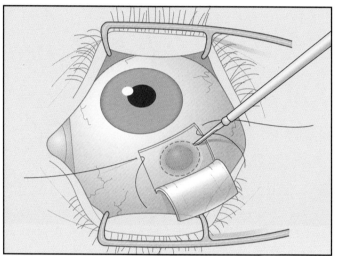

Figure 56-4. Schematic ab externo eye-wall biopsy.

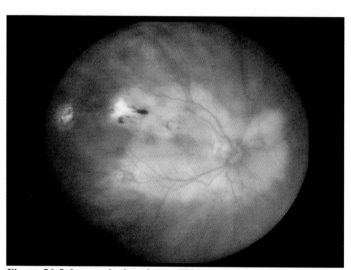

Figure 56-5. Intraocular lymphoma. This case had a negative vitrectomy and FNAB result. Diagnosis was obtained with eye-wall biopsy.

Endoretinal Biopsy

In patients who require an endoretinal biopsy for a diffuse process, it is easier to operate on a detached retina at the junction of the involved and uninvolved retina in the upper temporal quadrant (for easier gas/fluid retinal tamponade). Johnston and colleagues used endocautery and then removed a 2 x 2 mm area of retina with vertical cutting scissors, grasped it with forceps, and did an air/fluid exchange and endolaser. Cataract can occur after this procedure, along with vitreous hemorrhage and retinal detachment. We and others have demonstrated that a diagnosis of retinoblastoma can be made with a fine needle biopsy, but it is rarely indicated. Biopsy for suspected retinoblastoma should be limited only to cases with atypical presentations. The last patient to undergo biopsy for retinoblastoma in our center was an 18-year-old who had 20/50 vision, diffuse uveitis, and no obvious tumor.

REFERENCES

1. Ljung B-M, Char DH, Miller TR, Deschenes J. Intraocular lymphoma. Cytologic diagnosis and the role of immunologic markers. *Acta Cytol.* 1988;32:840-847.
2. Glasgow BJ, Brown HH, Zargoza AM, Foos RY. Quantitation of tumor seeding from fine needle aspiration of ocular melanoma. *Am J Ophthalmol.* 1988;105:538-546.
3. Char DH, Miller TR, Ljung BM, Howes EL Jr, Stoloff A. Fine needle aspiration biopsy in uveal melanoma. *Acta Cytol.* 1989;33:599-605.
4. Onken MD, Worley LA, Davila RM, Char DH, Harbour JW. Prognostic testing in uveal melanoma by transcriptomic profiling of fine needle biopsy specimens. *J Mol Diagn.* 2006;8:567-573.
5. Char DH, Miller TR, Crawford JB. Uveal tumour resection. *Br J Ophthalmol.* 2001;85:1213-1219.

Retinal Vascular Tumors

Arun D. Singh, Paul Rundle, and Ian G. Rennie

INTRODUCTION

Retinal vascular tumors represent at least four distinct clinical entities, which include retinal capillary hemangioma, retinal cavernous hemangioma, retinal arteriovenous communications (Wyburn-Mason syndrome), and retinal vasoproliferative tumors (Table 57-1).

RETINAL CAPILLARY HEMANGIOMA

Clinical Features

Retinal capillary hemangioma (RCH) are multiple in about one third of patients, and up to half of the cases have bilateral involvement. The mean age at diagnosis of RCH in von Hippel-Lindau disease is approximately 25 years.[1] Ophthalmoscopically, a RCH appears as a circumscribed, round retinal lesion with an orange-red color and prominent feeder vessels (Figure 57-1). Intraretinal and subretinal exudation is often seen around the tumor or in the macula. The majority of retinal capillary hemangiomas are located in the supero- and inferotemporal peripheral retina.[1] Prominent retinal vessels emerging from the optic disc are highly suggestive of a peripherally located RCH. In contrast, juxtapapillary RCH are not associated with visible prominent feeder vessels.

Treatment

There are several methods of treating a RCH and the choice is determined by the size, location, and associated findings of the subretinal fluid, retinal traction, and visual potential of the eye.[2] The treatment can be challenging owing to the presence of mul-

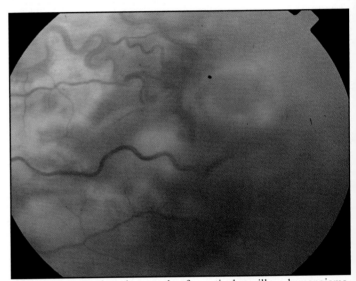

Figure 57-1. Fundus photograph of a retinal capillary hemangioma. Prominent feeder vessels, retinal exudation, and subretinal fluid are present. (Reproduced with permission from Bakri SJ, Sears JE, Singh AD. Transient closure of a retinal capillary hemangioma with verteporfin photodynamic therapy. *Retina.* 2005;25:1103-1134.)

tiple tumors in both eyes and the potential for the development of new tumors.

Laser photocoagulation applied over many sessions is effective in tumors that are 1.5 mm or smaller.

Cryotherapy is preferable to photocoagulation when the RCH is located anteriorly and is less than 3.0 mm in diameter.

Type	Appearance	Location	Feeder Vessels	Exudation	Systemic Association
Capillary hemangioma	Round red mass	Juxtapapillary/peripheral	Prominent	Present	VHL disease
Cavernous hemangioma	Grape-like clusters	Non-specific	Absent	Absent	CNS hemangioma
Arteriovenous malformations	Dilated/tortuous retinal vessels	Near the disc	Absent	Absent	Wyburn-Mason syndrome
Vasoproliferative tumor	Globular pale mass	Periphery	Absent	Present	Absent

Table 57-1. Diagnostic Features of Retinal Vascular Tumors

VHL, von Hippel-Lindau disease.

Photodynamic therapy has been reported to induce the occlusion of juxtapapillary and peripheral RCH.[3]

CAVERNOUS HEMANGIOMA OF THE RETINA

Cavernous hemangioma of the retina (CHR) are composed of multiple, thin-walled, dilated vascular channels with surface gliosis. Two forms of CHR are recognized: sporadic and syndromic. Retinal lesions appear as grape-like clusters of blood-filled saccular spaces in the inner layers of the retina or on the surface of the optic disc (Figure 57-2).[4] The size and location of the tumor are variable, but epiretinal membranes are usually present. There are no prominent feeder vessels, and there is a lack of subretinal or intraretinal exudation.

Treatment

In general, CHR are non-progressive, may undergo spontaneous thrombosis, and rarely cause vitreous hemorrhage. No effective treatment is known, or indeed required.

WYBURN-MASON SYNDROME

Wyburn-Mason syndrome is a rare sporadic disorder characterized by congenital arteriovenous malformations, principally of the retina and brain (Figure 57-3). Other involved tissues may include the skin, bones, kidneys, muscles, and gastrointestinal tract.[5]

Treatment

Retinal vascular malformations are usually not amenable to therapy.

VASOPROLIFERATIVE RETINAL TUMOR

Vasoproliferative retinal tumors (VPRT) were initially termed *presumed acquired retinal hemangiomas* to differentiate them from capillary hemangiomas.[6] At present, vasoproliferative retinal tumor is the preferred terminology. VPRT may be primary (74%) or secondary to a pre-existing ocular disease (26%). VPRT tumors appear as a globular, yellowish-pink vascular mass in the peripheral retina (Figure 57-4). The lesions lack the dilated, tortuous feeder vessels typically seen in RCH.

VPRT have a predilection for the inferior retina. Subretinal exudation, which may be extensive, is common, occurring in more than 80% of cases.[7] Exudative retinal detachment, retinal and vitreous hemorrhage, and vitreous cells are frequent associated findings. Most vasoproliferative retinal tumors can be treated successfully with triple freeze–thaw transconjunctival cryotherapy, although repeated treatments may be required.[7] Other treatment options include plaque brachytherapy,[7] laser photocoagulation,[7] and photodynamic therapy.

REFERENCES

1. Webster AR, Maher ER, Moore AT. Clinical characteristics of ocular angiomatosis in von Hippel-Lindau disease and correlation with germline mutation. *Arch Ophthalmol.* 1999;117:371-378.
2. Singh AD, Nouri M, Shields CL, Shields JA, Perez N. Treatment of retinal capillary hemangioma. *Ophthalmology.* 2002;109:1799-1806.

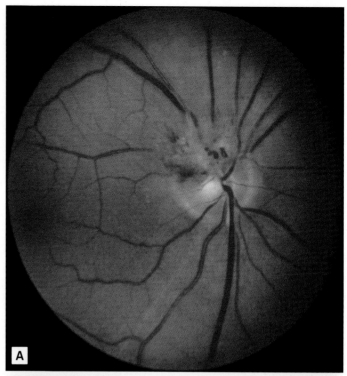

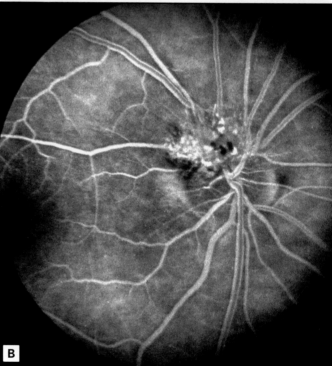

Figure 57-2. Fundus photograph of a peripapillary cavernous hemangioma of the retina. Note the absence of retinal exudation (A). On fluorescein angiography, characteristic hyperfluorescent saccular dilatations are evident (B). (Reprinted from Singh AD, Rundle PA, Rennie IG. Retinal vascular tumors. *Ophthalmol Clin North Am.* 2005;18:167-176.)

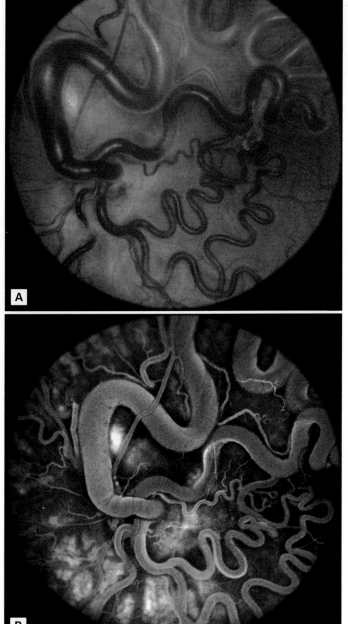

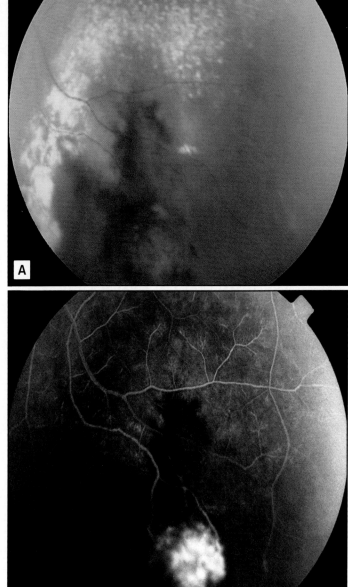

Figure 57-3. Fundus appearance of a typical retinal arteriovenous malformation (A). On fluorescein angiography, arteries and veins appear undistinguishable (B). (Reprinted from Singh AD, Rundle PA, Rennie IG. Retinal vascular tumors. *Ophthalmol Clin North Am.* 2005;18:167-176.)

Figure 57-4. Fundus appearance of a vasoproliferative retinal tumor (A). Diffuse hyperfluorescence in the late phase of the fluorescein angiogram (B). (Reprinted from Singh AD, Rundle PA, Rennie IG. Retinal vascular tumors. *Ophthalmol Clin North Am.* 2005;18:167-176.)

3. Atebara NH. Retinal capillary hemangioma treated with verteporfin photodynamic therapy. *Am J Ophthalmol.* 2002;134:788-790.
4. Dobyns WB, Michels VV, Groover RV, et al. Familial cavernous malformations of the central nervous system and retina. *Ann Neurol.* 1987;21:578-583.
5. Wyburn-Mason R. Arteriovenous aneurysm of midbrain and retina, facial nevi and mental changes. *Brain Dev.* 1943;66:163-203.
6. Shields JA, Decker WL, Sanborn GE, Augsburger JJ, Goldberg RE. Presumed acquired retinal hemangiomas. *Ophthalmology.* 1983;90:1292-1300.
7. Shields CL, Shields JA, Barrett J, De Potter P. Vasoproliferative tumors of the ocular fundus. Classification and clinical manifestations in 103 patients. *Arch Ophthalmol.* 1995;113:615-623.

Coats' Disease

Thomas M. Aaberg, Jr

INTRODUCTION

In 1908, George Coats, curator of the Royal London Ophthalmic Hospital, described an ophthalmic disease that was typically unilateral, had a predilection for healthy males, and resulted in focal deposition of exudates within the fundus and "peculiar" retinal vascular findings.[1]

CLINICAL FEATURES

The most common presenting signs in an affected child are strabismus and leukocoria. There is a gender predilection for Coats' disease, which affects males eight times more often than females. Although the majority of cases are unilateral, bilateral disease has been reported in up to 10% of cases.[2] Clinical findings vary depending on the stage of the disease. Early in the disease process, vascular telangiectasia occurs focally within the retina, most often near or anterior to the equator (Figure 58-1). The entire retinal vasculature (arteries, veins, and capillaries) appears to be affected. The caliber of the involved vessels varies as aneurysmal dilation and progressive telangiectasia occurs. The aneurysms may be saccular (sausage shaped) or bulbous (often described as having a light-bulb appearance).

DIFFERENTIAL DIAGNOSIS

The diagnosis of early stage Coats' disease is often straightforward. Foremost in the differential diagnosis is retinoblastoma, thereby making the stakes of an accurate diagnosis high (Table 58-1). Vitreoretinal traction rarely occurs in Coats' disease. In contrast, it frequently occurs in many childhood vitreoretinopathies that are associated retinal telangiectasia, such as familial exudative vitreoretinopathy, retinopathy of prematurity, persistent hyperplastic primary vitreous, incontinentia pigmenti, Norrie's disease, and retinal capillary hemangioma.

TREATMENT

The first line of treatment is laser photocoagulation and/or cryotherapy. The goal is to ablate the nonperfused retina and areas of telangiectasia. The entire area of retinal telangiectasia needs to be treated. The laser photocoagulation can only be performed in cases of absent or minimal exudative retinal detachment. Cases with a shallow exudative retinal detachment can be successfully

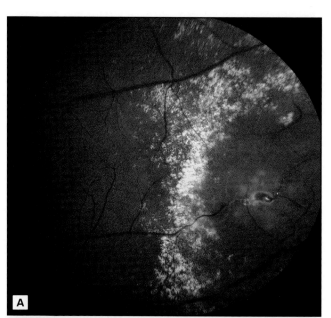

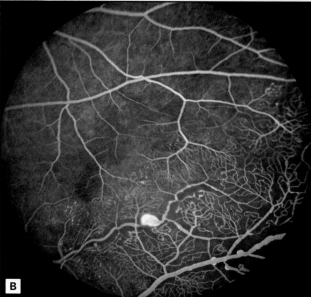

Figure 58-1. Fundus photograph of the left eye demonstrates the circinate lipid exudation surrounding retinal telangiectasia (A). Fluorescein angiography demonstrates the area of bulbous aneurysms, vascular telangiectasia, and areas of capillary nonperfusion (B).

Table 58-1. Coats' Disease and Retinoblastoma

Feature			Coats' Disease	Retinoblastoma
Demographic		Mean age at diagnosis	5 years	1.5 years
		Male	76%	50%
		Family history	0%	10%
Ophthalmic		Unilateral	95%	60%
		Retinal vessels	Irregular dilation with telangiectasia	Regular dilation and tortuosity
		Retinal mass	Absent	Present
		Retinal exudation	Present	Absent
		Vitreous seeds	Absent	Present
Diagnostic		USG	Retinal detachment	Retinal detachment with calcification
		CT scan	Calcification absent	Calcification present
		MRI	Retinal detachment	Retinal detachment with enhancing mass

USG, ultrasonography; CT, computed tomography; MRI, magnetic resonance imaging. (Adapted from Shields JA, Shields CL. Differentiation of Coats' disease and retinoblastoma. *J Pediatr Ophthalmol Strabismus*. 2001;38:262-266.)

treated with double freeze–thaw cryotherapy. Multiple treatment sessions every 3 months are usually necessary with either laser or cryotherapy.

PROGNOSIS

The natural history is usually of a progressive disease (Figure 58-2). Between 64% and 80% of eyes will become phthisical and develop advanced glaucoma or retinal detachment. Overall, it can be expected that roughly 75% of patients will have an anatomic improvement or stabilization of the affected eye with treatment.[3]

REFERENCES

1.　Coats G. Forms of retinal disease with massive exudation. *R Lond Ophthalm Hosp Rep.* 1908;17:440-525.
2.　Shields JA, Shields CL, Honavar SG, Demirci H. Clinical variations and complications of Coats disease in 150 cases: the 2000 Sanford Gifford Memorial Lecture. *Am J Ophthalmol.* 2001;131:561-571.
3.　Shields JA, Shields CL, Honavar SG, et al. Classification and management of Coats disease: the 2000 Proctor Lecture. *Am J Ophthalmol.* 2001;131:572-583.

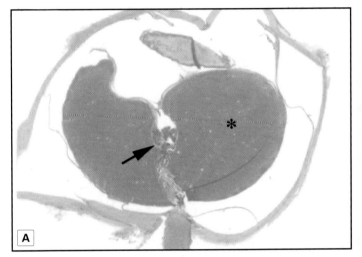

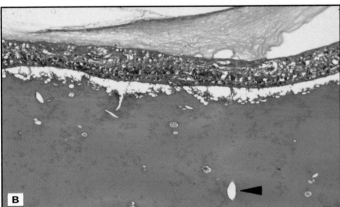

Figure 58-2. Enucleated eye with Coats' disease. Note the total exudative retinal detachment (arrow) and the subretinal exudate (asterisk) (Low-power, hematoxylin and eosin.) (A). Cystic degeneration, disorganization, and deposition of PAS-positive material in the outer retina. Cholesterol clefts are seen in the subretinal exudate (arrowhead). (High-power, hematoxylin and eosin.) (B).

Retinal Astrocytic Tumors

Mehryar Taban, Mehran Taban, and Arun D. Singh

INTRODUCTION

Retinal astrocytic tumors represent two distinct types of benign retinal astrocytic tumor: astrocytic hamartoma and "acquired" retinal astrocytoma. Retinal astrocytic hamartomas are more common and have a known association with tuberous sclerosis. Acquired retinal astrocytomas are rare astrocytic tumors that develop at any age, have no family history, and are not associated with tuberous sclerosis or other systemic syndromes.

RETINAL ASTROCYTIC HAMARTOMA

The astrocytic hamartoma of the retina and optic disc is a benign tumor that typically occurs in patients with tuberous sclerosis, although it can be seen in those with neurofibromatosis, retinitis pigmentosa, or as an isolated finding (Chapter 63).[1] Three ophthalmoscopic variants of retinal astrocytic hamartoma are recognized: the more common subtle, flat, round, semitranslucent lesion; the large, elevated, nodular, and calcified mulberry lesion; and the mixed type of lesion possessing features of the other two, being calcified in the central portion and semitranslucent in the periphery (Figure 59-1).

Differential Diagnosis

Despite the characteristic ophthalmoscopic features listed above, certain entities can closely resemble astrocytic hamartoma. Retinoblastoma, retinocytoma, myelinated nerve fibers, massive gliosis of the retina, retinal capillary hemangioma, and optic disc drusen can be difficult to differentiate ophthalmoscopically from astrocytic hamartoma (Table 59-1).

Treatment

Even though the great majority of retinal astrocytic hamartomas are asymptomatic, nonprogressive, and do not require treatment, ocular examination should be performed on an annual basis for possible associated exudative retinal detachment that may extend into the fovea. In these cases, laser photocoagulation can be employed. A patient with retinal astrocytic hamartomas should also be followed for other manifestations of tuberous sclerosis.

Association With Tuberous Sclerosis

The exact prevalence of retinal astrocytic hamartoma in tuberous sclerosis is not known. Approximately one third to half of patients with tuberous sclerosis have retinal or optic nerve hamartoma, and in half of these the hamartoma occur bilaterally (Chapter 63).[2]

Table 59-1. Differential Diagnosis of Astrocytic Hamartoma							
Diagnosis	Appearance	Calcification	Feeder Vessels	Exudation	RPE	Growth*	Association
Astrocytic hamartoma	Translucent or white mass	Present, yellow, spherical	Absent	Usually absent	Normal	Absent	Tuberous sclerosis
Retinoblastoma Retinocytoma	White mass	Present, white, chunky	Present Absent	Absent Absent	Normal Proliferation	Present Absent	13 q deletion syndrome
Myelinated nerve fibers	White patch, no mass	Absent	Vessels obscured	Absent	Normal	Absent	None
Massive gliosis of retina	White mass	May be present	Absent	May be present	Atrophy and proliferation	Absent	None
Retinal capillary hemangioma	Round red mass	Absent	Prominent	Present	Normal	May be present	VHL disease
Optic disc drusen	White mass	Present	Absent	Absent	Normal	Absent	Retinitis pigmentosa

*Short-term growth observed over weeks to months. RPE, retinal pigment epithelium; VHL, von Hippel-Lindau disease.

SECTION 5 Tumors of the Retina and Retinal Pigment Epithelium

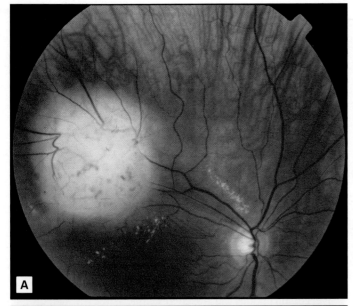

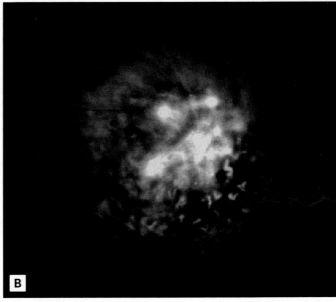

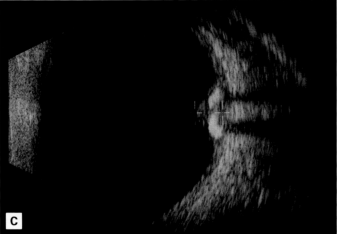

Figure 59-1. Fundus appearance of calcified large astrocytic hamartoma. Note surrounding retinal exudation (A). Fluorescein angiogram (arteriovenous phase) reveals fine intrinsic vessels (B). B-scan ultrasonograph indicative of intrinsic calcification (C). (Reproduced with permission from Giles J, Singh AD, Rundle PA, Noe KP, Rennie IG. Retinal astrocytic hamartoma with exudation. *Eye.* 2005;19:724-725.)

Prognosis

Although most astrocytic hamartomas remain stable, some become calcified over time.[3] In general, astrocytic hamartomas are silent, with an excellent visual prognosis. They are not known to undergo malignant transformation and have no tendency to metastasize. However, rarely, they have been associated with degenerative necrosis leading to vitreous seeding, vitreous or subretinal hemorrhage, and subretinal exudation or detachment.[4]

REFERENCES

1. Williams R, Taylor D. Tuberous sclerosis. *Surv Ophthalmol.* 1985;30:143-154.
2. Robertson DM. Ophthalmic manifestations of tuberous sclerosis. *Ann NY Acad Sci.* 1991;615:17-25.
3. Zimmer-Galler IE, Robertson DM. Long-term observation of retinal lesions in tuberous sclerosis. *Am J Ophthalmol.* 1995;119:318-324.
4. Shields JA, Eagle RC, Shields CL, et al. Aggressive retinal astrocytomas in 4 patients with tuberous sclerosis complex. *Arch Ophthalmol.* 2005;123:856-863.

Tumors of the Retinal Pigment Epithelium

Elias I. Traboulsi, Martin Heur, and Arun D. Singh

INTRODUCTION

Tumors of the retinal pigment epithelium (RPE) may be classified as reactive, hypertrophic, hamartomatous, and neoplastic (Table 60-1).[1] Those present at birth can be associated with systemic conditions such as familial adenomatous polyposis (FAP) or neurofibromatosis 2 (NF2). Acquired RPE tumors include benign and malignant lesions that are sometimes difficult to differentiate from choroidal neoplasms.

CONGENITAL HYPERTROPHY OF THE RETINAL PIGMENT EPITHELIUM

Congenital hypertrophy of the retinal pigment epithelium (CHRPE) is a round, darkly pigmented, flat lesion of the ocular fundus located at the level of the retinal pigment epithelium. In the older literature, CHRPE was classified as a benign melanoma of the retinal pigment epithelium (Figure 60-1).[2] CHRPE are isolated sporadic congenital lesions with no known underlying genetic basis. Punched-out hypopigmented or depigmented lacunae may be present, and occasionally the whole CHRPE patch is depigmented (albinotic patch of the fundus).

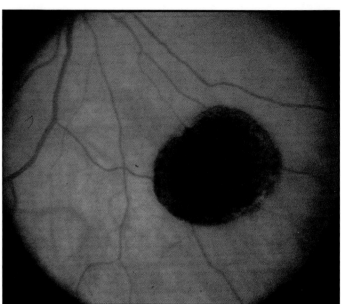

Figure 60-1. Solitary CHRPE. A sharply demarcated pigmented flat retinal lesion representing solitary CHRPE. The lighter area represents lacunae, which may enlarge slowly over many years.

Table 60-1. Classification of RPE Lesions				
Type	Subtype	Variants	Other Terminology	Association
Reactive	Hyperplasia			Trauma
	Metaplasia			Inflammation
				Toxicity
Hypertrophic	Solitary	Pigmented	Retinal nevus	None
		Non-pigmented	Benign melanoma of RPE	
	Grouped	Pigmented	Bear tracks	None
		Non-pigmented	Polar bear tracks	
	POFLs		Atypical CHRPE	Gardner syndrome
				Turcot syndrome
Hamartoma	RPE	Superficial	Congenital hamartoma	None
		Full-thickness		
		With intrinsic vascularization		
	RPE and retina		Combined hamartoma	Neurofibromatosis type 2
Neoplastic	Adenoma			CHRPE (rare)
	Adenocarcinoma			

RPE, retinal pigment epithelium; CHRPE, congenital hypertrophy of the retinal pigment epithelium; POFL, pigmented ocular fundus lesion.

Table 60-2. Differentiating Features of CHRPE and POFLs

Feature	CHRPE	Grouped Pigmentation	POFLs
Shape	Round	Variable	Oval
Depigmentation	Lacunae	Absent	Tail/lacunae
Size (basal diameter)	0.2-13 mm	Variable	0.15-4.5 mm
Laterality	Unilateral	Unilateral/ bilateral	Bilateral
Number	Solitary or grouped	Numerous	Four or more
Growth	Frequent but minimal	Unknown	Unknown
Malignant transformation	Rare	Never	Never
Histopathology (RPE changes)	Hypertrophy Hyperplasia	Hypertrophy	Hypertrophy Hyperplasia Hamartoma
Systemic association	None	None	Gardner syndrome, Turcot syndrome

RPE, retinal pigment epithelium; CHRPE, congenital hypertrophy of the retinal pigment epithelium; POFL, pigmented ocular fundus lesion.

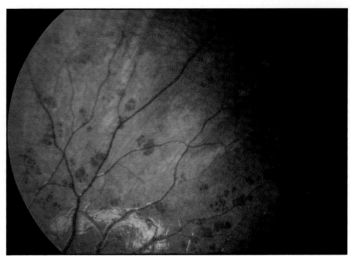

Figure 60-2. Multiple grouped pigmented lesions (grouped CHRPE) reminiscent of bear tracks.

Treatment is not necessary except for the very rare instance in which neovascularization develops at the edge of the CHRPE lesion.

Prognosis

CHRPE is a benign lesion that does not enlarge significantly, except in rare instances.[3] The development of nodules at the edge of CHRPE lesions, suggestive of RPE adenoma, has been rarely observed.[4]

CONGENITAL GROUPED PIGMENTATION OF THE RETINAL PIGMENT EPITHELIUM

Multiple areas of circumscribed and flat retinal pigmentation arranged in clusters are described as congenital grouped pigmentation of the RPE.[5] Such an appearance is suggestive of animal footprints—so-called bear tracks or animal tracks (Figure 60-2). In the majority of cases, involvement is unilateral (84%) and is limited to one sector.

PIGMENTED OCULAR FUNDUS LESIONS

Pigmented ocular fundus lesions (POFL) is a descriptive term that refers to fundus lesions observed in patients with Gardner syndrome and Turcot syndrome (Figure 60-3).[6]

There are distinct ophthalmoscopic features that distinguish CHRPE from POFL (Table 60-2).

SIMPLE HAMARTOMA OF THE RETINAL PIGMENT EPITHELIUM

Simple hamartoma of the RPE is a discrete, small (0.5 to 1.0 mm), black nodule in the macular area.

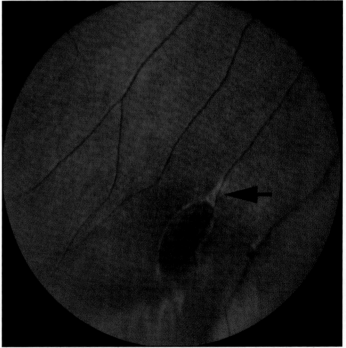

Figure 60-3. POFLs in the right eye of a patient with Gardner syndrome. Two oval pigmented retinal lesions are evident. Note depigmentation along the posterior margin (arrow).

ADENOMA AND ADENOCARCINOMA OF THE RETINAL PIGMENT EPITHELIUM

These are rare acquired tumors of the RPE. The differentiation between adenoma and adenocarcinoma can only be made on the basis of histopathologic findings because of similar clinical findings in both types of tumors.[7] The tumors are usually dark brown to black in color (Figure 60-4). Prominent retinal feeder vessels and exudative retinal detachment are usually present. The presence of surrounding retinal hard exudates is an important diagnostic feature, as it is almost never associated with untreated choroidal melanoma.

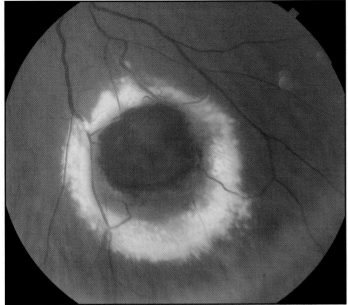

Figure 60-4. RPE adenoma. A circumscribed, dark, elevated nodular lesion involving the retina. (This figure was published in Singh AD. CHRPE and other pigmented RPE lesions. In: Huang D, Kaiser P, Lowder CY, Traboulsi EI, eds. *Retinal Imaging*, 519-523. © Elsevier 2006.)

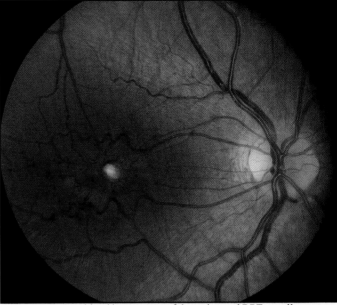

Figure 60-5. Combined hamartoma of the retina and RPE usually appears as a unilateral gray-black colored lesion with epiretinal membrane.

COMBINED HAMARTOMA OF THE RETINA AND RETINAL PIGMENT EPITHELIUM

Combined hamartoma of the retina and RPE (CHR), a term first coined by Gass, is a rare developmental disorder involving the retina and the RPE.[8] The tumor is gray-black in color and typically has an epiretinal membrane that may cause retinal traction (Figure 60-5).

REFERENCES

1. Gass JD. Focal congenital anomalies of the retinal pigment epithelium. *Eye.* 1989;3:1-18.
2. Jones IS, Reese AB. Benign melanomas of the retinal pigment epithelium. *Am J Ophthalmol.* 1956;42:207-212.
3. Shields CL, Mashayekhi A, Ho T, et al. Solitary congenital hypertrophy of the retinal pigment epithelium: clinical features and frequency of enlargement in 330 patients. *Ophthalmology.* 2003;110:1968-1976.
4. Shields JA, Shields CL, Singh AD. Acquired tumors arising from congenital hypertrophy of the retinal pigment epithelium. *Arch Ophthalmol.* 2000;118:637-641.
5. Santos A, Humayun M, Traboulsi EI. Congenital abnormalities of the retinal pigment epithelium. In: Traboulsi EI, ed. *Genetic Diseases of the Eye.* New York, NY: Oxford Press; 1998.
6. Traboulsi EI, Krush AJ, Gardner EJ, et al. Prevalence and importance of pigmented ocular fundus lesions in Gardner's syndrome. *N Engl J Med.* 1987;316:661-667.
7. Shields JA, Shields CL, Gunduz K, Eagle RC Jr. Neoplasms of the retinal pigment epithelium: the 1998 Albert Ruedemann Sr, memorial lecture, part 2. *Arch Ophthalmol.* 1999;117:601-608.
8. Gass JD. An unusual hamartoma of the pigment epithelium and retina simulating choroidal melanoma and retinoblastoma. *Trans Am Ophthalmol Soc.* 1973;71:171-183; discussions 184-185.

Tumors of the Ciliary Pigment Epithelium

Javier Elizalde, María de la Paz, and Rafael I. Barraquer

INTRODUCTION

Tumors arising from the ciliary epithelium may be grouped as congenital and acquired (Table 61-1).[1]

CONGENITAL TUMORS OF CILIARY EPITHELIUM

These tumors arise from the primitive medullary epithelium, before its differentiation into its various adult derivatives. Thus, they tend to become clinically apparent in young children and have an embryonic appearance histologically.

Glioneuroma is perhaps the rarest tumor in the group, with only a few cases reported in the literature.[2]

MEDULLOEPITHELIOMA

Clinical Features

Medulloepithelioma is typically a disease of childhood that becomes clinically apparent during the first decade of life.[3,4] The tumor is an irregular, variably sized white or gray translucent mass arising from the ciliary region (Figure 61-1). The presence of cysts within the tumor is of diagnostic importance (Figure 61-2).[3,4] Iris neovascularization is a common and early finding in eyes with medulloepithelioma.[5]

Pathology

According to Zimmerman's classification, medulloepithelioma may be divided into non-teratoid and teratoid types, and either may have benign or malignant cytologic features (see Table 61-1). The nonteratoid medulloepithelioma contains multilayered sheets of cords of poorly differentiated neuroepithelial cells that are histologically similar to the embryonic retina and ciliary epithelium. In contrast, the teratoid type demonstrates variable degrees of heteroplasia (hyaline cartilage, rhabdomyoblasts, undifferentiated mesenchymal cells resembling embryonal sarcoma).

Management

Because most of these tumors are cytologically malignant and infiltrate the adjacent vitreous, enucleation is usually advisable. In carefully selected small tumors (<3 clock hours), local removal by iridocyclectomy or brachytherapy may be a good option.[6]

Table 61-1. Classification of Ciliary Epithelium Tumors				
Congenital	Glioneuroma			
	Medulloepithelioma	Teratoid	Benign	
			Malignant	
		Non-teratoid	Benign	
			Malignant	
Acquired	Pseudoadenomatous hyperplasia	Reactive		
		Age-related (Fuchs' or coronal adenoma)		
	Adenoma			
	Adenocarcinoma			

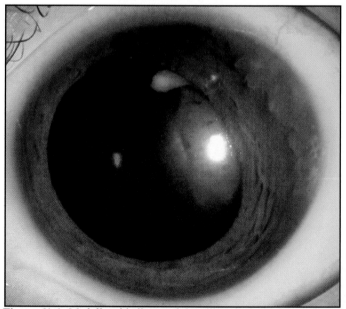

Figure 61-1. Medulloepithelioma of the ciliary body. Note translucent mass behind the iris and invading the anterior chamber through the iris root.

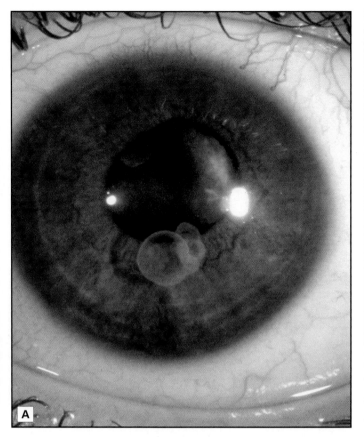

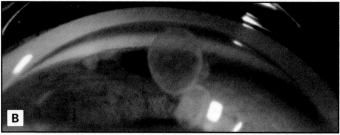

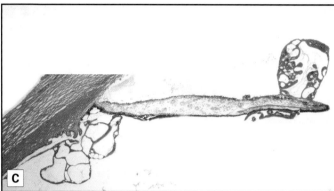

Figure 61-2. Anterior chamber cysts secondary to medulloepithelioma of the ciliary body (A). Multiple cysts within the anterior chamber and emerging through the pupil (gonioscopic photographs) (B). Histopathologic composite photograph showing a cyst adherent to the anterior border layer of the iris, another one behind the iris, and some cysts near the ciliary body (Hematoxylin and eosin x35) (C).

ACQUIRED TUMORS OF THE CILIARY EPITHELIUM

Pseudoadenomatous Hyperplasia (Reactive Proliferation)

Age-Related Hyperplasia (Fuchs' or Coronal Adenoma)

This is commonly observed as an opaque white mass, usually confined to a ciliary process in eyes removed surgically or post mortem with little clinical significance.[7]

Reactive Hyperplasia

The nonpigmented ciliary epithelium contributes to the development of a cyclitic membrane.

Adenoma and Adenocarcinoma of the Ciliary Epithelium

True acquired neoplasms of the pigmented or non-pigmented ciliary epithelium are relatively rare. Similar tumors arise from the pigment epithelium in the region of the iris and from the retinal pigment epithelium (Chapter 60).

REFERENCES

1. Zimmerman LE. The remarkable polymorphism of tumours of the ciliary epithelium. *Trans Aust Coll Ophthalmol.* 1970;2:114-125.
2. Kivela T, Kauniskangas L, Miettinen P, Tarkkanen A. Glioneuroma associated with colobomatous dysplasia of the anterior uvea and retina. A case simulating medulloepithelioma. *Ophthalmology.* 1989;96:1799-1808.
3. Broughton WL, Zimmerman LE. A clinicopathologic study of 56 cases of intraocular medulloepitheliomas. *Am J Ophthalmol.* 1978;85:407-418.
4. Shields JA, Eagle RC Jr, Shields CL, Potter PD. Congenital neoplasms of the nonpigmented ciliary epithelium (medulloepithelioma). *Ophthalmology.* 1996;103:1998-2006.
5. Singh A, Singh AD, Shields CL, Shields JA. Iris neovascularization in children as a manifestation of underlying medulloepithelioma. *J Pediatr Ophthalmol Strabismus.* 2001;38:224-228.
6. Balmer A, Munier F, Uffer S, et al. Medullo-epithelioma: presentation of 3 cases. *Klin Monatsbl Augenheilkd.* 1996;208:377-380.
7. Zaidman GW, Johnson BL, Salamon SM, Mondino BJ. Fuchs' adenoma affecting the peripheral iris. *Arch Ophthalmol.* 1983;101:771-773.

Lymphoma of the Retina and Central Nervous System

Arun D. Singh, Hilel Lewis, Andrew P. Schachat, and David Peereboom

INTRODUCTION

Primary lymphoma of the central nervous system (CNS) is now considered to be a variant of extranodal non-Hodgkin's lymphoma (NHL) that arises from specific sites such as the brain, spinal cord, meninges, or eyes, and is called primary CNS lymphoma (PCNSL).[1] Primary intraocular lymphoma (PCNSL-O) is a variant of PCNSL with predominantly ophthalmic involvement. Ophthalmic involvement with other forms of lymphoma is usually orbital, conjunctival, or uveal, in contrast to vitreoretinal involvement in PCNSL-O.

CLINICAL FEATURES

PCNSL is typically a disease of the elderly, with a mean age of about 60 years.[2,3] Intraocular involvement may precede, occur simultaneously, or follow the CNS disease. In general, intraocular involvement is the presenting feature in PCNSL-O and subsequent CNS involvement occurs in 56% to 85% of patients over a period of months to years. Conversely, about 20% of patients with PCNSL have concurrent intraocular involvement.

Ophthalmic

The most frequent symptoms are of painless blurred vision, floaters, or both. Bilateral involvement occurs in up to 80% of cases.[4] Owing to the nonspecific nature of the ophthalmic manifestations, a diagnosis of PCNSL-O is difficult to make on clinical grounds alone, and a delay in diagnosis is common. The most common manifestations are of a posterior uveitis or vitritis (50%), combined anterior and posterior uveitis (22%), and chorioretinitis, or subretinal pigment epithelial infiltrates (18%) (Figures 62-1 and 62-2).[5]

Central Nervous System

The brain, spinal cord, and meninges, either separately or in various combinations, can be involved. The lesions in the CNS tend to be periventricular in location, thus allowing access to cerebrospinal fluid (CSF) and meninges.

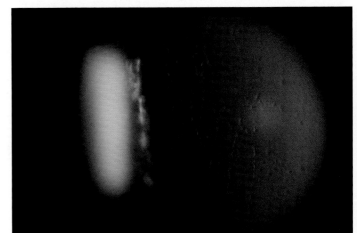

Figure 62-1. Slit-lamp photograph (retroillumination) showing vitreous cellular infiltrate.

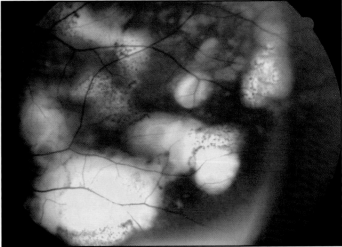

Figure 62-2. Fundus photograph of the left eye demonstrating multiple creamy subretinal pigment epithelial deposits. These deposits regressed following external beam radiotherapy (45 Gy).

This chapter is modified from Singh AD, Lewis H, Schachat AP. Primary lymphoma of the central nervous system. *Ophthalmol Clin North AM.* 2005;18:199-207.

David Peereboom, MD, has received research support from Novartis and Schering Plough and is on the speakers' bureau of Schering Plough.

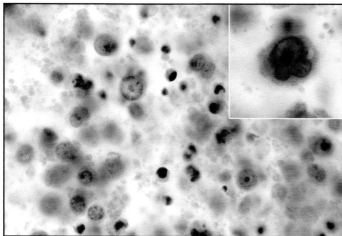

Figure 62-3. Vitrectomy sample containing large atypical lymphocytes, necrotic lymphoid cells, and nuclear debris. Inset shows characteristic nuclear membrane protrusions and a prominent nucleolus (main figure, Millipore filter, hematoxylin and eosin, original magnification x250).

DIAGNOSTIC EVALUATION

It is imperative that all cases of PCNSL-O be thoroughly evaluated to exclude CNS involvement at the initial diagnosis, and periodically thereafter. Conversely, periodic ophthalmic examinations should be part of the diagnostic evaluation and subsequent management of a patient diagnosed with PCNSL.

Ophthalmic

Diagnostic vitrectomy should be considered in middle-aged or older patients with "idiopathic" unilateral or bilateral recurrent uveitis, or uveitis that is unresponsive to steroids. Neoplastic cells can be identified by an experienced cytologist using an array of techniques, such as liquid-based cytology, cytospin, and cell-block preparations stained with modified Papanicolaou, Giemsa, or standard hematoxylin and eosin stains (Figure 62-3).

Central Nervous System

Ophthalmic craniospinal magnetic resonance imaging (MRI) with gadolinium is the diagnostic procedure of choice. Cranial lesions appear as multiple isointense nodules on T1-MRI and demonstrate characteristic dense and diffuse contrast enhancement (Figure 62-4). Meningeal enhancement with gadolinium is indicative of meningeal involvement. The presence of malignant lymphocytes in the CSF is confirmatory. The CSF shows lymphocytic pleocytosis, raised protein concentration, and normal or low glucose.

TREATMENT

As PCNSL is very sensitive to corticosteroids, treatment should be withheld in suspected cases until a tissue diagnosis is obtained. The treatment of PCNSL is still evolving, and some of the guiding principles are discussed below (Figure 62-5).

Ophthalmic

Traditional therapy with ocular radiation (40 Gy in divided doses) controls ocular involvement in the majority of cases,[6] but most progress to develop CNS disease (see Figure 62-4).[4] Irradia-

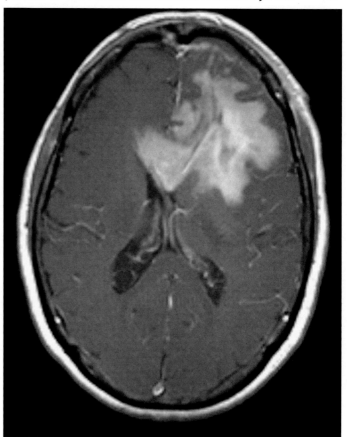

Figure 62-4. T1-weighted MRI scan of the brain with gadolinium, showing a diffusely enhancing area in the left frontal lobe.

tion of both eyes (because of the high incidence of bilaterality) should be strongly considered for patients with proven PCNSL-O. Because radiation therapy to the brain may have significant side effects, its use for prophylaxis in patients without proven CNS involvement is not advisable. Instead, high-dose methotrexate (8 g/m²) in combination with intrathecal methotrexate and other agents may be considered.[7,8] Intravitreal methotrexate as an initial treatment, or for those with recurrence following ocular radiation therapy, has been investigated in a small number of patients with encouraging results.[9]

Central Nervous System

Until recently, whole-brain radiotherapy was the mainstay of treatment, which improved the median survival from 4 months to about 12 to 18 months in untreated patients.[10]

As the blood–brain barrier is a limiting factor that restricts drug entry into the CNS, various strategies to circumvent it have been developed. These include the use of high doses, intrathecal drug delivery, intraventricular drug delivery by a reservoir, and temporary disruption of the blood–brain barrier with mannitol infusion.[2,7] Preliminary data suggest that a median survival of about 50 months, which is comparable to that achieved with a combination of radiation therapy and chemotherapy, can be achieved by chemotherapy alone.[11] However, the treatment of PCNSL is still evolving and is currently being investigated within a framework of international multidisciplinary collaborative studies.

PROGNOSIS

Most patients die within 2 years of diagnosis as a result of progressive or recurrent CNS disease.

REFERENCES

1. Hochberg FH, Miller DC. Primary central nervous system lymphoma. *J Neurosurg.* 1988;68:835-853.
2. Char DH, Ljung BM, Miller T, Phillips T. Primary intraocular lymphoma (ocular reticulum cell sarcoma) diagnosis and management. *Ophthalmology.* 1988;95:625-630.
3. Whitcup SM, de Smet MD, Rubin BI, et al. Intraocular lymphoma. Clinical and histopathologic diagnosis. *Ophthalmology.* 1993;100:1399-1406.
4. Peterson K, Gordon KB, Heinemann MH, DeAngelis LM. The clinical spectrum of ocular lymphoma. *Cancer.* 1993;72:843-849.
5. Freeman LN, Schachat AP, Knox DL, et al. Clinical features, laboratory investigations, and survival in ocular reticulum cell sarcoma. *Ophthalmology.* 1987;94:1631-1639.
6. Margolis L, Fraser R, Lichter A, Char DH. The role of radiation therapy in the management of ocular reticulum cell sarcoma. *Cancer.* 1980;45:688-692.
7. Sandor V, Stark-Vancs V, Pearson D, et al. Phase II trial of chemotherapy alone for primary CNS and intraocular lymphoma. *J Clin Oncol.* 1998;16:3000-3006.
8. Hormigo A, DeAngelis LM. Primary ocular lymphoma: clinical features, diagnosis, and treatment. *Clin Lymphoma.* 2003;4:22-29.
9. Singh AD, Lewis H, Schachat AP. Primary lymphoma of the central nervous system. *Ophthalmol Clin North Am.* 2005;18:199-207.
10. Deangelis LM, Hormigo A. Treatment of primary central nervous system lymphoma. *Semin Oncol.* 2004;31:684-692.
11. Pels H, Schmidt-Wolf IG, Glasmacher A, et al. Primary central nervous system lymphoma: results of a pilot and phase II study of systemic and intraventricular chemotherapy with deferred radiotherapy. *J Clin Oncol.* 2003;21:4489-4495.

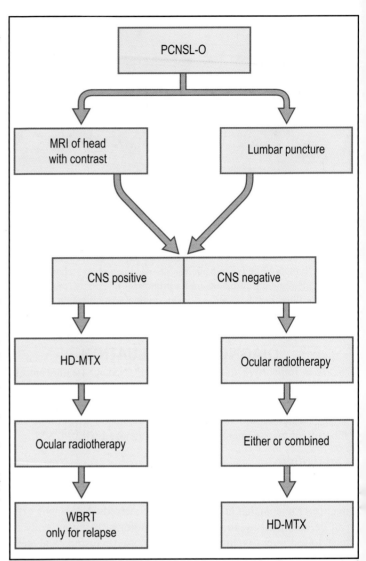

Figure 62-5. Schema outlining our current approach of management of patients with PCNSL-O. HD-MTX, high-dose methotrexate; WBRT, wholebrain radiation therapy.

Ocular Paraneoplastic Diseases

Rishi P. Singh and Arun D. Singh

INTRODUCTION

Paraneoplastic disorders are defined as syndromes in which the end-organ effect is not a direct consequence of the mass or of distant metastasis.[1] Instead, an autoimmune response to the primary tumor causes end-organ disorder and dysfunction. The temporal relationship of paraneoplastic illnesses can occur before, at the time of diagnosis, and even after the identification of the primary malignancy, and in rare cases the primary may never be discovered.

Ocular paraneoplastic diseases include a wide range of clinical manifestations, ranging from color deficiencies to complete blindness. Their diagnosis is complicated by the fact that cancers can by themselves cause remote ocular effects due to toxicity from antineoplastic agents, nutritional deficiencies, and direct opportunistic infections. This chapter summarizes the salient features of cancer-associated retinopathy (CAR), melanoma-associated retinopathy (MAR), bilateral diffuse uveal melanocytic proliferation (BDUMP), paraneoplastic optic neuropathy, and opsoclonus manifesting as paraneoplastic ocular disease (Table 63-1).[2]

CANCER-ASSOCIATED RETINOPATHY

CAR is most commonly associated with small cell carcinoma of the lung, followed by gynecological and breast carcinomas.

Clinical Features

Cancer-associated retinopathy is characterized by painless progressive visual loss over weeks to months. Initial complaints are of dimming of vision and positive visual phenomena, such as shimmering lights. Early in the course, the eye may appear to be entirely normal. Posterior segment findings predominate and include narrowing of the retinal vessels, chorioretinal atrophy, and optic nerve atrophy. Vitritis, periphebitis, and arteriolar sheathing occur later in the disease course.[2]

Diagnostic Evaluation

On visual field testing, the most common finding is a constriction within the central 20 degrees of visual fields. Electroretinographic studies are confirmatory. The classic pattern is of suppressed phototopic and scotopic responses (Figure 63-1).[3] It is also possible to obtain serum assays for several antiretinal antibodies, such as anti-recoverin antibodies and anti-enolase antibodies from commercial laboratories.[4]

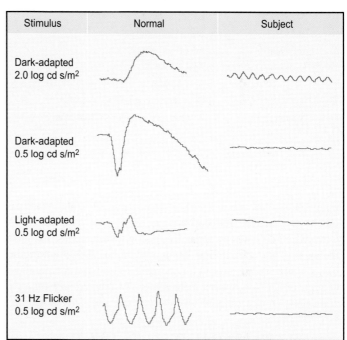

Stimulus	Normal	Subject
Dark-adapted 2.0 log cd s/m²		
Dark-adapted 0.5 log cd s/m²		
Light-adapted 0.5 log cd s/m²		
31 Hz Flicker 0.5 log cd s/m²		

Figure 63-1. A 67-year-old man with a known history of lung cancer presented with halos in both eyes. Electroretinograms recorded from a normal control subject and from the patient. Responses recorded from the two eyes of the patient were averaged together. Extinguished ERG responses in the patient were suggestive of cancer-associated retinopathy. (Courtesy of Neal Peachey, PhD.)

Treatment

Intravenous high-dose methylprednisone and, less commonly, oral steroids have shown benefit in reversing the visual changes seen early in the illness. Once photoreceptor degeneration has begun, steroid use only stabilizes vision.[5]

MELANOMA-ASSOCIATED RETINOPATHY

MAR typically occurs after diagnosis, when metastatic disease is present.[6] As with CAR, patients with MAR have antibodies toward tumor antigens that cross-react with antigens on bipolar cells.[7] Patients typically report shimmering, flickering photopsias, peripheral scotomas, acute-onset night blindness, and slowly progressive visual loss. Patients typically have near-normal visual acuity, color vision, and central visual fields. Few patients

SECTION 5   Tumors of the Retina and Retinal Pigment Epithelium

Table 63-1. Paraneoplastic Retinopathies

Feature	CAR	MAR	BDUMP
Symptoms	Bilateral visual loss Positive visual phenomenon Nyctalopia	Near normal acuities Normal color vision Normal central visual fields	Severe visual loss Cutaneous/mucosal focal melanocytic proliferation
Fundus examination	Vessel attenuation, chorioretinal atrophy, optic atrophy	Majority have normal appearance Few have vascular attenuation, RPE changes, and vitreous cells	Multiple elevated uveal melanocytic tumors Exudative retinal detachment
Visual field	Central/paracentral scotoma	Paracentral scotoma	Central/paracentral scotomas
ERG findings	Depressed scotopic and photopic response	Negative ERG	Depressed scotopic and photopic response
Associated malignancy	Lung carcinoma (small cell) Gynecological carcinoma Breast carcinoma	Cutaneous melanoma	Small cell carcinoma and others
Antibodies	Anti-recoverin Anti-enolase Anti-65-kDA Heat shock cognate protein 70	Rod bipolar on cells	Not known
Prognosis	Progression to severe visual loss	Progression to severe visual loss	Progression to severe visual loss

CAR, cancer-associated retinopathy; MAR, melanoma-associated retinopathy; BDUMP, bilateral diffuse uveal melanocytic proliferation.

manifest fundus changes. MAR manifests ERG abnormalities, including absent or reduced b-waves even after dark adaptation with preserved a-waves. A positive history of cutaneous malignant melanoma and circulating immunoglobulin (Ig)-G antibodies directed toward human rod bipolar cells establishes the diagnosis (Figure 63-2). Aggressive management of the primary tumor in addition to immunosuppressive therapy are under investigation.

BILATERAL DIFFUSE UVEAL MELANOCYTIC PROLIFERATION (PARANEOPLASTIC MELANOCYTIC PROLIFERATION)

BDUMP is a rare but recognized paraneoplastic disorder that causes bilateral painless visual loss in patients with systemic carcinomas. The primary tumor can arise from numerous sites, but gynecological neoplasms, including those of the ovary, cervix, and uterus, predominate.[2] It is believed that production of hormonal or other oncogenic stimulus by the primary carcinoma causes activation and proliferation of pre-existing nevus cells within the uveal tract, mucosal membranes, and skin.[8] As the proliferation of melanocytes is not limited to the uvea, paraneoplastic melanocytic proliferation may be a better descriptive term.[8] Patients typically manifest severe progressive visual loss over months to years. The typical fundus pattern consists of multiple elevated red round patches at the level of the retinal pigment epithelium (Figure 63-3).[9]

Diagnostic Evaluation

The angiographic findings consist of early hyperfluorescence due to focal destruction of the pigment epithelium and sparing of the choriocapillaris. In late frames, there is marked choroidal hyperfluorescence with patches of hypofluorescence.[9]

Treatment

No treatment has been shown to prevent severe visual loss in patients with BDUMP.

PARANEOPLASTIC OPTIC NEUROPATHIES

Paraneoplastic optic neuropathies occur within the clinical spectrum of cerebellar and brainstem paraneoplastic disorders.[10]

OPSOCLONUS

Opsoclonus is part of a larger group of ocular disorders caused by paraneoplastic cerebellar degeneration.[11]

REFERENCES

1. Sawyer RA, Selhorst JB, Zimmerman LE, Hoyt WF. Blindness caused by photoreceptor degeneration as a remote effect of cancer. *Am J Ophthalmol.* 1976;81:606-613.
2. Chan JW. Paraneoplastic retinopathies and optic neuropathies. *Surv Ophthalmol.* 2003;48:12-38.
3. Scholl HP, Zrenner E. Electrophysiology in the investigation of acquired retinal disorders. *Surv Ophthalmol.* 2000;45:29-47.
4. Thirkill CE, Keltner JL, Tyler NK, Roth AM. Antibody reactions with retina and cancer-associated antigens in 10 patients with cancer-associated retinopathy. *Arch Ophthalmol.* 1993;111:931-937.

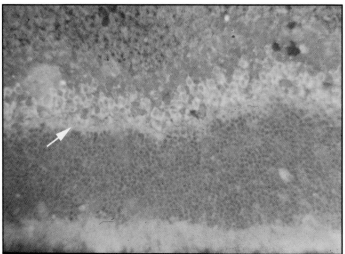

Figure 63-2. A 64-year-old man with a history of malignant melanoma of the maxillary sinus presented with photopsia, difficulty with night vision, and reduced peripheral visual field OU. An electroretinogram showed marked reduction in the b-wave amplitude under scotopic testing conditions to a bright flash. Indirect immunofluorescence was performed on cryosections of unfixed human retina using serum and IgG from the patient. Fluorescein isothiocyanate-labeled antihuman IgG and IgM were used as secondary antibodies. A weak but specific labeling of bipolar cells was observed (arrow). (Reprinted from Singh AD, Milam AH, Shields CL, et al. Melanoma-associated retinopathy. *Am J Ophthalmol.* 1995;119:369-370.)

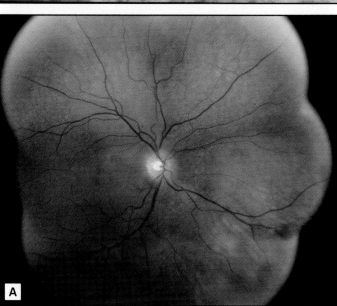
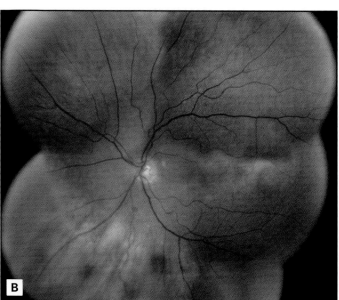

Figure 63-3. A 56-year-old woman presented with progressive deteriorating vision in both eyes for the past 6 months. The onset of visual symptoms coincided with the diagnosis of large cell carcinoma of the lung. She was not known to have metastases and was receiving chemotherapy. The corrected visual acuity was 20/40 in the right eye and 20/60 in the left. Anterior segment examination was unremarkable. On ophthalmoscopic examination, the choroid was diffusely thickened in both eyes (A, right eye; B, left eye). (Reproduced with permission from Singh AD, Rundle PA, Slater DN, et al. Uveal and cutaneous involvement in paraneoplastic melanocytic proliferation. *Arch Ophthalmol.* 2003;121:1637-1640. Copyright © 2003 American Medical Association. All rights reserved.)

5. Keltner JL, Thirkill CE, Tyler NK, Roth AM. Management and monitoring of cancer associated retinopathy. *Arch Ophthalmol.* 1992;110:48-53.

6. Singh AD, Milam AH, Shields CL, et al. Melanoma-associated retinopathy. *Am J Ophthalmol.* 1995;119:369-370.

7. Milam AH, Saari JC, Jacobson SG, et al. Autoantibodies against retinal bipolar cells in cutaneous melanoma-associated retinopathy. *Invest Ophthalmol Vis Sci.* 1993;34:91-100.

8. Singh AD, Rundle PA, Slater DN, et al. Uveal and cutaneous involvement in paraneoplastic melanocytic proliferation. *Arch Ophthalmol.* 2003;121:1637-1640.

9. Gass JD, Gieser RG, Wilkinson CP, et al. Bilateral diffuse uveal melanocytic proliferation in patients with occult carcinoma. *Arch Ophthalmol.* 1990;108:527-533.

10. Cross SA, Salomao DR, Parisi JE, et al. Paraneoplastic autoimmune optic neuritis with retinitis defined by CRMP-5-IgG. *Ann Neurol.* 2003;54:38-50.

11. Luque FA, Furneaux HM, Ferziger R, et al. Anti-Ri: an antibody associated with paraneoplastic opsoclonus and breast cancer. *Ann Neurol.* 1991;29:241-251.

Material presented in this chapter was published in Singh AD, Damato BE, Pe'er J, Murphree AL, Perry JD. *Clinical Ophthalmic Oncology.* © Elsevier 2007.

Neuro-Oculocutaneous Syndromes (Phakomatoses)

Arun D. Singh, Elias I. Traboulsi, and Lynn Schoenfield

INTRODUCTION

The term *phakomatoses* is derived from the Greek word phakos, which means birth mark.[1] Common features of the phakomatoses include a predominance of neural and ocular involvement, with variable cutaneous and visceral manifestations (Table 64-1). The characteristic systemic manifestations of the phakomatoses are due to the development of hamartomas, which are benign tumors arising from tissues normally present in a specific organ (Box 64-1). Advances in molecular genetics have led to the identification of genes responsible for von Hippel-Lindau disease, tuberous sclerosis, and neurofibromatosis, and have allowed molecular genetic diagnosis (Table 64-2).

NEUROFIBROMATOSIS TYPE 1

Several distinct forms of neurofibromatosis have now been recognized. The most frequent type is neurofibromatosis type 1 (von Recklinghausen's disease), followed by neurofibromatosis type 2 (also called central neurofibromatosis). Other rare types include multiple meningiomatosis, spinal schwannomatosis, and segmental neurofibromatosis.

NF1 is one of the most common genetic disorders, with protean manifestations involving neural tissues (Figure 64-1).[2] The disease has a prevalence of about 1/3000, with equal distribution in various ethnic groups.[1,2] The National Institutes of Health Consensus Development Conference has suggested clinical criteria diagnostic for NF1 (Table 64-3). Significant ocular findings in NF1 are summarized in Table 64-4.

NEUROFIBROMATOSIS TYPE 2

NF2 is also called "central NF" because the majority of its manifestations are related to central nervous system involvement. Unlike NF1, cutaneous findings are not a predominant feature of NF2. In contrast to neurofibromas, which are hallmarks of NF1, schwannomas are the characteristic tumors of NF2 (Table 64-5).

Bilateral vestibular schwannomas (VS) are diagnostic of NF2 (Figure 64-2).[3] Ocular abnormalities are present in more than two thirds of cases and include cataracts, retinal hamartomas, and ocular motility disorders (Box 64-2).[4]

Box 64-1. The Characteristic Features of Phakomatoses

- Neuro-oculocutaneous syndrome
- Systemic hamartomatoses
- Familial predisposition to cancer
- Autosomal dominant inheritance (few exceptions)

VON HIPPEL-LINDAU DISEASE

It was not until 1964 that Melmon and Rosen established the clinical spectrum of von Hippel-Lindau disease (VHL) when they reported cases of von Hippel's disease and Lindau's disease with overlapping manifestations.[5]

VHL disease is a multisystem disorder with a predilection for the retina and central nervous system (CNS). Significant clinical manifestations of VHL disease are included in the diagnostic criteria (Table 64-6). Retinal capillary hemangiomas (RCHs) occur in less than 75% of cases, CNS hemangiomas in more than 50% of cases, renal carcinomas in less than 50% of cases, and pheochromocytomas in less than 25% (Figure 64-3).[6]

TUBEROUS SCLEROSIS COMPLEX

The term *tuberous sclerosis* is based on the neuropathologic observations of multiple potato-like (tubers) lesions in the brain.[7] TSC includes two genetic diseases (TSC1 and TSC2) with dominant inheritance and high penetrance (95%).[8]

The hamartomas in the brain (astrocytoma and ependymoma) lead to childhood seizures and mental retardation. The skin manifestations (facial angiofibromas, subungual fibromas, hypomelanotic macules, and shagreen patches) are mainly of diagnostic significance (Figure 64-4). The ocular involvement is limited to the retina. Visceral hamartomas most commonly involve the lungs, kidney, and heart.[8] The classic triad of epilepsy, mental retardation, and adenoma sebaceum is present in only one third of cases (Table 64-7).[9]

Table 64-1. Organ System Involvement in Various Phakomatoses

Disorder	Clinical Features			
	Neurological	Ocular	Cutaneous	Visceral
Neurofibromatosis 1	Present	Present	Present	Absent
Neurofibromatosis 2	Present	Absent	Absent	Absent
Von Hippel-Lindau disease	Present	Present	Absent	Present
Tuberous sclerosis complex (I)	Present	Present	Present	Present
Tuberous sclerosis complex (II)	Present	Present	Present	Present
Sturge-Weber syndrome	Present	Present	Present	Absent
Wyburn-Mason syndrome	Present	Present	Absent	Absent
Retinal cavernous hemangioma	Present	Present	Absent	Absent
Sebaceous nevus syndrome	Present	Present	Present	Absent
Ataxia-telangiectasia	Present	Present	Present	Present
Neurocutaneous melanosis	Present	Variable	Present	Absent
Phakomatosis pigmentovascularis	Variable	Variable	Present	Absent

Table 64-2. Inheritance Pattern of Various Phakomatoses

Disorder	Inheritance	Genetic Locus	Gene	Protein	Function
Neurofibromatosis 1	Autosomal dominant	17q11	NF1	Neurofibromin	Inhibits ras activity
Neurofibromatosis 2	Autosomal dominant	22q12	NF2	Merlin/ Schwannomin	Links cytoskeletal proteins and cell membrane
Von Hippel-Lindau disease	Autosomal dominant	3p25	VHL	pVHL	Inhibits mRNA elongation
Tuberous sclerosis complex (I)	Autosomal dominant	9q34	TSC1	Hamartin	Regulates vesicular movement
Tuberous sclerosis complex (II)	Autosomal dominant	16p13	TSC2	Tuberin	Inhibits GTP binding proteins
Sturge-Weber syndrome	Sporadic	-	-	-	-
Wyburn-Mason syndrome	Sporadic	-	-	-	-
Retinal cavernous hemangioma	Autosomal dominant	3q, 7p, 7q	-	-	-
Sebaceous nevus syndrome	Sporadic	-	-	-	-
Ataxia-telangiectasia	Autosomal recessive	11q22	ATM	ATM protein	Protein kinase
Neurocutaneous melanosis	Sporadic	-	-	-	-
Phakomatosis pigmentovascularis	Sporadic	-	-	-	-

Table 64-3. Criteria for the Clinical Diagnosis of NF1

The presence of any two or more of the following is diagnostic

Café-au-lait spots (6 or more)	>5mm in diameter in prepubertal individuals
	>15mm diameter in postpubertal individuals
Neurofibroma	Any type: 2 or more or
	Plexiform: 1 or more
Axillary and inguinal freckles	
Optic nerve glioma	1 or more
Lisch nodules	2 or more
A distinctive osseous lesion	Sphenoid wing dysplasia or congenital bowing or thinning of long bone cortex, with or without pseudoarthrosis
First-degree relative with NF1	

(Adapted from National Institutes of Health Consensus Development Conference. *Arch Neurol*. 1988;45:575-578.)

Table 64-4. Ophthalmic Manifestations of NF1

Location	Lesion	Frequency (%)
Eyelid	Nodular neurofibroma	18
	Plexiform neurofibroma	5
	Café-au-lait spots	3
Conjunctiva	Neurofibroma	5
Cornea	Prominent corneal nerves	6-22
	Posterior embryotoxon	3-5
Angle	Congenital glaucoma	50
Uvea	Lisch nodules	70-92
	Choroidal hamartoma	51
	Choroidal nevus	3-5
Optic nerve	Pilocytic astrocytoma	2-12
	Optic disc drusen	1

(Adapted from Lewis RA, Riccardi VM. Von Recklinghausen neurofibromatosis. Incidence of iris hamartomata. *Ophthalmology*. 1981;88:348-354.)

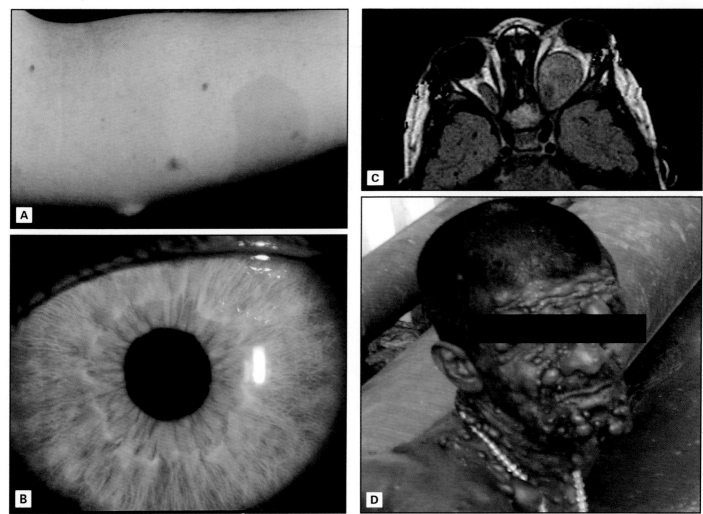

Figure 64-1. Common manifestations of NF1. Café-au-lait spots (A). Multiple Lisch nodules (B). Magnetic resonance image of optic nerve glioma (C). Multiple neurofibromas (D).

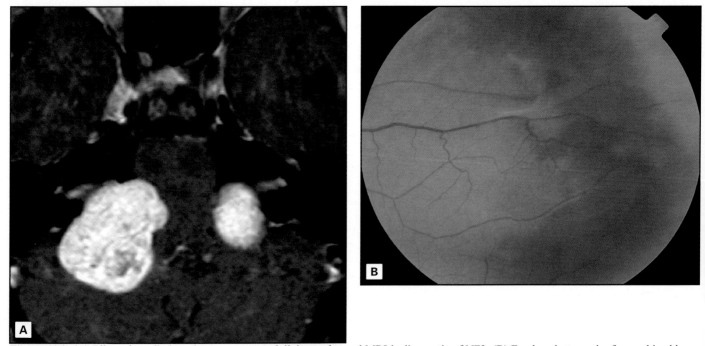

Figure 64-2. (A) Bilateral vestibular schwannoma on gadolinium-enhanced MRI is diagnostic of NF2. (B) Fundus photograph of a combined hamartoma of the retina and retinal pigment epithelium.

Table 64-5. Criteria for the Diagnosis of NF2

Presence of any one of the following features

Bilateral vestibular schwannoma		
First-degree relative with NF2	PLUS	Unilateral vestibular schwannoma <30 years
First-degree relative with NF 2	PLUS	Any two of the following: meningioma, glioma, schwannoma, juvenile posterior subcapsular lenticular opacities/juvenile cortical cataract

(Adapted from National Institutes of Health Consensus Development Conference. Neurofibromatosis: Conference Statement. *Arch Neurol.* 1988;45:575-578.)

Table 64-6. Diagnostic Criteria for VHL Disease

Family History*	Required Feature
	Any one of the following
Positive	One or more retinal capillary hemangiomas
	One or more CNS hemangiomas
	One or more visceral lesions**
Negative	Two or more retinal capillary hemangiomas
	Two or more CNS hemangiomas
	One retinal hemangioma with a visceral lesion
	One CNS hemangioma with a visceral lesion

*Family history of retinal hemangioma, CNS hemangioma, or visceral lesion.

**Visceral lesions include renal cysts, renal carcinoma, pheochromocytoma, pancreatic cysts, islet cell tumors, epididymal cystadenoma, endolymphatic sac tumor, adnexal papillary cystadenoma of probable mesonephric origin.

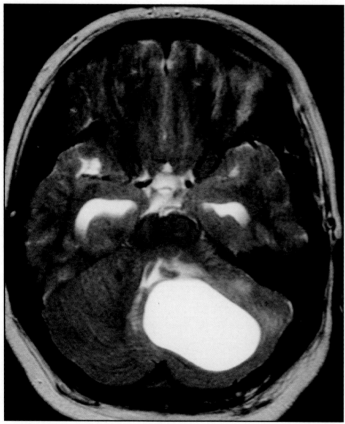

Figure 64-3. MRI scan (T2-weighted) of a cerebellar hemangioma appearing as a cystic lesion.

Box 64-2. The Ocular Abnormalities in NF2

- Cataracts: posterior subcapsular, capsular, cortical, mixed
- Retinal hamartoma
- Epiretinal membrane
- Ocular motility disorders

STURGE-WEBER SYNDROME

The triad of leptomeningeal hemangioma, choroidal hemangioma, and cutaneous hemangioma has been called Sturge-Weber syndrome (SWS) (Table 64-8, Figure 64-5). In the absence of CNS involvement, patients should only be given a diagnosis of port-wine stain or facial angioma to avoid the stigmata associated with a diagnosis of Sturge-Weber syndrome.

WYBURN-MASON SYNDROME

Wyburn-Mason syndrome is a non-hereditary sporadic disorder. Unlike other phakomatoses, there is no cutaneous involvement in Wyburn-Mason syndrome.[10] The incidence of intracranial arteriovenous malformations in patients with retinal arteriovenous malformations is 30% (Figure 64-6). Conversely, 8% of cases with intracranial arteriovenous malformations have retinal arteriovenous malformations (Table 64-9).[11]

RETINAL CAVERNOUS HEMANGIOMA

Retinal cavernous hemangiomas can be associated with cerebral cavernous malformations as an autosomal dominant syndrome with high penetrance and variable expressivity.[12]

NEVUS SEBACEOUS SYNDROME

Nevus sebaceous syndrome (of Jadassohn) is a distinct clinical disorder within the spectrum of epidermal nevus syndrome (of Solomon) characterized by cutaneous sebaceous nevus and extracutaneous manifestations.[13]

ATAXIA-TELANGIECTASIA

Ataxia-telangiectasia is a childhood neurodegenerative disorder with neural, ocular, and cutaneous manifestations associated with immune dysfunction. In addition to some of the features outlined below, premature aging, chromosomal instability, and hypersensitivity to ionizing radiation are also important aspects of this disorder (Table 64-10).[14]

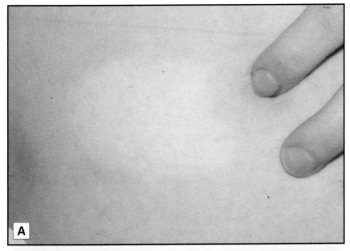

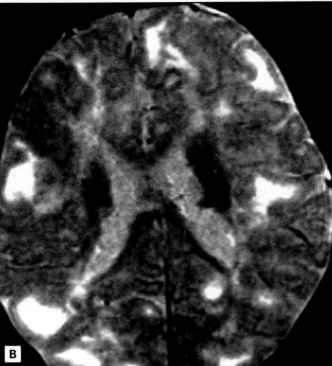

Figure 64-4. Common manifestations of TSC. The hypomelanotic macules ("ash-leaf" sign) (A). Subcortical tubers on T2-weighted axial MR image of the brain appear as multiple subcortical high signal intensity areas (B). (Reproduced with permission from Seki I, Singh AD, Longo S. Pathological case of the month: congenital cardiac rhabdomyoma. *Arch Pediatr Adolesc Med.* 1996;150:877-878. Copyright © 1996 American Medical Association. All rights reserved.)

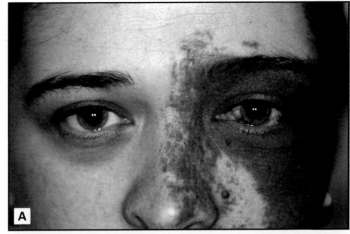

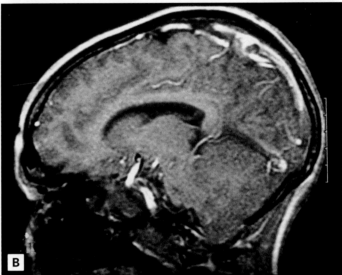

Figure 64-5. (A) Typical facial distribution of cutaneous hemangioma. (B) Leptomeningeal hemangioma in Sturge-Weber syndrome.

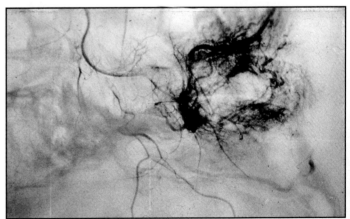

Figure 64-6. The intracranial arteriovenous malformation seen on arteriography.

Table 64-7. Revised Diagnostic Criteria for Tuberous Sclerosis Complex

Definite diagnosis	Two major features
Probable diagnosis	One major feature plus two minor features
	One major feature plus one minor feature
Possible diagnosis	One major feature
	Two minor features

Major Features	Minor Features
Facial angiofibroma or forehead plaque	Multiple dental enamel pits
Ungual/periungual fibroma	Hamartomatous rectal polyps
Hypomelanotic macules (3 or more)	Bone cysts
Shagreen patch	Cerebral white matter migration lines
Multiple retinal hamartomas	Gingival fibromas
Cortical tuber	Nonrenal hamartoma
Subependymal nodule	Retinal achromic patch
Subependymal giant cell astrocytoma	"Confetti" skin lesions
Cardiac rhadomyoma (1 or more)	Multiple renal cysts
Lymphangiomyomatosis	
Renal angiomyolipoma	

(Adapted from Roach ES, Gomez MR, Northrup H. Tuberous Sclerosis Complex Consensus Conference: revised clinical diagnostic criteria. *J Child Neurol.* 1998;13:624-628.)

Table 64-8. Sturge-Weber Syndrome

Organ System	Clinical Features
Central nervous system	Leptomeningeal angiomatosis*
	Cortical atrophy
	Seizures
	Developmental delay
	Behavioral problems
Eye and adnexa	Nevus flammeus
	Prominent episcleral vessels
	Glaucoma
	Diffuse choroidal hemangioma*
Cutaneous	Nevus flammeus*

*Any two of three features essential for diagnosis.

Table 64-9. Wyburn-Mason Syndrome

Organ System	Clinical Features
Central nervous system	Racemose hemangioma
Retina	Racemose hemangioma
Orbit	Racemose hemangioma

Table 64-10. Ataxia-Telangiectasia

Clinical Features	Laboratory Features
Progressive cerebellar ataxia	Elevated serum a-fetoprotein after 2 years of age
Oculocutaneous telangiectasia	
Hypotonic facies	Elevated plasma carcinoembryonic antigen
Oculomotor apraxia	
Dysplasia of the thymus gland	Low serum antibody levels (IgA, IgG-2, IgE)
Recurrent pulmonary infections	Spontaneous chromosome breaks and rearrangements (in vitro studies)
Susceptibility to neoplasia	
Endocrine abnormalities	
Progeric changes	Increased sensitivity to ionizing radiation

NEUROCUTANEOUS MELANOSIS

Neurocutaneous melanosis (NCM) is a non-familial phakomatosis characterized by multiple and large congenital cutaneous nevi in association with meningeal melanosis or melanoma.[15]

REFERENCES

1. Van der Hoeve J. The Doyne Memorial Lecture. Eye symptoms in phakomatoses. *Trans Ophthalmol Soc UK.* 1932;52:380-401.
2. Riccardi VM. *Neurofibromatosis: Phenotype, Natural History, and Pathogenesis.* 2nd ed. Baltimore, MD: Johns Hopkins University Press; 1992.
3. Antinheimo J, Sankila R, Carpen O, et al. Population-based analysis of sporadic and type 2 neurofibromatosis-associated meningiomas and schwannomas. *Neurology.* 2000;54:71-76.
4. Ragge NK, Baser ME, Klein J, et al. Ocular abnormalities in neurofibromatosis 2. *Am J Ophthalmol.* 1995;120:634-641.
5. Melmon KL, Rosen SW. Lindau's disease. *Am J Med.* 1964;36:595-617.
6. Singh AD, Shields CL, Shields JA. von Hippel-Lindau disease. *Surv Ophthalmol.* 2001;46:117-142.
7. Gomez MR. History of the tuberous sclerosis complex. *Brain Dev.* 1995;17:55-57.
8. Kwiatkowski DJ, Short MP. Tuberous sclerosis. *Arch Dermatol.* 1994;130:348-354.
9. Webb DW, Fryer AE, Osborne JP. On the incidence of fits and mental retardation in tuberous sclerosis. *J Med Genet.* 1991;28:395-397.
10. Wyburn-Mason R. Arteriovenous aneurysm of midbrian and retina, facial nevi and mental changes. *Brain Dev.* 1943;66:163-203.
11. Theron J, Newton TH, Hoyt WF. Unilateral retinocephalic vascular malformations. *Neuroradiology.* 1974;7:185.
12. Dobyns WB, Michels VV, Groover RV, et al. Familial cavernous malformations of the central nervous system and retina. *Ann Neurol.* 1987;21:578-583.
13. Solomon LM, Fretzin DF, Dewald RL. The epidermal nevus syndrome. *Arch Dermatol.* 1968;97:273-285.
14. Boder E. Ataxia-telangiectasia: some historic, clinical and pathologic observations. *Birth Defects: Original Article Series.* 1975;11:255-270.
15. Makkar HS, Frieden IJ. Neurocutaneous melanosis. *Semin Cutan Med Surg.* 2004;23:138-144.

Chapter

65

Retinoblastoma and Cancer Genetics

Alfred G. Knudson, Jr

INTRODUCTION

For the pediatrician-in-training of more than 50 years ago, retinoblastoma was a rare curiosity, of interest because of its embryonal origin, sometimes hereditary predisposition, and frequent lethality. Here I discuss a personal view of these developments from the point of view of cancer genetics.

EVIDENCE FOR THE ROLE OF GENETICS IN THE ORIGIN OF CANCER

Early Evidence

Although a heritable predisposition to cancer has long been known, the first specific proposal for a role of genetics in the origin of cancer was set forth by Boveri[1] in his heuristic volume of 1914. Impressed by the finding of von Hansemann of aberrant mitoses in cancer cells,[2] Boveri proposed that some chromosomes might stimulate cell division and that others might inhibit it, anticipating the much later discovery of oncogenes and tumor suppressor genes. When Muller[3] later discovered that ionizing radiation could induce mutation of genes, he proposed, knowing that such radiation is carcinogenic, that specific gene mutations initiate a process whose later progress entailed spontaneous mutations in other genes until some requisite number of mutations was reached, thus explaining the typical latent periods of radiogenic cancer.[4] Nordling[5] first proposed that the number of such "hits" might be six for colon cancer. This conclusion provided a satisfying theory, but no means for discovery of specific mutations. Such cancers were clearly too complicated at that time, with contemporaneous tools.

Cytogenetic Evidence

An encouraging discovery was that by Nowell and Hungerford of the Philadelphia chromosome, Ph1, in chronic myelocytic leukemia cells with no other visible cytogenetic abnormality.[6] Could such a single genetic defect be characterized? The answer at that time was no; the ability to localize a gene had not been discovered.

Number of Events as Evidence

If an induced hit could be the first on the path to cancer, so could an inherited hit, such as is found with a dominantly inher-

ited predisposition to specific cancers. There should not be "one-hit" hereditary cancer because cancer would be too common in a corresponding non-hereditary form. One might expect, then, that the smallest number of hits would be two, the second being somatic. If two hits were sufficient, then the resulting cancer might occur in very early life. This possibility caused my attention to be focused on retinoblastoma, which in its heritable form can be found even in newborn babies. One hit was clearly insufficient, for all retinoblasts would form tumors, yet the mean number of tumors observed was approximately three.[7] Non-hereditary tumors, although rare, would occur following two hits, because a clone of somatically mutant retinoblasts could give rise to a cell with a second hit that would create a single tumor. Such tumors should on average occur later than those arising in genetically predisposed persons, as is indeed the case.

Implications for the Nature of the Gene(s) Mutated

Such a scenario had important implications for the nature of the gene(s) mutated. The two hits could occur in one copy of each of two separate genes, ie, in co-dominant fashion, or in both alleles of a single gene, in recessive fashion. The first scenario would support Boveri's notion of a genetic change that stimulated cell division; the second would support his notion of loss of a suppressor of cell division. At that time, there was no means of discriminating between these alternatives. However, in an analysis of fusion of cancer cells with normal cells, Harris and colleagues[8] found that the fusion product was not cancerous until it lost one or more chromosomes, from which they concluded that cancer, at least in some cases, involved loss of a tumor suppressor. I favored the latter possibility and suggested that the gene might code for a cell surface protein involved in signal transduction,[9] whereas Comings[10] proposed that it might encode a nuclear protein that inhibits the activation of what we now call a proto-oncogene, a prediction very close to what was later found.

With the recessive mechanism, the second event could be one of several kinds, including mutation, loss by deletion, loss of a whole chromosome, or mitotic recombination.[11] A search for these could be undertaken if the locations of the inherited and second hits were known. The location of the inherited mutation was revealed by a few cases of congenital deletions in band q14 of chromosome 13.[12,13]

ROLE OF OPHTHALMOLOGISTS IN THE DISCOVERY OF THE RB1 GENE

Three ophthalmologists, Linn Murphree, Brenda Gallie, and Thaddeus Dryja, were important participants in the discovery of the RB1 gene as the first tumor suppressor gene. Robert Sparkes,[14] together with Murphree and others, discovered a close linkage between RB1 and the esterase D gene (EsD). In persons heterozygous for a variant allele or for hemizygosity of the normal allele of EsD, these investigators and their colleagues were able to show allele loss in some tumors, supporting the recessive hypothesis.[15,16] Then, all of them joined with Webster Cavenee, who had discovered multiple polymorphic markers (restriction fragment length polymorphisms or RFLPs) on chromosome 13, to demonstrate the predicted multiple mechanisms of the second events in support of recessiveness.[17] These tools and findings were then employed by Friend et al[18] to use a DNA marker to clone the RB1 gene.

The cloning of RB1 was almost immediately followed by the cloning of other dominantly heritable cancer genes, including WT1, NF1, and APC. In virtually every case, a two-hit tumor was demonstrated, in keeping with recessiveness, making retinoblastoma a model for many tumors. However, in most cases, these tumors are benign, and further genetic changes are necessary for malignancy, as anticipated by Muller and Nordling. Now there are some 40 to 50 hereditary cancers that follow the model of two hits established for retinoblastoma.

THE RB1 GENE AND ITS IMPORTANCE FOR CANCER BIOLOGY

The RB1 gene has an importance for cancer biology far beyond expectation. It was soon discovered that its encoded protein interacts with an E2F transcription factor to regulate the cell cycle.[19-23] Indeed, the Rb protein is a major regulator of the cell cycle in all dividing cells, an observation that raises the question "Why is RB1 a retinoblastoma gene?" Of course, we now know, thanks to high cure rates and long-term follow-up of survivors, that it is not only a retinoblastoma gene. In fact, most cancers seem to be mutant for RB1 or for genes closely related to it metabolically. This phenomenon has been exploited by "smart" DNA tumor viruses, including simian virus 40, human papillomavirus, and some adenoviruses, each of which produces a protein that inactivates Rb protein.

The critical importance of RB1 is also demonstrated by the effect of homozygosity for inactivating mutations. In mice, the homozygous state is lethal to the developing embryo, with multiple defects, especially in the brain. Of further interest is the fact that homozygosity for most tumor suppressor genes associated with hereditary cancer results in fetal lethality. If we did not know these genes for their predisposition to cancer in the heterozygous mutant state, we would know them as recessive developmentally lethal genes, thereby proving the long-suspected relationship between cancer and development.

REFERENCES

1. Boveri T. Zur frage der entstehung maligner tumoren. Jena: Gustav Fischer, 1914. English translation: Boveri M. *The Origin of Malignant Tumors.* Baltimore, MD: Williams & Wilkins; 1929.
2. von Hansemann D. Über asymmetrische Zellteilung in Epithelkrebsen und deren biologische Bedeutung. *Virchow's Arch Path Anat.* 1890;119:299-326.
3. Muller HJ. Artificial transmutation of the gene. *Science.* 1927;46:84-87.
4. Muller HJ. Radiation damage to the genetic material. *Sci Progr.* 1951;7:93-165, 481-493.
5. Nordling CE. A new theory on the cancer-inducing mechanism. *Br J Cancer.* 1953;6:68-72.
6. Nowell PC, Hungerford DA. A minute chromosome in human chronic granulocytic leukemia. *Science.* 1960;132:1497.
7. Knudson AG. Mutation and cancer: statistical study of retinoblastoma. *Proc Natl Acad Sci USA.* 1971;68:820-823.
8. Harris H, Miller OJ, Klein G, et al. Suppression of malignancy by cell fusion. *Nature.* 1969;223:363-368.
9. Knudson AG. Mutation and human cancer. *Adv Cancer Res.* 1973;17:317-352.
10. Comings DE. A general theory of carcinogenesis. *Proc Natl Acad Sci USA.* 1973;70:3324-3328.
11. Knudson AG. Retinoblastoma: a prototypic hereditary neoplasm. *Semin Oncol.* 1978;5:57-60.
12. Francke U, Kung F. Sporadic bilateral retinoblastoma and 13q- chromosomal deletion. *Med Pediatr Oncol.* 1976;2:379-385.
13. Knudson AG Jr, Meadows AT, Nichols WW, et al. Chromosomal deletion and retinoblastoma. *N Engl J Med.* 1976;295:1120-1123.
14. Sparkes RS, Sparkes MC, Wilson MG, et al. Regional assignment of genes for human esterase D and retinoblastoma to chromosome band 13q14. *Science.* 1980;208:1042-1044.
15. Benedict WF, Murphree AL, Banerjee A, et al. Patient with 13 chromosome deletion: evidence that the retinoblastoma gene is a recessive cancer gene. *Science.* 1983;219:973-975.
16. Godbout R, Dryja TP, Squire J, et al. Somatic inactivation of genes on chromosome 13 is a common event in retinoblastoma. *Nature.* 1983;304:451-453.
17. Cavenee WK, Dryja TP, Phillips RA, et al. Expression of recessive alleles by chromosomal mechanisms in retinoblastoma. *Nature.* 1983;305:779-784.
18. Friend SH, Bernards R, Rogelj S, et al. A human DNA segment with properties of the gene that predisposes to retinoblastoma and osteosarcoma. *Nature.* 1986;323:643-646.
19. Bagchi S, Weinmann R, Raychaudhuri P. The retinoblastoma protein copurifies with E2F-I, an E1A-regulated inhibitor of the transcription factor E2F. *Cell.* 1991;65:1063-1072.
20. Chellappan SP, Hiebert S, Mudryj M, et al. The E2F transcription factor is a cellular target for the RB protein. *Cell.* 1991;65:1053-1061.
21. Helin K, Lees JA, Vidal M, et al. A cDNA encoding a pRB-binding protein with properties of the transcription factor E2F. *Cell.* 1992;70:337-350.
22. Kaelin WG, Krek W, Sellers WR, et al. Expression cloning of a cDNA encoding a retinoblastoma-binding protein with E2F-like properties. *Cell.* 1992;70:351-364.
23. Shirodkar S, Ewen M, DeCaprio JA, et al. The transcription factor E2F interacts with the retinoblastoma product and a p107-cyclin A complex in a cell cycle-regulated manner. *Cell.* 1992;68:157-166.

Chapter

66

Genetic and Cellular Events in Retinoblastoma

Michael A. Dyer and J. William Harbour

INTRODUCTION

Tumorigenesis is a multistep process that involves sequential genetic alterations.[1] Preneoplastic cells must overcome their dependence on extrinsic mitogenic signals, evade apoptosis, prevent degradation of life-span limiting telomeres, recruit vasculature, and acquire invasive properties to become malignant tumor cells.[1]

RETINOBLASTOMA TUMORIGENESIS: KNUDSON'S TWO-HIT HYPOTHESIS

By studying the inheritance pattern of retinoblastoma, Knudson proposed a "two-hit" model to explain how a mutant "tumor suppressor" gene could be inherited as a dominant trait in which inactivation of the second, normal allele occurred in a susceptible somatic tissue such as the developing retina.[2] The Knudson hypothesis was confirmed by the cloning of the RB1 gene from retinoblastomas in 1986 by a team headed by Weinberg and Dryja.[3] Surprisingly, RB1 mutations subsequently were found in many other tumors unrelated to retinoblastoma, such as lung and breast cancer,[4,5] indicating that the Rb pathway is broadly important as a tumor suppressor.[6]

MOUSE MODELS OF RETINOBLASTOMA

The first genetically engineered animal model of spontaneous retinoblastoma was a transgenic mouse line in which the oncogenic T antigen from the SV40 virus was expressed in the retina.[7] Several groups generated mice in which one copy of the RB1 gene was nonfunctional, thereby replicating the situation with patients with heritable retinoblastoma.[8] Surprisingly, these mice developed pituitary tumors but none developed retinoblastoma.[8] Loss of RB1 in the mouse (but not humans) is compensated by up-regulation of p107,[9] thus explaining the apparent contradiction between mouse and human susceptibility to retinoblastoma. These findings led to the generation of the first true knockout mouse model of retinoblastoma.[10]

CELL OF ORIGIN

There are at least four possible cells of origin for retinoblastoma: (1) retinal stem cell, (2) differentiated neuron or glial cell, (3) retinal progenitor cell, or (4) a newly postmitotic cell committed or biased toward a particular retinal fate (Figure 66-1).[10]

EVENTS IN RETINOBLASTOMA PROGRESSION

While the initiating genetic event in retinoblastoma—biallelic inactivation of the RB1 gene—is well established, until recently, little was known about the subsequent genetic events that contribute to retinoblastoma formation and progression.[11]

Circumventing Apoptosis

New research has shown that amplification of the MDMX and MDM2 genes suppress the p53 pathway in human retinoblastoma[11] and that these tumor do not arise from intrinsically death-resistant cells as previously believed.[12]

Is Retinoblastoma a Unique Exception?

Comprehensive analysis of human retinoblastomas has found that the p53 pathway is inactivated by the amplification of the MDMX and MDM2 genes and that these genetic changes suppress the p53 oncogenic stress response allowing RB1-deficient retinoblasts to clonally expand.[11]

CLINICAL IMPLICATIONS

With the identification of the target for chemotherapy, researchers have been able to specifically activate p53-induced cell death in retinoblastoma cells with a small molecule inhibitor (nutlin-3a) of the MDMX-p53 and MDM2-p53 interaction.[11] By combining nutlin-3a with a topoisomerase inhibitor (topotecan) that induces a p53 DNA damage response, synergistic killing of retinoblastoma cells with MDMX amplifications was achieved.[11] In addition, by administering nutlin-3 and topotecan to the eye with subconjunctival injections, the intraocular concentrations were sufficient to block MDMX and MDM2 from interacting with p53 that led to synergistic killing of retinoblastoma cells.[13] More importantly, this local delivery of targeted chemotherapy bypassed all of the toxicity associated with systemic administration of broad-spectrum chemotherapy (etoposide, carboplatin, vincristin) that is widely used to treat retinoblastoma.

REFERENCES

1. Hahn WC, Weinberg RA. Modelling the molecular circuitry of cancer. *Nat Rev Cancer*. 2002;2:331-341.
2. Knudson A. Mutation and cancer: statistical study of retinoblastoma. *PNAS*. 1971;68:820-823.

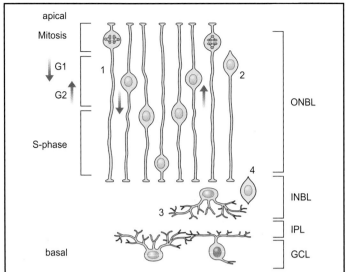

Figure 66-1. Retinoblastoma: cell of origin. Retinoblastoma could arise from four different cell populations. The first potential cell of origin is a proliferating retinal progenitor cell. Multipotent retinal progenitor cells undergo interkinetic nuclear migration as they transition through the cell cycle. Rb inactivation is believed to occur during DNA replication; however, it is not necessarily required to prevent deregulated proliferation. It is expected that the tumors arising from this cell would express progenitor cell markers and possibly differentiation markers. The second possibility is a newly postmitotic cell that is committed to a particular cell fate but fails to complete the differentiation program. It is expected that the tumors arising from this cell would express markers characteristic of this committed cell type. An extension of this hypothesis is the possibility that a more mature differentiated retinal cell gives rise to retinoblastoma by re-entering the cell cycle. Stem cells have been identified in the ciliary marginal zone (CMZ) of the retina but not the neural retina.

3. Friend SH, Bernards R, Rogelj S, et al. A human DNA segment with properties of the gene that predisposes to retinoblastoma and osteosarcoma. *Nature.* 1986;323:643-646.

4. Harbour JW, Lai SL, Whang-Peng J, Gazdar AF, Minna JD, Kaye FJ. Abnormalities in structure and expression of the human retinoblastoma gene in SCLC. *Science.* 1988;241:353-357.

5. Lee EY, To H, Shew JY, Bookstein R, Scully P, Lee WH. Inactivation of the retinoblastoma susceptibility gene in human breast cancers. *Science.* 1988;241:218-221.

6. Sherr CJ, McCormick F. The RB and p53 pathways in cancer. *Cancer Cell.* 2002;2:103-112.

7. Windle JJ, Albert DM, O'Brien JM, et al. Retinoblastoma in transgenic mice. *Nature.* 1990;343:665-669.

8. Lee EY, Chang CY, Hu N, et al. Mice deficient for Rb are nonviable and show defects in neurogenesis and haematopoiesis. *Nature.* 1992;59:288-294.

9. Robanus-Maandag E, Dekker M, van der Valk M, et al. p107 is a suppressor of retinoblastoma development in pRb-deficient mice. *Genes Dev.* 1998;12:1599-1609.

10. Zhang J, Schweers B, Dyer MA. The first knockout mouse model of retinoblastoma. *Cell Cycle.* 2004;3:952-959.

11. Laurie NA, Donovan SL, Shih C-S, et al. Inactivation of the p53 pathway in retinoblastoma. *Nature.* 2006;444:61-66.

12. Chen D, Livne-Bar I, Vanderluit JL, Slack RS, Agochiya M, Bremner R. Cell-specific effects of RB or RB/p107 loss on retinal development implicate an intrinsically death-resistant cell-of-origin in retinoblastoma. *Cancer Cell.* 2004;5:539-551.

13. Laurie NA, Gray JK, Zhang J, et al. Topotecan combination chemotherapy in two new rodent models of retinoblastoma. *Clin Cancer Res.* 2005;11:7569-7578.

Geographic and Environmental Factors

Greta R. Bunin and Manuela Orjuela

GEOGRAPHIC VARIATION IN INCIDENCE

The incidence in North America and much of Europe is relatively uniform, is somewhat higher in Central and South America, and varies more widely in Asia and Africa.[1] Overall, the rates are higher in less industrialized countries.

North America

The incidence of retinoblastoma in the United States did not change significantly between 1975 and 1995. Annual rates by race/ethnicity and region generally range from 10 to 14 per million children aged 0 to 4 years (Figure 67-1A).

Europe

Most countries have incidences in the range of 6 to 12 per million per year in children aged 0 to 4 years.

Central and South America

Population-based registries do not exist for all countries in Central and South America, and for some countries, rates are only available within selected cities (Figure 67-1B). However, even with these limitations there appear to be two groups in Central and South America: those regions with an incidence under 9.5 per million per year in children aged 0 to 4, and those with an incidence higher than 15 per million per year.[1]

Asia

Incidence also varies greatly in Asia (Figure 67-1C).[1]

Africa

In Africa, where there are few population-based registries, incidence is also quite variable (Figure 67-1D).[1]

Oceania

The incidence rate in Australia is similar to that in the United States and Canada (Figure 67-1E).[1]

ETIOLOGICAL FACTORS FOR HERITABLE RETINOBLASTOMA

Only a few epidemiologic studies have investigated possible risk factors for new germline mutations.[2] Moreover, such studies have been limited in scope, mostly focusing on paternal age.[3] The cohort studies of children of cancer survivors and of atomic bomb survivors have limited power to detect anything but large effects.

ETIOLOGICAL FACTORS FOR NONHERITABLE RETINOBLASTOMA

The data on such possible risk factors for nonheritable retinoblastoma are very limited. The findings cannot be considered conclusive.

Environmental Exposure

The mother's use of insect or garden sprays during pregnancy, diagnostic X-ray with direct fetal exposure, and father's employment as a welder, machinist, or related metal worker have been associated with an increased risk of non-heritable retinoblastoma.[2] The limited evidence suggests a role for diet and/or use of multivitamin supplements during pregnancy.[4] A study in The Netherlands estimated that children born after in vitro fertilization (IVF) had a 5- to 7-fold increased risk of retinoblastoma.

Maternal infection with human papillomavirus is hypothesized to contribute to the development of retinoblastoma.[5]

REFERENCES

1. Parkin DM, Kramarova E, Draper GJ, et al. *International Incidence of Childhood Cancer*. Lyon, France: International Agency for Research on Cancer; 1998.
2. Bunin GR, Meadows AT, Emanuel BS, et al. Pre- and post-conception factors associated with heritable and non-heritable retinoblastoma. *Cancer Res.* 1989;49:5730-5735.
3. Pellie C, Briard M-L, Feingold J, Freza J. Parental age in retinoblastoma. *Humangenetik.* 1973;20:59-62.
4. Orjuela MA, Titievsky L, Liu X, et al. Fruit and vegetable intake during pregnancy and risk for development of sporadic retinoblastoma. *Cancer Epidemiol Biomarkers Prev.* 2005;14:1433-1440.
5. Orjuela M, Ponce Castaneda V, Ridaura C, et al. Presence of human papilloma virus in tumor tissue from children with retinoblastoma: an alternative mechanism for tumor development. *Clin Cancer Res.* 2000;6:4010-4016.

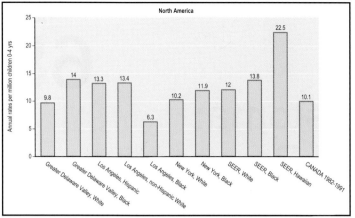

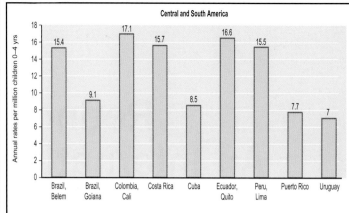

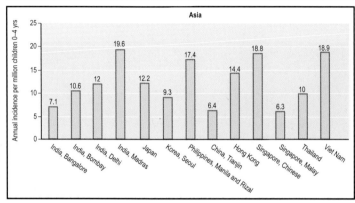

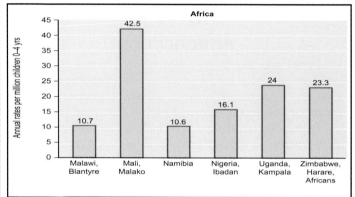

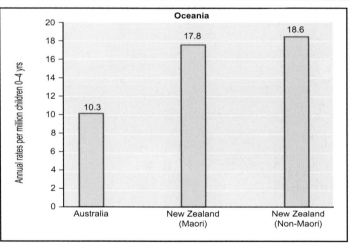

Figure 67-1. Incidence of retinoblastoma in children aged 0 to 4 years in North America (A), Central and South America (B), Asia (C), Africa (D), and Oceania (E). (Data derived from Parkin DM, Kramarova E, Draper GJ, et al. *International Incidence of Childhood Cancer.* Lyon, France: International Agency for Research on Cancer; 1998.)

Retinoblastoma:
An International Perspective

Guillermo L. Chantada and Carlos Leal-Leal

INTRODUCTION

In the previous chapter (Chapter 67), Bunin and Orjuela introduced evidence that the incidence of nonheritable retinoblastoma may be higher in some developing countries, especially among the poorer populations of tropical Brazil and Namibia.[1,2]

Retinoblastoma represents a challenge in developing countries. Whereas in affluent societies more than 90% of affected children survive, many fewer children living in developing nations outlive this disease.

CLINICAL FEATURES

Strabismus, a presenting sign in 20% of children in the United States, is not recognized as a presenting sign in central Africa.[3,4] Proptosis due to orbital extension of retinoblastoma, which is rarely a presenting sign of retinoblastoma in the United States, is the second most common sign in the Congo (Figure 68-1). An intermediate situation is observed in countries such as Mexico, Argentina, and some parts of India, where leukocoria is the most common presenting sign.

DELAYED DIAGNOSIS

Patient-Related Factors

These include the lack of symptoms of retinoblastoma in young children, who are unable to express visual disturbances, together with the lack of awareness of the general population that ocular abnormalities such as strabismus and leukocoria may be signs of cancer.

Physician-Related Factors

Pediatricians frequently do not detect leukocoria because of limited ophthalmic examination with an undilated pupil. Therefore, they rarely recognize the significance of the parents' complaints on the first visit.[5]

SURVIVAL

Survival With Retinoblastoma Is Lower in Developing Countries

Survival rates lower than 50% have been reported in some Latin American and African countries. As more than 80% of the world's children live in developing countries, globally there may be more children dying of retinoblastoma than surviving.

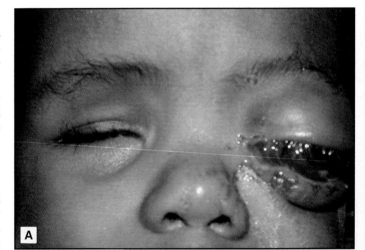

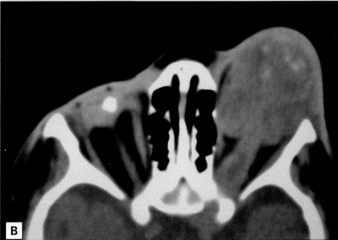

Figure 68-1. Patient with bilateral retinoblastoma and overt extraocular extension OS (A), which is confirmed by computed tomography (B).

Steps to Improve Survival

An improvement in the survival of retinoblastoma patients in developing countries should not depend on better treatment for extraocular disease. Rather, early detection and reduction in systemic dissemination, a coordinated multistep approach involving public education, professional education screening, and socioeconomic development are necessary. To be effective, resources must also be aimed at reducing treatment refusal.

DEVELOPMENTS THAT PROVIDE HOPE FOR THE FUTURE

Creation of Cooperative Groups

Cooperative groups for the treatment of childhood cancer are difficult to establish in developing countries because of limited financial support and infrastructure. Recently, the Children's Oncology Group in North America has launched clinical trial protocols that provide the framework for international applications (Chapter 81). In addition, cooperative groups for the treatment of retinoblastoma have been created in Mexico, Brazil, India, and Central America. These developments should provide evidence-based treatment guidelines that will benefit children from developing countries.

International Collaborative Efforts

Collaborative efforts between retinoblastoma centers in the northern and southern hemispheres have proved successful in improving outcomes in pediatric oncology.[6] Transfer of knowledge and resources is the main purpose of these programs, the first of which included cooperation between New York City institutions, sponsored by the Fund for Ophthalmic Knowledge, and Buenos Aires, Argentina. This cooperation included donations of teaching material, participation in common research studies, and financial support for laboratory research. The International Network for Cancer Treatment and Research (www.inctr.org) created a retinoblastoma group involving researchers from many different countries. Its ambitious program aims to develop a common treatment protocol for participating institutions. An outreach program of the St Jude Children's Research Center (www.stjude.org) supports the treatment of retinoblastoma in Central America based on Internet transmission of RetCam images, as well as an active teaching program. Other programs include cooperation between national groups (Children's Oncology Group and India) and hospitals (Childrens Hospital Los Angeles and Mexico City; Institut Curie, Paris and Algeria).

Efforts in Developing Countries

A multicentric study was started in Central America under the sponsorship of St Jude's hospital. Chemoreduction protocols are being successfully implemented. New drug (ifosfamide, idarubicin, topotecan, irinotecan) testing has also been actively pursued in developing countries.

SUMMARY

Retinoblastoma presents unique challenges to treating physicians in developing countries. The burden of caring for 80% of the world's retinoblastoma cases falls to individuals and national healthcare systems with limited resources where caring for children with extraocular disease is relatively common. Retinoblastoma specialists from developing countries have taken the lead in creating a new international staging system for extraocular retinoblastoma. Understanding the cause(s) of nonheritable or environmental retinoblastoma will probably take place in countries outside North America and Europe. The need for the cost containment will lead to more effective and less expensive approaches. Initiatives in developing countries will be a valuable contribution to the rest of the world.

REFERENCES

1. Antoneli CB, Steinhorst F, de Cassia Braga Ribeiro K, et al. Extraocular retinoblastoma: a 13-year experience. *Cancer.* 2003;98:1292-1298.
2. Wessels G, Hesseling PB. Incidence and frequency rates of childhood cancer in Namibia. *S Afr Med J.* 1997;87:885-889.
3. Abramson DH, Frank CM, Susman M, et al. Presenting signs of retinoblastoma. *J Pediatr.* 1998;132:505-508.
4. Kaimbo WK, Mvitu MM, Missotten L. Presenting signs of retinoblastoma in Congolese patients. *Bull Soc Belge Ophtalmol.* 2002;283:37-41.
5. Chantada G, Fandino A, Manzitti J, Urrutia L, Schvartzman E. Late diagnosis of retinoblastoma in a developing country. *Arch Dis Child.* 1999;80(2):171-174.
6. Ribeiro RC, Pui CH. Saving the children—improving childhood cancer treatment in developing countries. *N Engl J Med.* 2005;352:2158-2160.

Staging and Grouping of Retinoblastoma

A. Linn Murphree and Guillermo L. Chantada

INTRODUCTION

A commonly used tumor classification is essential in order to plan initial treatment, determine prognosis, assess treatment response, compare outcomes, and plan clinical trials.[1]

REESE-ELLSWORTH CLASSIFICATION

In the 1960s, Reese and Ellsworth[2] proposed a preoperative grouping system as a way to assess the likelihood of salvaging the eye (Table 69-1).

International Retinoblastoma Classification: Staging System

At the International Symposium on Retinoblastoma held in Paris in May 2003, a committee of retinoblastoma experts from large centers worldwide drafted yet another staging system. Investigators from centers in South and North America, Europe, and South Africa edited this draft into a consensus document.[3] This staging system was designed to be used in conjunction with the new intraocular grouping system that was also under development at the same time. This staging system combines clinical and pathologic staging and has a single end point—survival of the patient with retinoblastoma. Patients are classified according to extent of disease, including the presence of microscopic or overt extraocular extension and metastatic extension (Table 69-2). Roman numerals are used for stage assignment.

International Retinoblastoma Classification: Grouping System

Eyes are classified according to the extent of disease and dissemination of intraocular tumor (Table 69-3).[4] The grouping is based on the natural history of this eye disease as well as the probability of salvaging the eye(s). Each group may contain elements of preceding groups, but is defined by the most advanced tumor in the eye (Figures 69-1 through 69-5, Box 69-1).

REFERENCES

1. Fleming I. Staging of pediatric cancers: problems in the development of a national system. *Semin Surg Oncol.* 1992;8:94–97.
2. Ellsworth RM. The practical management of retinoblastoma. *Trans Am Ophthalmol Soc.* 1969;67:462–534.
3. Chantada G, Doz F, Antonelli CB, et al. A proposal for an international retinoblastoma staging system. *Pediatr Blood Cancer.* 2005. Epub.
4. Murphree AL. Intraocular retinoblastoma: the case for a new group classification. *Ophthalmol Clin North Am.* 2005;18:41–53.

Table 69-1. Reese-Ellsworth Classification

Group	Subgroup	Descriptor	Prognosis
Group I	Ia	Solitary tumor <4 DD at or behind the equator	Very favorable
	Ib	Multiple tumors, none >4 DD, all at or behind the equator	
Group II	IIa	Solitary tumor, 4 to 10 DD, all at or behind the equator	Favorable
	IIb	Multiple tumors, 4 to 10 DD, behind the equator	
Group III	IIIa	Any lesion anterior to the equator	Doubtful
	IIIb	Solitary tumors larger than 10 DD behind the equator	
Group IV	IVa	Multiple tumors, some larger than 10 DD	Unfavorable
	IVb	Any lesion extending anteriorly to the ora serrata	
Group V	Va	Massive tumors involving over half the retina	Very unfavorable
	Vb	Vitreous seeding	

Table 69-2. Staging System for Patients in International Retinoblastoma Classification

Stage	Substage		Descriptor	Comments
Stage 0			Intraocular tumor only	No evidence of regional or metastatic disease; patient may not have had an enucleation
Stage I			Tumor completely removed by enucleation	Retinoblastoma may be present in the non-enucleated eye. High-risk pathology may be present within the enucleated specimen
Stage II			Residual orbital tumor	Microscopic tumor present in the optic nerve at the site of surgical resection (cut end of nerve)
Stage III	a. Overt orbital extension		Overt regional disease	Orbital or node involvement diagnosed clinically or by neuroimaging
	b. Preauricular or cervical lymph node extension			
Stage IV	a. Hematogenous metastasis without CNS disease	1. Single lesion	Metastatic Disease	
		2. Multiple lesions		
	b. CNS disease	1. Prechiasmatic lesion		
		2. CNS mass		
		3. Leptomeningeal disease		

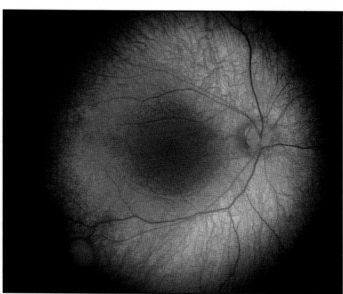

Figure 69-1. Group A retinoblastoma. Small round tumor(s) located away from the fovea and disc. No tumor may be larger than 3 mm in any diameter (base or height). Tumor(s) must be 2 DD (3 mm) or more from the fovea and must be 1 DD (1.5 mm) or more from the optic disc. No vitreous seeding is allowed. (Reprinted from Murphree AL. Intraocular retinoblastoma: the case for a new group classification. *Ophthalmol Clin North Am.* 2005;18:41-53.)

Table 69-3. Grouping System for Eyes in International Retinoblastoma Classification

Group	Descriptor
Group A	Small[1] round tumor(s) located away from the fovea[2] and disc[3]
Group B	All eyes without tumor dissemination[4] not in Group A[5]
Group C	Local[6] tumor dissemination
Group D	Diffuse[7] tumor dissemination
Group E	Unsalvageable eyes[8]

[1]No tumor may be larger than 3 mm in any diameter (base or height). No vitreous seeding allowed.
[2]Tumor(s) must be 2 DD (3 mm) or more from the fovea.
[3]Tumor(s) must be 1 DD (1.5 mm) or more from the optic disc.
[4]Tumor dissemination is defined to include both vitreous seeding and the presence of subretinal fluid even if subretinal seeding is not clinically apparent. A cuff of subretinal fluid extending no more than 5 mm from the base of the tumor is allowed in Group B. No vitreous seeding of any extent is allowed.
[5]Tumors may be of any size, shape, or location. Current or RPE evidence of previous detachment of 1 quadrant or less is allowed.
[6]Vitreous or subretinal seeding may extend no more than 3 mm from tumor.
[7]Vitreous seeding may be large, diffuse, and/or "greasy." Avascular masses of tumor may be present in the vitreous. Subretinal dissemination may consist of fine seeds, large avascular plaques on the underside of the detached retina, or extensive subretinal masses (exophytic disease).
[8]See Box 69-1 for features that confer Group E status.

Box 69-1. Clinical Features That Confer Group E Status

- Neovascular glaucoma
- Massive intraocular hemorrhage
- Blood-stained cornea
- Massive tumor necrosis associated with aseptic orbital cellulitis
- Phthisis or pre-phthisis
- Tumor anterior to anterior vitreous face
- Anterior segment tumor
- Tumor touching the lens
- Diffuse infiltrating retinoblastoma

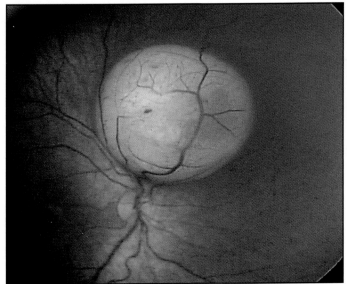

Figure 69-2. Group B retinoblastoma. All eyes without tumor dissemination not in Group A. A cuff of subretinal fluid extending no more than 5 mm from the base of the tumor is allowed. Tumors may be of any size, shape, or location, but vitreous seeding or subretinal fluid of any extent is not allowed. (Reprinted from Murphree AL. Intraocular retinoblastoma: the case for a new group classification. *Ophthalmol Clin North Am.* 2005;18:41-53.)

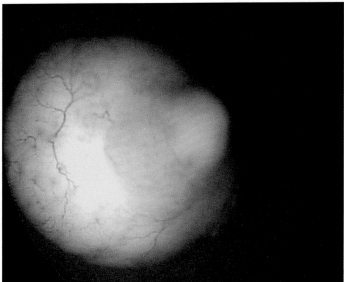

Figure 69-3. Group C retinoblastoma. Local tumor dissemination. Vitreous or subretinal seeding may extend no more than 3 mm from tumor. Current or RPE evidence of previous detachment of one quadrant or less is allowed. Note the "nipple" that is the likely source of the vitreous seeding. (Reprinted from Murphree AL. Intraocular retinoblastoma: the case for a new group classification. *Ophthalmol Clin North Am.* 2005;18:41-53.)

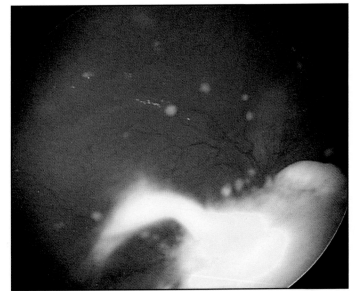

Figure 69-4. Group D retinoblastoma. Diffuse tumor dissemination. Vitreous seeding may be large, diffuse, and/or "greasy." Avascular masses of tumor may be present in the vitreous. Subretinal dissemination may consist of fine seeds or large avascular plaques on the underside of the detached retina or extensive subretinal masses (exophytic disease). (Reprinted from Murphree AL. Intraocular retinoblastoma: the case for a new group classification. *Ophthalmol Clin North Am.* 2005;18:41-53.)

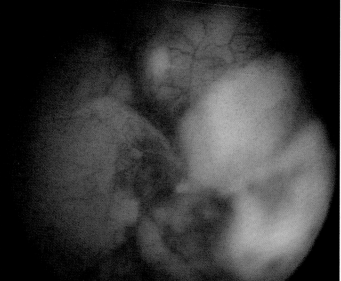

Figure 69-5. Group E retinoblastoma. Unsalvageable eyes include those displaying any one or more of the following features: neovascular glaucoma, massive intraocular hemorrhage, bloodstained cornea, massive tumor necrosis associated with aseptic orbital cellulites, phthisis or prephthisis, tumor anterior to anterior vitreous face, anterior segment tumor, tumor touching the lens, or diffuse infiltrating retinoblastoma. (Reprinted from Murphree AL. Intraocular retinoblastoma: the case for a new group classification. *Ophthalmol Clin North Am.* 2005;18:41-53.)

Heritable Retinoblastoma: The RB1 Cancer Predisposition Syndrome

A. Linn Murphree and Arun D. Singh

INTRODUCTION

Terms commonly used in the literature to refer to the group of patients genetically predisposed to retinoblastoma include *bilateral*, *hereditary*, *heritable*, and *familial* (Table 70-1). None of these terms is always accurate or precise when referring to the group as a whole. At least 15% of all unilateral retinoblastoma cases carry an RB1 germline mutation (Figure 70-1). Fully two thirds of all patients with RB1 germline mutations did not inherit the mutant allele from a parent (Chapter 67). Most are the result of endogenous germline mutations in RB1. Although these endogenously derived new or "founder" RB1 mutations are not inherited, they are heritable (capable of being transmitted to offspring).

RBI CANCER PREDISPOSITION SYNDROME

Phenotype

Compared to the single phenotype (unifocal unilateral retinoblastoma) seen in non-heritable retinoblastoma, more than 10 clinical phenotypes may result from a germline RB1 mutation. Not all patients with a genetic predisposition to retinoblastoma develop tumors in both eyes, or even in one eye. Each does, however, share a 50% probability of passing the predisposition-to-cancer trait to each of their children. Each of the families of those children deserves to know that their children may be at risk. They should also know that their growing children should be watched carefully for unexplained "bumps, lumps, or sore spots" that do not resolve spontaneously within 2 weeks. Such findings may be early signs of osteosarcoma or soft tissue sarcoma. They should avoid sunburn (increases risk for melanoma) and second-hand tobacco smoke (increases risk for carcinoma of the lung and bladder in the fourth and fifth decades of life). Clinical clues to the presence of the RB1 cancer predisposition syndrome include all familial cases (parent, grandparent, child, or sibling with retinoblastoma), bilateral retinoblastoma, trilateral retinoblastoma (Chapter 72), 13q deletion syndrome (Chapter 73), and the presence of or a positive family history of non-ocular malignant neoplasms (Box 70-1) (Chapter 71).

Table 70-1. Terms Currently Used to Define Genetic Predisposition to Retinoblastoma

Terminology			
Laterality	Inheritance	Family History	RB1 Cancer Predisposition Syndrome
Bilateral	Inherited from a parent	+	+
	Negative family history	-	+
Unilateral[1]	Inherited from a parent	+	+
	Negative family history	-	+
	Non-heritable[2]	-	-

[1]15% to 20% of unilateral patients have an RB1 germline mutation; 80% to 85% do not.
[2]A diagnosis of non-heritable unilateral Rb can only be made with certainty if the RB1 gene test is normal.

Genotype

A variety of genetic changes at RB1 predisposes to retinoblastoma and other cancers in the RB1 cancer predisposition syndrome. About 20% of the changes are deletions larger than 1 kb; 30% consist of small deletions or insertions; and about 45% are point mutations. Mutations have been found in 25 of the 27 coding exons and in promoter elements. More than 930 RB1 mutations published by 2005 were gathered into a searchable database by Valverde and colleagues. Their meta-analysis revealed that the retinoblastoma protein is most commonly inactivated by deletions and nonsense mutations. In contrast, most genetic diseases are caused by missense mutations. Almost 40% of RB1 gene mutations are recurrent and occur in 16 hot spots, and include 12 nonsense, two missense, and three splicing mutations. The remainder of the mutations are scattered along RB1, but are most common in exons 9, 10, 14, 18, 20, and 23. There is some clustering by country of origin, suggesting the involvement of a predisposing ethnic background.

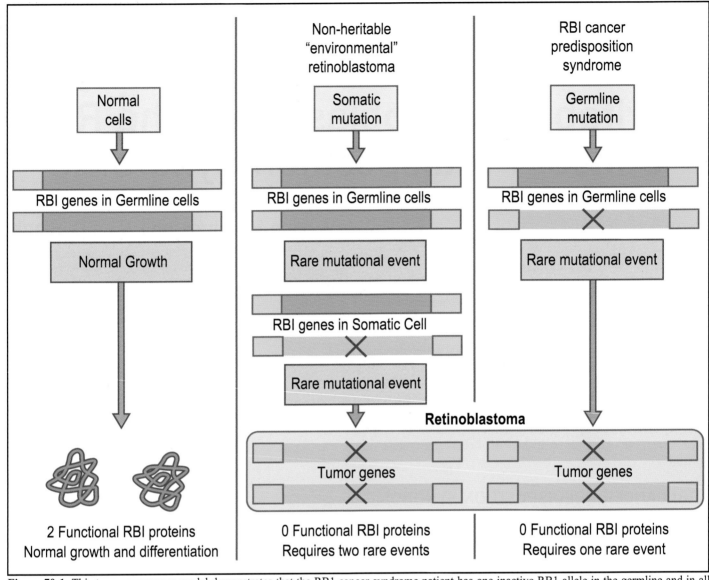

Figure 70-1. This tumor suppressor model demonstrates that the RB1 cancer syndrome patient has one inactive RB1 allele in the germline and in all somatic cells. A single rare, second event is all that is required for reduction to homozygosity at the RB1 locus and for retinoblastoma to be created in a retinoblast. Additional mutations may be required for nonocular cancer to arise. The two rare mutational events occur in somatic cells. For retinoblastoma to appear, both alleles in a single retinoblast must be inactivated. Environmental pressure would be expected to have an impact on nonheritable retinoblastoma.

SUMMARY

Nonheritable retinoblastoma is a diagnosis of exclusion and can only be made with certainty if RB1 gene testing is negative (Chapter 73). The new assumption must be that each newly diagnosed retinoblastoma patient, regardless of age at diagnosis, laterality, or lack of a positive family history, has the RB1 cancer predisposition syndrome until that diagnosis is actively disproved.

Box 70-1. Clinical Clues to the Presence of RB1 Cancer Predisposition Syndrome

- Family history of retinoblastoma (parent, grandparent, child, or sibling)
- Bilateral retinoblastoma
- Trilateral retinoblastoma
- 13q deletion syndrome
- Second malignant neoplasm

Material presented in this chapter was published in Singh AD, Damato BE, Pe'er J, Murphree AL, Perry JD. *Clinical Ophthalmic Oncology.* © Elsevier 2007.

Non-Ocular Tumors

Cari E. Lyle, Carlos Rodriguez-Galindo, and Matthew W. Wilson

INTRODUCTION

Retinoblastoma must be seen as more than an intraocular cancer representing a prototypical hereditary cancer in humans. Children with an RB1 germline mutation who survive heritable retinoblastoma (all familial cases, all bilateral cases, and about 15% of unilateral cases) are at an exceptionally high risk for developing and dying from subsequent primary tumors, particularly osteosarcomas and soft tissue sarcomas. The most feared non-ocular tumor is the intracranial primitive neuroectodermal tumor that arises in the pineal gland, the pinealoblastoma (Chapter 72). Those patients with heritable retinoblastoma who survive through childhood without developing trilateral retinoblastoma are still at increased risk for developing a variety of second non-ocular malignancies (Chapter 70).

PATHOGENESIS

Genetic Susceptibility

Although nonheritable retinoblastoma makes up the vast majority of cases of this disease, it is those patients with the heritable form who are far more likely to develop second non-ocular malignancies (Figure 71-1A). The high rate of subsequent cancers in heritable retinoblastoma is attributed to the presence of germline mutations in the retinoblastoma tumor suppressor gene, RB1.

Effects of Radiation Therapy

In addition to increasing the incidence of non-ocular tumors, radiation therapy also influences the age of onset, location, and type of non-ocular cancer (Figure 71-1B).[1] Receiving radiation treatment in the first year of life may place the patient at a greater risk of second tumors within the field of radiation.[2]

INCIDENCE

In the United States, more retinoblastoma patients die of non-ocular cancers than from the initial eye tumor. Reports of the cumulative incidence of second cancers in patients with germline RB1 mutations vary, but it is believed to be approximately 1% per year of life.[3] The heritable patients had a cumulative risk of 36% of developing a new cancer 50 years after diagnosis.

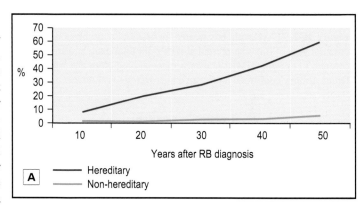

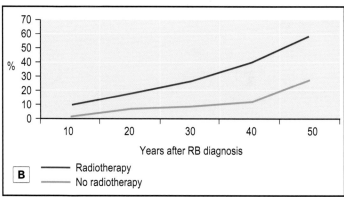

Figure 71-1. Cumulative incidence of second malignancy following diagnosis of retinoblastoma in patients with hereditary and nonhereditary retinoblastoma (A) and in the hereditary retinoblastoma with and without radiation treatment (B). (Data derived from Wong FL, Boice JD, Abramson DH, et al. Cancer incidence after retinoblastoma. Radiation dose and sarcoma risk. *JAMA.* 1997;278:1262-1267.)

CLINICAL FEATURES

A wide variety of neoplasms have been described in survivors of retinoblastoma. The most common second malignancy is osteosarcoma, which accounts for approximately one third of cases.[4] During adolescence, osteosarcomas are the most common and tend to occur predominantly in the field of radiation. Soft tissue sarcomas and melanomas are second in frequency, accounting for 20% to 25% of the cases (Figure 71-2).

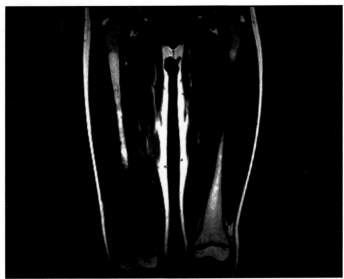

Figure 71-2. A 7-year-old boy treated for bilateral retinoblastoma during the fi rst year of life who presented with right thigh pain and swelling. A coronal T1-weighted MRI shows a mass arising from the right distal femur. Biopsy confirmed a primitive neuroectodermal tumor.

TREATMENT

The treatment of the different types of non-ocular tumors is highly variable, depending on the tumor's cell of origin as well as its location and extent. Radical resection, often combined with preoperative chemotherapy, is the treatment modality of choice. Avoidance of further radiation to potentially radiation-induced second malignancies is desirable.[5]

PREVENTION

Screening children for second malignancies is a lifelong process. The most important aspect of screening starts with educating the family about common signs of non-ocular cancers.

SCREENING

The morbidity and mortality of patients with non-ocular tumors are high.[6]

REFERENCES

1. Wong FL, Boice JD, Abramson DH, et al. Cancer incidence after retinoblastoma. Radiation dose and sarcoma risk. *JAMA.* 1997;278:1262-1267.
2. Abramson DH, Frank CM. Second nonocular tumors in survivors of bilateral retinoblastoma. A possible age effect on radiation-related risk. *Ophthalmology.* 1998;105:573-580.
3. Kleinerman RA, Tarone RE, Abramson DH, et al. Hereditary retinoblastoma and risk of lung cancer. *J Natl Cancer Inst.* 2000;92:2037-2039.
4. Moll AC, Imhof SM, Schouten-Van Meeteren AY, et al. Second primary tumors in hereditary retinoblastoma: a register-based study, 1945-1997: is there an age effect on radiation-related risk? *Ophthalmology.* 2001;108:1109-1114.
5. Eng G, Li FP, Abramson DH, et al. Mortality from second tumors among long-term survivors of retinoblastoma. *J Natl Cancer Inst.* 1993;85:1121-1128.
6. Aerts I, Pacquement H, Doz F, et al. Outcome of second malignancies after retinoblastoma: a retrospective analysis of 25 patients treated at the Institut Curie. *Eur J Cancer.* 2004;40:1522-1529.

Trilateral Retinoblastoma

Cari E. Lyle, Carlos Rodriguez-Galindo, and Matthew W. Wilson

INTRODUCTION

Trilateral retinoblastoma (TRB) refers to the association of bilateral retinoblastoma with an asynchronous intracranial tumor representing multicentric tumorigenesis in patients with the RB1 cancer predisposition syndrome.[1-3]

NATURE OF THE MIDLINE INTRACRANIAL TUMORS

TRB tumors are primitive neuroectodermal tumors exhibiting varying degrees of neuronal or photoreceptor differentiation.[4] The majority of these tumors are pineoblastomas, but 20% to 25% of cases are suprasellar or parasellar.

INCIDENCE OF TRILATERAL RETINOBLASTOMA

The incidence of TRB is approximately 3% in all patients with retinoblastoma and is estimated at around 5% to 6% in patients with bilateral retinoblastoma; the incidence may be as high as 10% to 15% in patients with familial retinoblastoma.[3] The median age at diagnosis of TRB is 23 to 48 months,[3] and the interval between the diagnosis of bilateral retinoblastoma and the diagnosis of the brain tumor is usually more than 20 months.[1,5]

SCREENING FOR TRILATERAL RETINOBLASTOMA

The children at highest risk for developing TRB are those with bilateral disease and a family history of retinoblastoma. Because of the poor prognosis of TRB, screening the midline lesions with neuroimaging is a common practice, although the screening recommendations are somewhat controversial (Figure 72-1).[6]

TREATMENT AND PROGNOSIS

The rare survivors are usually those diagnosed during neuroimaging. Despite treatment with intensive chemotherapy + craniospinal irradiation,[1] patients usually die of disseminated neuroaxis disease in less than 9 months.[1,5]

REFERENCES

1. Kivelä T. Trilateral retinoblastoma: a meta-analysis of hereditary retinoblastoma associated with primary ectopic intracranial retinoblastoma. *J Clin Oncol.* 1999;17:1829-1837.

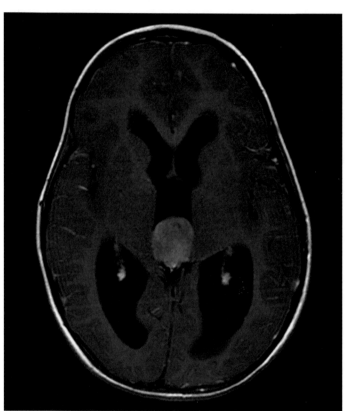

Figure 72-1. Brain MRI of a 3-year-old girl with trilateral retinoblastoma. Axial sequence shows a pineal tumor with secondary hydrocephalus. Resection and subsequent histopathologic evaluation confirmed a pinealoblastoma.

2. Amoaku WMK, Willshaw HE, Parkes SE, Shah KJ, Mann JR. Trilateral retinoblastoma: a report of five patients. *Cancer.* 1996;78:858-863.
3. Blach LE, McCormick B, Abramson DH, Ellsworth RM. Trilateral retinoblastoma—incidence and outcome: decade of experience. *Int J Radiat Oncol Biol Phys.* 1994;29:729-733.
4. Marcus DM, Brooks SE, Leff G, et al. Trilateral retinoblastoma: insights into histogenesis and management. *Surv Ophthalmol.* 1998;43:59-70.
5. Paulino AC. Trilateral retinoblastoma: is the location of the intracranial tumor important? *Cancer.* 1999;86:135-141.
6. Singh AD, Shields CL, Shields JA. New insights into trilateral retinoblastoma. *Cancer.* 1999;86:3-5.

Genetic Testing and Counseling

Robin D. Clark and Nancy C. Mansfield

INTRODUCTION

All patients with bilateral retinoblastoma have a germline mutation in RB1. However, for those with unilateral retinoblastoma, genetic counseling is less straightforward as only about 15% to 20% will have a germline mutation. Determining which patients have germline RB1 gene mutations allows genetic counseling for future reproduction, and it also allows the ophthalmologist and oncologist to make treatment and surveillance decisions tailored specifically to the patient's risk status.

Pedigree or Family History

The family history, documented in a three-or-more-generation pedigree, is the fundamental working tool for the geneticist.

Chromosome 13q14 Deletions

Deletion of chromosome 13q14, the site of the RB1 gene, and neighboring regions on the long arm of chromosome 13 can lead to mental retardation and retinoblastoma. Developmental delay or mental retardation may be appreciated before retinoblastoma is diagnosed (Figure 73A-1).

Mosaicism in which the RB1 mutation is present in some but not all cells of the affected child, is common in the first affected member of a family with retinoblastoma (Figure 73A-2).[1]

Low-penetrance mutations and variable expressivity are often due to missense mutations in RB1 that do not truncate the protein product.[2]

THE ISOLATED CASE OF UNILATERAL RETINOBLASTOMA

It is the isolated case of unilateral retinoblastoma (URb) that is most problematic for the genetic counselor. The lack of a family history and an older age at onset of unilateral sporadic retinoblastoma does not exclude a germline RB1 mutation.[3]

Mutation Detection

In the ideal situation, a small sample of fresh frozen tumor will be saved at the time of enucleation to be used later for mutation detection. When both blood and tumor samples are submitted for DNA testing, it will be apparent when the test fails to detect the mutation as all tumors should have 2 RB1 mutations. When DNA testing shows an abnormal result, the parents and other first-degree relatives should be tested for the same mutation. Unaf-

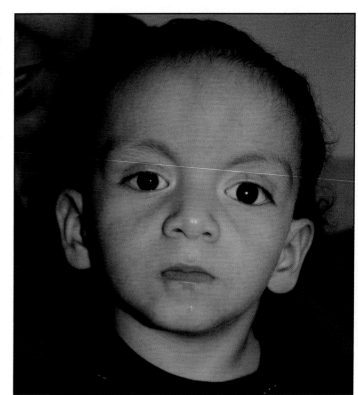

Figure 73A-1. It is the isolated case of unilateral retinoblastoma (URb) that is most problematic for the genetic counselor. The lack of a family history and an older age at onset of unilateral sporadic retinoblastoma does not exclude a germline RB1 mutation.

fected relatives may have the same RB1 mutation without ever having had retinoblastoma.

Normal Results

False-negative results are a concern because even in the best laboratories, using a variety of DNA techniques, RB1 gene analysis yields a detection rate of about 92% (Table 73A-1). Therefore, normal results should always be interpreted with caution, and patients should be counseled that sensitivity for mutation detection is not 100%.

Linkage analysis is an indirect form of DNA testing in which the actual mutation is not detected, but nearby DNA markers, some of which may be within the RB1 gene itself, can be tracked

Table 73A-1. Retinoblastoma Gene Testing Techniques: Limitations and Detection Rates

	Technique	Limitations	Detection Rate (%)
Cytogenetic analysis	Chromosome analysis	Limited to detection of chromosome 13 translocations, rearrangements, and very large deletions	5
		Should be done in conjunction with FISH for 13q14	
	FISH for 13q14	Limited to detection of large RB1 gene deletions	
		Should be done in conjunction with chromosome analysis	
Direct DNA analysis	RB1 gene sequence analysis	Limited to detection of small sequence variations	70
		Detects small deletions, insertions, point mutations	
		Does not reliably detect mosaicism or splice site changes deep within introns	
	RB1 quantitative multiplex PCR	Limited to detection of deletions and gene rearrangements	20
	RB1 allele-specific PCR	Limited to cases in which familial mutation is known and mosaicism is suspected	
	Methylation of RB1 promoter	Limited to nonhereditary, sporadic, unilateral retinoblastoma	11
Indirect DNA analysis	Linkage analysis	Limited to multigenerational families	
		Mosaicism in proband can lead to false-positive result for unaffected offspring	

RB1, retinoblastoma gene; FISH, fluorescence in situ hybridization; PCR, polymerase chain reaction.

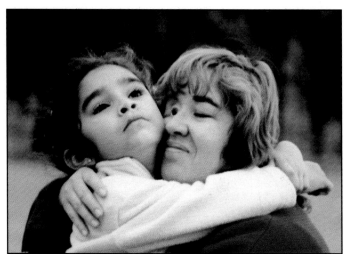

Figure 73A-2. The mother in this photograph had unilateral retinoblastoma. After her daughter was diagnosed with bilateral retinoblastoma, the mother was found to be mosaic for the germline mutation in RB1 that caused the daughter's disease. This family illustrates the point that when retinoblastoma is caused by a new sporadic mutation, the founder individual may be mosaic for the RB1 mutation (ie, it can occur at some point after conception and the first cell division). When searching for the mutation in a two-generation family, the second generation should always be tested first, if possible. Also, this family confirms comments in the text that a negative DNA test for a germline mutation in a unilateral patient may fail to detect low-level mosaicism.

through affected relatives. Linkage analysis should be used with caution in prenatal diagnosis as undetected mosaicism in the first affected case can lead to false-positive results in unaffected offspring.

REFERENCES

1. Dudin G, Nasr A, Traboulsi E, et al. Hereditary retinoblastoma and 13q-mosaicism. *Cytogenet Cell Genet.* 1984;38:235-237.
2. Lohmann DR, Brandt B, Hopping W, et al. Distinct RB1 gene mutations with low penetrance in hereditary retinoblastoma. *Hum Genet.* 1994;94:349-354.
3. Brichard B, Heusterspreute M, De Potter P, et al. Unilateral retinoblastoma, lack of familial history and older age does not exclude germline RB1 gene mutation. *Eur J Cancer.* 2006;42:65-72.

Family Counseling

Nancy C. Mansfield and Robin D. Clark

INTRODUCTION

The counselor should understand the special significance that retinoblastoma has, not only for the affected child or adult survivor, but for the entire family. Even when the facts and information are absorbed by the family, genetic counseling for retinoblastoma is complicated by the psychological and emotional aspects of this disorder. Geneticists, ophthalmologists, psychologists, social workers, and other mental health professionals work best when they work together to help families grapple with the lifelong implications of the information they have been given.

THE FAMILY/PATIENT'S REACTION TO THE DIAGNOSIS

Often family members experience one or more common feelings (Box 73B-1). These responses are all coping mechanisms that many of us use at one time or another to allow us to handle difficult situations. It is normal for parents to experience one or more of these reactions. The successful counselor will anticipate these responses and help families find ways to cope effectively.

ANXIETY ABOUT HAVING MORE CHILDREN

The ability to reproduce effectively goes to the core of our view of ourselves. Most couples want to have a family. If they have a child with retinoblastoma, the parent can also feel that they are somehow defective or abnormal.

HOW TO GIVE BAD NEWS

Arguably, there is no right way to give bad news, but it seems that there are many wrong ways. Most of us are uncomfortable when we give bad news, and few feel that we do this part of our job particularly well. In these difficult situations, it may be easy to rationalize doing it quickly, but taking more time is always preferable (Box 73B-2).

Box 73B-1. Common Emotional Reactions

Denial	Intellectualization	Anger
Depression	Guilt	Blaming
Shock	Helplessness	Anxiety
Worry	Flat affect	Doubt over results
Negation of the information	Unwillingness to follow through with recommended tests	Questioning every piece of information

---

Box 73B-2. How to Communicate Effectively With Patients When Delivering Bad News

- Allow enough time: Often an hour or more is needed.
- Arrange for a face-to-face appointment. This is not to be done over the phone.
- Follow the "Golden Rule" and treat others as you would wish to be treated.
- Demonstrate kindness, respect, dignity, acceptance, and validation.
- Sit down when speaking.
- If giving bad news, say you are "Sorry to report . . ."
- Offer tissues or a glass of water when patients are upset.
- Explain information clearly, concisely, and slowly.
- Make a drawing or create a list to reinforce your points.
- Have information repeated back to you to be sure you were understood.
- Plan to give information more than once.
- If in a teaching institution, involve your students either before or after seeing the family.
- Set up a follow-up appointment to go over the information and answer questions.
- Assume that much of the information will not be absorbed owing to anxiety.
- Accept the reaction of families even if you are surprised by their feelings.
- If necessary, offer referrals for support.
- Offer your assistance in the future when the need arises.
- Teach kindness to your staff, as they are your representatives.
- Expect the unexpected: we cannot predict reactions even from the most resourceful individuals.

Chemotherapy for Retinoblastoma: An Overview

Rima F. Jubran, Judith G. Villablanca, and Anna T. Meadows

INTRODUCTION

The management of patients with intraocular retinoblastoma has changed dramatically in the past 15 years with the introduction of primary systemic chemotherapy. In the early 1990s, several investigators from North America and Great Britain began using systemic agents to treat intraocular retinoblastoma (CEV regimen, comprising carboplatin, etoposide, and vincristine) that had been found to be successful in the treatment of central nervous system neoplasms.[1] Other indications for chemotherapy in a patient with retinoblastoma include prophylaxis against metastasis following enucleation in the presence of histopathologic high-risk features, extraocular retinoblastoma with local and/or regional spread, metastatic retinoblastoma with or without central nervous system (CNS) involvement, and trilateral retinoblastoma (Box 74-1).

RESPONSE TO SYSTEMIC CEV CHEMOTHERAPY COMBINED WITH LOCAL THERAPY

Good responses were noted when these agents were combined with local ophthalmic therapy (Chapter 75). The intention was to reduce the volume of intraocular tumor with systemic chemotherapy so as to allow better tumor kill with local laser photocoagulation and cryotherapy (Figure 74-1).

Response in Eyes With Early Disease

This approach was very successful in eyes with Reese–Ellsworth Stage I–III tumors (International Group A and Group B) using either six courses of low-dose or three courses of high-dose CEV.[2,3]

Response in Eyes With Advanced Disease

Although eyes with subretinal or vitreous seeds responded initially, the tumors usually recurred within 9 months of diagnosis.[2,4] This spurred the idea that increasing the doses of the CEV regimen (high-dose CEV) and adding subtenon or periocular carboplatin delivered locally might achieve higher drug concentrations in the vitreous, where blood supply was poor, and would improve the outcomes of patients with Reese–Ellsworth Group IV–V eyes (International Group C and D eyes). Preliminary studies with high-dose CEV and subtenon carboplatin have indeed resulted in improved ocular salvage rates.[5,6] However, toxicities reported with this therapy include periorbital fat atrophy associated with

mild to moderate cosmetic changes, limitation of extraocular movements, and rare cases of optic atrophy.[5]

OTHER SYSTEMIC CHEMOTHERAPY REGIMENS

They include carboplatin alone, carboplatin with vincristine, and carboplatin, etoposide/tenoposide, and vincristine. Furthermore, some have added cyclosporin in an effort to reduce chemotherapy resistance.[7]

CHEMOTHERAPY AGENTS

Carboplatin interrupts DNA replication and cell division by forming cross-links with DNA.

Etoposide is an epipodophyllotoxin and acts as a topoisomerase II inhibitor.

Vincristine is an alkaloid that disrupts microtubules inducing metaphase arrest.

CEV TOXICITY

Common Expected Toxicity

Myelosuppression is the most common toxicity, with blood product transfusion and uncomplicated febrile neutropenic hospital admissions as the result.

Uncommon Serious Toxicity

Toxicity associated with etoposide is the secondary acute myeloid leukemia.[8] There have been few reports of secondary

Box 74-1. Indications for Chemotherapy

- Intraocular retinoblastoma
- Prophylaxis against metastasis following enucleation in the presence of histopathologic high-risk features
- Extraocular retinoblastoma with local and/or regional spread
- Metastatic retinoblastoma with or without CNS involvement
- Trilateral retinoblastoma

leukemia in patients treated with systemic chemotherapy for intraocular retinoblastoma due to the lower cumulative doses of etoposide used in these patients compared to the pediatric oncology population at large.

PROPHYLAXIS FOR PATIENTS WITH HIGH-RISK HISTOPATHOLOGY

High-Risk Features

Common criteria include "massive" choroidal invasion, involvement of tumor past the lamina cribrosa, and tumor invading into the sclera (Chapter 77).

THERAPEUTIC APPROACHES TO EXTRAOCULAR RETINOBLASTOMA

The treatment of extraocular retinoblastoma is discussed in more detail in Chapters 78 (Orbital Retinoblastoma) and 79 (Metastatic Retinoblastoma).

REFERENCES

1. Kingston JE, Hungerford JL. Madreperla SA, et al. Results of combined chemotherapy and radiotherapy for advanced intraocular retinoblastoma. *Arch Ophthalmol.* 1996;114:1339-1343.
2. Freidman DL, Himelstein B, Shields CL, et al. Chemoreduction and local ophthalmic therapy for intraocular retinoblastoma. *J Clin Oncol.* 2000;22:12-17.
3. Jubran RF, Murphree AL, Villablanca JG. "High dose" CEV and local ophthalmic therapy for group B intraocular retinoblastoma. *Proceedings 12th International Symposium on Retinoblastoma.* 2005.
4. Shields CL, Honavar SG, Meadows AT, et al. Chemoreduction plus focal therapy for retinoblastoma: factors predictive of need for treatment with external beam radiotherapy or enucleation. *Am J Ophthalmol.* 2002;133:657-664.
5. Abramson DH, Frank CM, Dunkel IJ. A phase I/II study of subconjuctival carboplatin for intraocular retinoblastoma. *Ophthalmology.* 1999;106:1947-1950.
6. Villablanca JG, Jubran RF, Murphree AL. Phase I study of subtenon carboplatin with systemic high dose carboplatin/etoposide/vincristine for group C, D and E intraocular retinoblastoma. *Proceedings 12th International Symposium on Retinoblastoma.* 2005.
7. Chan HS, DeBoer G, Thiessen JJ, et al. Combining cyclosporine with chemotherapy controls intraocular retinoblastoma without requiring radiation. *Clin Cancer Res.* 1996;2:1499-1508.
8. Smith MA, Rubinstein L, Anderson JR, et al. Secondary leukemia or myelodysplastic syndrome after treatment with epipodophyllotoxins. *J Clin Oncol.* 1999;17:567.

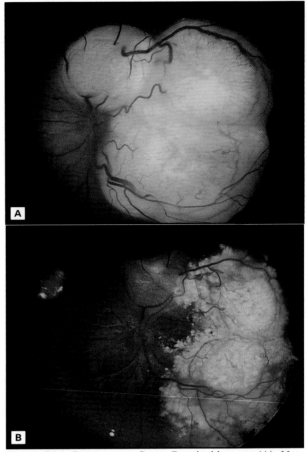

Figure 74-1. Pretreatment Group B retinoblastoma (A). Note reduction in tumor volume 3 weeks after the administration of the first cycle of carboplatin, etoposide, vincristine (B). Focal consolidation may start at this time (concurrently with the second cycle of chemotherapy) or at the beginning of the third cycle.

Local Therapy, Brachytherapy, and Enucleation

A. Linn Murphree

INTRODUCTION

The two most common surgical procedures used as part of the treatment of intraocular retinoblastoma are local therapy, either primary or for consolidation following systemic chemotherapy, and enucleation.

TERMINOLOGY

Local Treatment

Before primary systemic chemotherapy was introduced as treatment for intraocular retinoblastoma in the early 1990s, all intraocular retinoblastoma therapy, including photocoagulation, thermotherapy, chemothermotherapy, cryotherapy, brachytherapy, and external beam radiotherapy, could be considered local treatment (Table 75-1). External beam radiotherapy of retinoblastoma is discussed in Chapter 76.

Local Primary Treatment

Primary treatment refers to local treatment employed as the sole therapy for very small tumors (Group A).

Chemoreduction or Neoadjuvant Chemotherapy

The term *chemoreduction* is used to describe induction of tumor shrinkage as the function of primary systemic chemotherapy, implying the need for a subsequent consolidation treatment.

Consolidation Treatment

In today's treatment environment, local treatment is applied more frequently following primary systemic chemotherapy or chemoreduction. The term consolidation, as used in oncology, is a therapy that is used in tandem with primary therapy to "mop up" or eliminate the tumor cells that were resistant to, or were not inactivated by, the primary therapy. In the case of intraocular retinoblastoma, local consolidation consists of direct laser photocoagulation, hyperthermia, thermochemotherapy, thermotherapy, or cryotherapy. Brachytherapy is not routinely used for focal consolidation because of the very high risk of aggressive radiation retinopathy.

LOCAL PRIMARY TREATMENT

Group A eyes with small intraretinal lesions away from critical structures are candidates for local primary therapy, such as direct laser photocoagulation or cryotherapy (Chapter 69).

LOCAL CONSOLIDATION TREATMENT

Photocoagulation

Photocoagulation is useful in most situations for local consolidation after at least one cycle of systemic chemotherapy (Figure 75-1). Typically, the treatment is repeated every 3 to 4 weeks immediately before the next cycle of chemotherapy. Edge recurrence may appear if the laser consolidation is insufficient or significantly delayed.

Transpupillary Thermotherapy

Transpupillary thermotherapy (TTT) is a direct tumor cell killing system that couples large spot size (2 to 3 mm) and long burn duration (1 minute) with low power settings, applied to achieve the end point of gentle whitening in the treatment spot (Chapter 40).

Thermochemotherapy

The use of the infrared diode laser hyperthermia (42° to 45°C) to provide synergistic tumor killing with platinum-based chemotherapy, carboplatin, is referred to as thermochemotherapy.[1]

TRANS-SCLERAL CRYOTHERAPY

The indications for cryotherapy are similar to those for laser thermotherapy, but cryotherapy is more suitable for anterior tumors. At least 70% of carefully selected tumors can be treated with cryotherapy.[2] The treatment is repeated every 3 to 4 weeks. A flat chorioretinal scar is an acceptable end point (Figure 75-2).

BRACHYTHERAPY

The principles of brachytherapy (Chapter 8) and plaque design (Chapter 41) are discussed in other sections of the book. The standard apical dose for retinoblastoma is 45 Gy.[3]

Brachytherapy is rarely considered for routine focal consolidation because of the very high risk of aggressive radiation retinopathy. Instead, it is useful for either the primary treatment of an isolated Group B tumor at or anterior to the equator, or for the treatment of edge recurrences that are too large or extensive for laser or cryotherapy (Figure 75-3).

Table 75-1. Local Treatment of Retinoblastoma

Treatment	Indication	Complications
Photocoagulation	Primary treatment, consolidation treatment, and for tumor recurrence	Tumor seeding into vitreous
		Retinal fibrosis and traction
	Tumors not more than 3 mm in diameter, with no evidence of seeding, and located posterior to the equator	Retinal vascular occlusion
Thermotherapy	Primary treatment, consolidation treatment, and for tumor recurrence	Iris atrophy, focal cataracts
		Tumor seeding into vitreous
	Tumors not more than 3 mm in diameter, with no evidence of seeding, and located posterior to the equator	Retinal fibrosis and traction
		Retinal vascular occlusion
Thermochemotherapy	Consolidation treatment. Tumors not more than 12 mm in diameter, with no evidence of seeding, and located posterior to the equator	Iris atrophy, focal cataracts
		Tumor seeding into vitreous, transient retinal detachment, diffuse choroidal atrophy
Cryotherapy	Primary treatment, consolidation treatment, and for tumor recurrence	Large area of retinal atrophy, transient retinal detachment, retinal hole, retinal detachment
	Tumors not more than 3 mm in diameter, with no evidence of seeding, and located anterior to the equator "Cutting cryo" for posterior tumors	
Brachytherapy	Primary treatment, residual tumor following photocoagulation/thermotherapy thermochemotherapy/ cryotherapy, and for tumor recurrence	Radiation retinopathy, radiation optic neuropathy
	Tumor less than 15 mm in diameter Presence of diffuse vitreous seeding is contraindication	

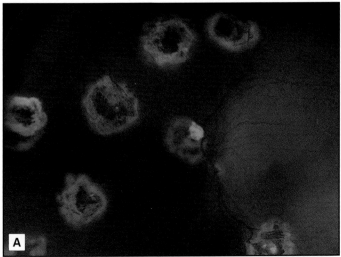 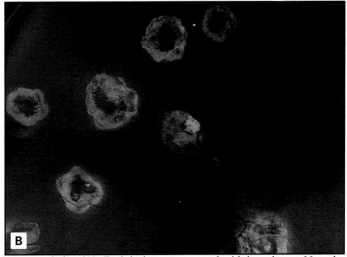

Figure 75-1. Image taken immediately after the third consolidation laser photocoagulation (A). Each lesion was covered with laser burns. Note the distinct gentle white burn at the lesion edge. There is differential energy uptake. Three weeks later, all lesions are flat with no clinical evidence of active disease (B). We recommend three complete coverage of lesions like these at 3- to 4-week intervals.

ENUCLEATION

Enucleation is the best choice for advanced disease present in only one eye. If an ocular "event" such as diffuse subretinal satellite tumors occurs, then enucleation may be the treatment of choice (Figure 75-4). Some of the principles and techniques of enucleation are discussed elsewhere (Chapter 98).

Attention to Surgical Closure and Prevention of Implant Extrusion

We pack fat and connective tissue (autologous orbital fat graft-AOFG) harvested from the back of the enucleated globe over the anterior surface of the implant. We then close the anterior Tenon's capsule with horizontal mattress sutures 4 to 5 mm posterior to the conjunctival edge using 5-0 Vicryl for good position and maintenance of the upper and lower cul-de-sac.

Meticulous intraoperative hemostasis (MIH) allows the surgery to be precise and controlled and facilitates the obtaining of a long section of optic nerve.

Long Optic Nerve Stump

Certain surgical steps can facilitate obtaining about a 15-mm long optic nerve stump in all cases of retinoblastoma (see Figure 75-4 and Chapter 78).[4]

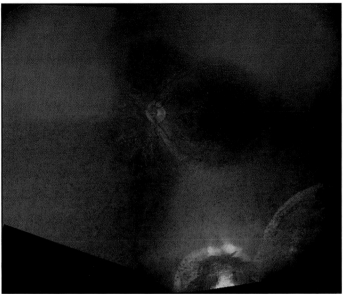

Figure 75-2. Two cryotherapy scars in the inferotemporal periphery. Note extensive destruction of the peripheral retina.

Harvest of Fresh Tumor for RB1 Testing or Other Research Uses

An 8.5- to 9.0-mm corneal trephine can be used to gently open a round "window" in the wall of the globe. Forceps and scissors are then used to remove a sample of the tumor.

REFERENCES

1. Murphree AL, Villablanca JG, Deegan WF 3rd, et al. Chemotherapy plus local treatment in the management of intraocular retinoblastoma. *Arch Ophthalmol.* 1996;114:1348-1356.
2. Abramson DH, Ellsworth RM, Rozakis GW. Cryotherapy for retinoblastoma. *Arch Ophthalmol.* 1982;100:1253-1256.
3. Shields CL, Shields JA, Cater J, et al. Plaque radiotherapy for retinoblastoma: long term tumor control and treatment complications in 208 tumors. *Ophthalmology.* 2001;108:2116-2121.
4. Moshfeghi DM, Moshfeghi AA, Finger PT. Enucleation. *Surv Ophthalmol.* 2000;44:277-301.

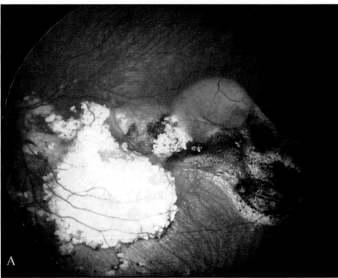

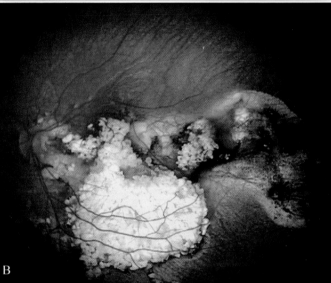

Figure 75-3. A Group C eye with solitary peripheral tumor that is a candidate for brachytherapy. A 12-month-old child with bilateral retinoblastoma treated with chemoreduction and consolidation. Note tumor recurrence within the chorioretinal scar from previous cryotherapy in the left eye (A). There was tumor regression within 4 weeks of brachytherapy (B). A 16-mm round ruthenium-106 plaque (apical dose 38.70 Gy, total duration 32 hours) was used for plaque radiotherapy.

Figure 75-4 (on page 192). Key steps in the successful enucleation of a Group E eye. Immediately after the peritomy, the Tenon's capsule is being spread widely and deeply between the rectus muscles with a curved Stephens' scissor (A). 2 mL of a 1:1 mixture of short- and long-acting local anesthesia is deposited in the retrobulbar space using an irrigating cannula (B). Dry orbit immediately after removing the iced saline-filled test tube that had provided gentle pressure to the apex for 10 minutes (C). 20-mm conical SST Medpor implant being inserted into the orbit (D). The predrilled holes and orientation for the rectus muscles are indicated by a skin marker. The four rectus muscles are attached to the predrilled implant (E). The previously harvested retrobulbar fat and connective tissue is placed over the exposed surface of the implant to provide a cushion between suture knots and Tenon's closure to assist in preventing postoperative implant extrusion (F). The first horizontal mattress suture (5-0 Vicryl) has been tied (G). Three to four more mattress sutures will be used to approximate the tissues. Six to eight vertical interrupted sutures across the horizontal mattress sutures will provide strength to the Tenon's closure. The appearance of the child immediately after the drape has been removed following the removal of the left eye (H). Note the lack of ecchymosis or lid edema. A simple patch will be used only for the first 24 hours.

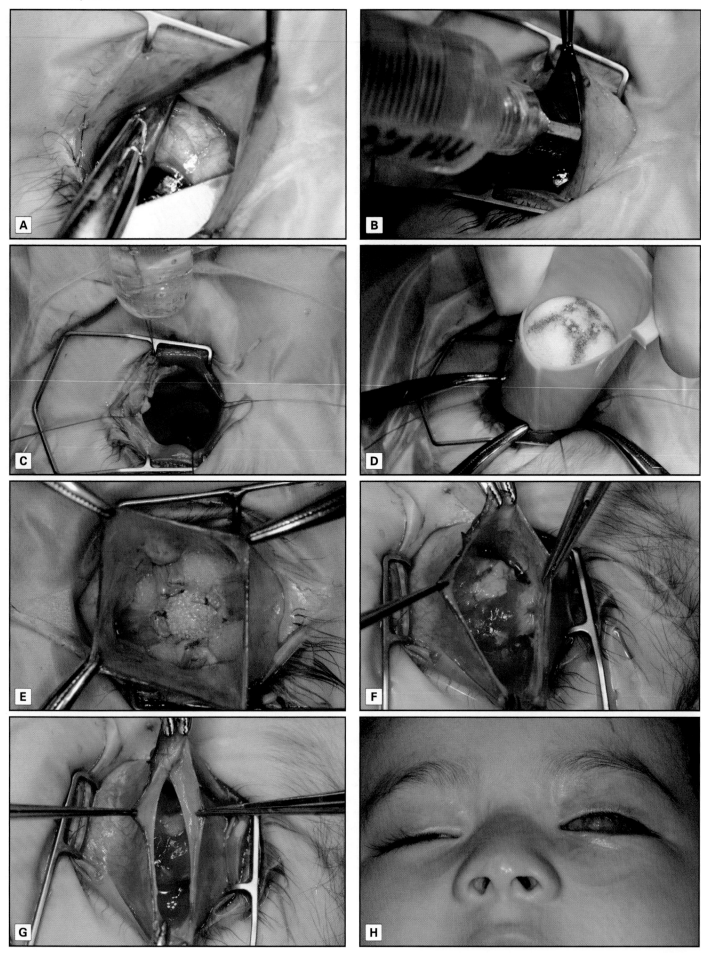

Teletherapy: Indications, Risks, and New Delivery Options

Thomas E. Merchant

INTRODUCTION

In the treatment of retinoblastoma, radiation therapy provides the benchmark for the evaluation of tumor control, for eye preservation, and for side effects. Its role has recently been diminished by the haunting prospect of long-term side effects and a move toward chemotherapy combined with local ophthalmic therapy (Chapter 74).[1]

EFFICACY

Radiation therapy, in its many forms, is a highly effective non-surgical treatment for retinoblastoma, but its effectiveness must be balanced against its potential side effects, because of the patients' young age and genetic susceptibility to further malignancy (Chapter 71).

Globe Preservation

Radiation therapy has an excellent track record in preserving the eye. In patients with Reese–Ellsworth Group I–II disease, tumor control rates measured at 5 years are in excess of 95%. In patients with more advanced disease (Reese–Ellsworth Groups III–IV), 5-year control rates reduce to approximately 50%, owing partly to the greater tumor burden and the intraocular extent of disease.[2] Patients with Reese–Ellsworth Group Vb disease have 5-year eye-preservation rates of approximately 53%.[3] Poor tumor control in advanced cases is often attributed to vitreous seeding.

Visual Acuity

Most patients are reported to have good visual acuity (20/20–20/40) after radiation therapy; the rest have at least some prospect of functional vision (20/50–20/400).[4,5] Final visual acuity and field are affected by tumor location, which often depends on the patient's age at the time of diagnosis: younger patients are more likely to have tumors in the macula (Figure 76-1).[6]

SIDE EFFECTS AND SECONDARY MALIGNANCIES

These side effects include ophthalmic complications, such as retinal detachment, vitreous hemorrhage, cataract formation, and glaucoma; somatic complications, such as orbital hypoplasia; and the most daunting of all, the second malignant neoplasm (Chapter 71).

REDUCING SIDE EFFECTS FROM RADIATION THERAPY

A number of measures may be taken to reduce the likelihood of second malignant neoplasms and radiation-related treatment effects in children with retinoblastoma: (1) delay radiation therapy until the patient is 12 months old; (2) reduce the total dose of radiation; (3) use episcleral plaque brachytherapy; and (4) apply new external beam treatment methods and modalities (Figure 76-2), including conformal radiation therapy, intensity-modulated radiation therapy, and proton beam radiation therapy (Box 76-1) (Chapter 8).

CURRENT RECOMMENDATIONS

Our recommendations for patients with newly diagnosed retinoblastoma include 36 Gy for Reese–Ellsworth Group I or II disease and standard dose irradiation (45 Gy) for more advanced (Reese–Ellsworth Group III–V) disease. For patients whose disease progresses after chemotherapy, our bias is to irradiate with standard doses (outside a protocol) and to use episcleral plaque brachytherapy when possible. We recommend defining the clinical target volume as the optic globe and the treatment planning target volume as the optic globe with a 3- to 5-mm margin. Additional individualized techniques include using a split beam to spare the lens and using electrons, conformal irradiation, IMRT, and proton beam radiation therapy.

REFERENCES

1. Wilson MW, Rodriguez-Galindo C, Haik BG, et al. Multiagent chemotherapy as neoadjuvant treatment for multifocal intraocular retinoblastoma. *Ophthalmology.* 2001;108:2106-2114; discussion 2114-2115.
2. Blach LE, McCormick B, Abramson DH. External beam radiation therapy and retinoblastoma: long-term results in the comparison of two techniques. *Int J Radiat Oncol Biol Phys.* 1996;35:45-51.

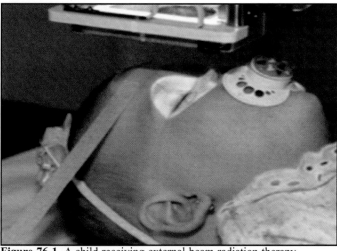

Figure 76-1. A child receiving external beam radiation therapy.

> **Box 76-1. Measures to Reduce Radiation-Related Treatment Effects in Children With Retinoblastoma**
>
> - Delay radiation therapy until the patient is 12 months old
> - Reduce the total dose of radiation
> - Use episcleral plaque brachytherapy (if applicable)
> - Consider new external beam treatment methods, including conformal radiation therapy, intensity-modulated radiation therapy, and proton beam radiation therapy

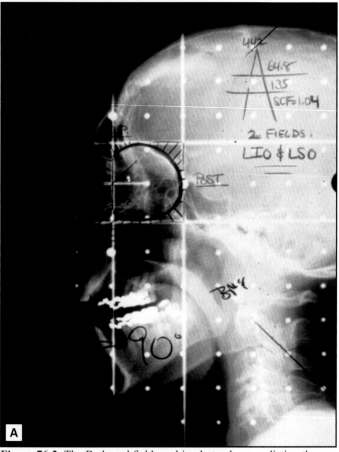

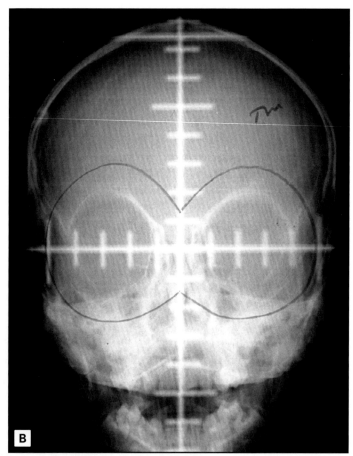

Figure 76-2. The D-shaped field used in photon beam radiation therapy (A). An en face bilateral electron field (B).

3. Abramson DH, Beaverson KL, Chang ST, et al. Outcome following initial external beam radiotherapy in patients with Reese-Ellsworth group Vb retinoblastoma. *Arch Ophthalmol.* 2004;122:1316-1323.

4. Egbert PR, Donaldson SS, Moazed K, Rosenthal AR. Visual results and ocular complications following radiotherapy for retinoblastoma. *Arch Ophthalmol.* 1978;96:1826-1830.

5. Hall LS, Ceisler E, Abramson DH. Visual outcomes in children with bilateral retinoblastoma. *J AAPOS.* 1999;3:138-142.

6. Brinkert AW, Moll AC, Jager MJ, et al. Distribution of tumors in the retina in hereditary retinoblastoma patients. *Ophthalm Genet.* 1998;19:63-67.

77

Histopathologic Features and Prognostic Factors

Patricia Chévez-Barrios, Ralph C. Eagle, Jr, and Eduardo F. Marback

INTRODUCTION

Retinoblastoma is a tumor that arises from the neuroblastic cells that comprise the nuclear layers of the retina.[1-4] Grossly, the tumor is classified by its pattern of growth into endophytic, exophytic, mixed, diffuse infiltrative, and necrotic variants.

GROSS FEATURES

Endophytic

Endophytic tumor grows from the retina into the vitreous cavity and disperses small pieces of tumor into the vitreous called vitreous seeds (Figure 77-1A).

Exophytic

Exophytic tumor grows toward the choroid into the subretinal space, detaching the retina and forming subretinal tumor seeds, which are prone to choroidal invasion (Figure 77-1B).

Mixed

This growth pattern is the most common and displays both endophytic and exophytic patterns (Figure 77-1C).

Diffuse Infiltrative

Another growth pattern of clinical importance is the diffuse infiltrative type, which typically presents in older children. Diffuse tumors infiltrate the retina without forming an obvious retinal mass and often invade the anterior segment, forming a pseudohypopyon of tumor cells mistaken clinically for an inflammatory process.[2]

Necrotic

Finally, an extensively necrotic retinoblastoma can present clinically as an inflammatory process that mimics orbital cellulitis with chemosis and proptosis.[1,5,6]

HISTOPATHOLOGIC FEATURES

The characteristic histopathologic findings in retinoblastoma include a tumor that replaces the retina with medium-sized cells that have a high nuclear:cytoplasmic ratio, marked apoptotic and mitotic activity, and foci of necrosis with calcification (Figure 77-2A, B). The areas of necrosis typically surround vessels that are cuffed by a layer of viable cells measuring 90 to 100 μm in radius (Figure 77-2C). The active turnover of the tumor often releases DNA from the cells, which forms basophilic deposits on basement membranes. Most of the tumor grows as sheets or large foci of undifferentiated cells.[1] Occasionally, there are areas of tumor differentiation evident as rosettes and fleurettes. The most differentiated tumors exhibit actual photoreceptor differentiation that are seen as bouquet-like aggregates of cells called fleurettes, which lack mitoses or necrosis. A tumor composed solely of fleurettes is designated retinocytoma or retinoma—the benign counterpart of retinoblastoma (Chapter 80).[1-3] Flexner–Wintersteiner rosettes comprise a ring of nuclei surrounding an empty lumen analogous to the subretinal space. The cells are joined by intercellular attachments similar to those found between photoreceptors. Primitive Homer Wright rosettes are formed by a rim of nuclei with a center filled by tangles of cytoplasmic filaments.

HISTOPATHOLOGIC FACTORS THAT MAY BE PROGNOSTIC

Multivariate statistical analysis has suggested the correlation of certain histopathologic findings and prognostic risk factors (see Table 81-2).[7-9] Multicenter prospective trials are underway to evaluate the value of adjuvant chemotherapy based on the known histopathologic risk factors (Chapter 81).

CONCLUSION

Perhaps the question of which child with an enucleated eye containing retinoblastoma is at risk for disease dissemination will be best answered when we begin to understand other indicators of tumor behavior and when we use these indicators in combination with the traditional prognostic factors. Animal models, and collaborative clinical trials, will ultimately allow the use of targeted therapies to prevent metastasis and death from retinoblastoma.

REFERENCES

1. McLean IW, Burnier M, Zimmerman L, Jakobiec F. Tumors of the retina. In: McLean IW, Burnier MN, Zimmerman LE, et al, eds. *Atlas of Tumor Pathology. Tumors of the Eye and Ocular Adnexa.* Washington, DC: Armed Forced Institute of Pathology; 1994: 100-135.

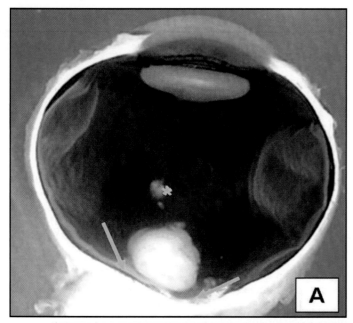

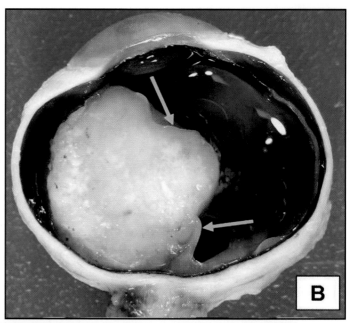

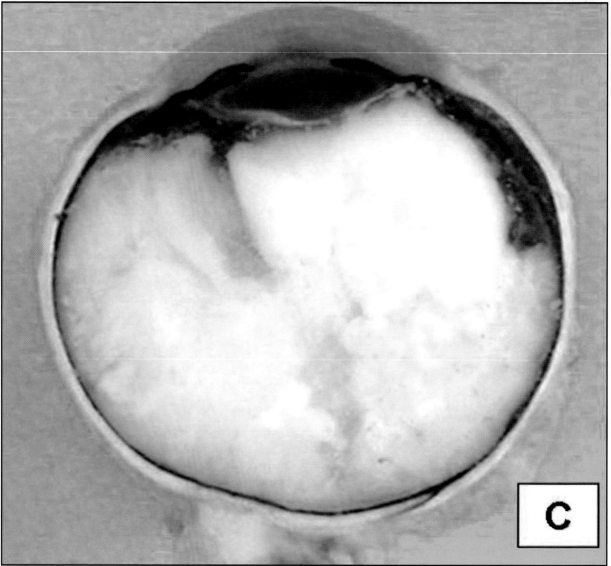

Figure 77-1. Patterns of tumor growth. Endophytic growth pattern with tumor arising from retina (arrows) and invading into the vitreous (A). Notice the formation of vitreous seeds (*), which are small pieces of tumor floating in the vitreous. Exophytic growth pattern with tumor arising from retina (arrows) and invading into the subretinal space (B). Mixed growth pattern is a combination of endophytic and exophytic where the retina is mostly replaced by tumor (C).

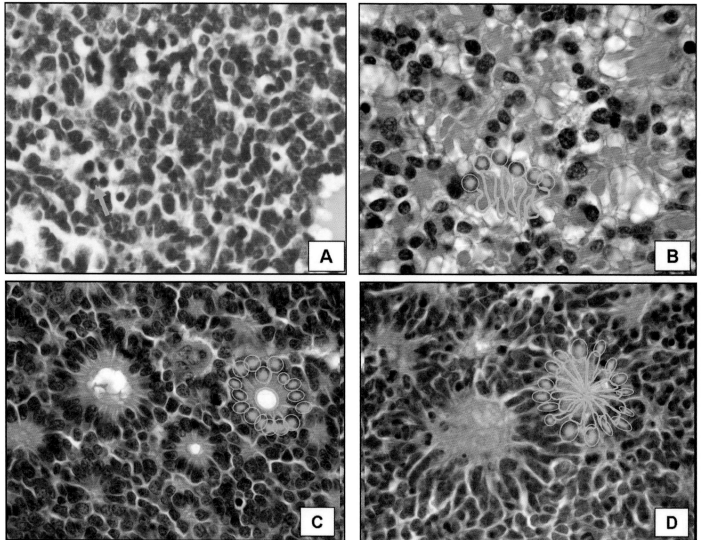

Figure 77-2. Retinoblastoma is composed of small blue cells and arises from the retina (ret); the tumor cell alternates with geographic areas of necrosis (N) and invades the vitreous (vit) (A). (Original magnification x2.) Higher magnification shows necrosis (N) and calcifications (Ca++) (B). Flexner–Wintersteiner rosettes are tumor cells forming a round structure with a clear center rimmed by a membrane like the outer limiting membrane in the retina (C). Homer Wright rosettes have a lumen filed by cytoplasmic prolongations of the tumor cells (D). (Original magnification x40.)

2. Hurwitz RL, Chévez-Barrios P, Chintagumpala M, Shields C, Shields J. Retinoblastoma. In: Pizzo PA, Poplack D, eds. *Principles and Practice of Pediatric Oncology.* 5th ed. Philadelphia, PA: Lippincott-Raven; 2006:825-846.

3. Sang DN, Albert DM. Retinoblastoma: clinical and histopathologic features. *Hum Pathol.* 1982;13:133-147.

4. Augsburger JJ, Oehlschlager U, Manzitti JE. Multinational clinical and pathologic registry of retinoblastoma. Retinoblastoma International Collaborative Study report 2. *Graefes Arch Clin Exp Ophthalmol.* 1995;233:469-475.

5. Andersen SR, Jensen OA. Retinoblastoma with necrosis of central retinal artery and vein and partial spontaneous regression. *Acta Ophthalmol.* 1974;52:183-193.

6. Mullaney PB, Karcioglu ZA, Huaman AM, al-Mesfer S. Retinoblastoma associated orbital cellulitis. *Br J Ophthalmol.* 1998;82:517-521.

7. Kopelman JE, McLean IW, Rosenberg SH. Multivariate analysis of risk factors for metastasis in retinoblastoma treated by enucleation. *Ophthalmology.* 1987;94:371-377.

8. Messmer EP, Heinrich T, Hopping W, et al. Risk factors for metastases in patients with retinoblastoma. *Ophthalmology.* 1991;98:136-141.

9. Singh AD, Shields CL, Shields JA. Prognostic factors in retinoblastoma. *J Pediatr Ophthalmol Strabismus.* 2000;37:134-141.

Orbital Retinoblastoma

Santosh G. Honavar

INTRODUCTION

Orbital retinoblastoma is relatively more common in developing countries. In a recent large multicenter study from Mexico, 18% of 500 patients presented with an orbital retinoblastoma.[1]

CLINICAL MANIFESTATIONS

Primary orbital retinoblastoma is clinically or radiologically detected orbital extension of an intraocular retinoblastoma at the initial presentation, with or without proptosis or a fungating mass (Figure 78-1).

Secondary orbital retinoblastoma is orbital recurrence following uncomplicated enucleation for intraocular retinoblastoma.

Accidental orbital retinoblastoma is inadvertent perforation, fine needle aspiration biopsy, or intraocular surgery in an eye with unsuspected intraocular retinoblastoma.

Overt orbital retinoblastoma is previously unrecognized extrascleral or optic nerve extension discovered during enucleation.

Microscopic orbital retinoblastoma is orbital extension of retinoblastoma not evident clinically but observed histopathologically.

DIAGNOSTIC EVALUATION

A thorough clinical evaluation paying attention to the subtle signs of orbital retinoblastoma is necessary. Magnetic resonance imaging (preferably) or CT scan of the orbit and brain in axial and coronal orientations with 2-mm slice thickness helps confirm the presence of orbital retinoblastoma and determine its extent. Systemic evaluation, including a detailed physical examination, palpation of the regional lymph nodes, fine needle aspiration biopsy if involved, imaging of the orbit and brain, chest X-ray, ultrasonography of the abdomen, bone marrow biopsy, and cerebrospinal fluid cytology are necessary to stage the disease.

MANAGEMENT

Orbital retinoblastoma has been managed in the past with orbital exenteration, chemotherapy, or external beam radiotherapy in isolation or in sequential combination with variable results.[2-4] It is well known that local treatments have a limited effect on the course of this advanced disease. We have developed a treatment protocol (Table 78-2) comprising initial triple-drug (vincristine, etoposide, carboplatin) high-dose chemotherapy (three to six cycles) followed by surgery (enucleation, extended enucleation, or orbital exenteration as appropriate), orbital radiotherapy, and an additional 12-cycle standard dose chemotherapy (Table 78-1).[5] There is concern about the long-term carcinogenic effects of high-dose etoposide as it is known to cause leukemia. Considering that these patients had an otherwise extremely poor prognosis for survival, such risks may be acceptable.

Table 78-1. Chemotherapy Drugs, Dose (mg/kg body weight) and Schedule for Orbital Retinoblastoma

Drugs	Standard Dose		High Dose	
	Day 1	Day 2	Day 1	Day 2
Vincristine	0.05		0.025	
Etoposide	5.0	5.0	12.0	12.0
Carboplatin	18.6		28.0	

REFERENCES

1. Leal-Leal C, Flores-Rojo M, Medina-Sanson A, et al. A multicentre report from the Mexican Retinoblastoma Group. *Br J Ophthalmol.* 2004;88:1074-1077.
2. Doz F, Khelfaoui F, Mosseri V, et al. The role of chemotherapy in orbital involvement of retinoblastoma. The experience of a single institution with 33 patients. *Cancer.* 1994;74:722-732.
3. Kiratli H, Bilgic S, Ozerdem U. Management of massive orbital involvement of intraocular retinoblastoma. *Ophthalmology.* 1998;105:322-326.
4. Goble RR, McKenzie J, Kingston JE, et al. Orbital recurrence of retinoblastoma successfully treated by combined therapy. *Br J Ophthalmol.* 1990;74:97-98.
5. Honavar SG, Singh AD. Management of advanced retinoblastoma. *Ophthalmol Clin North Am.* 2005;18:65-73.

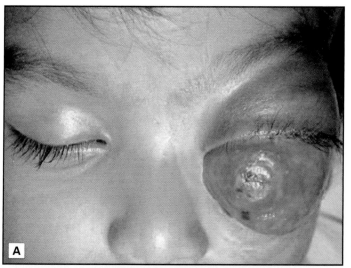
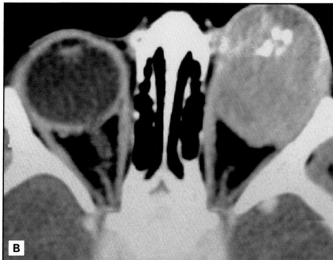
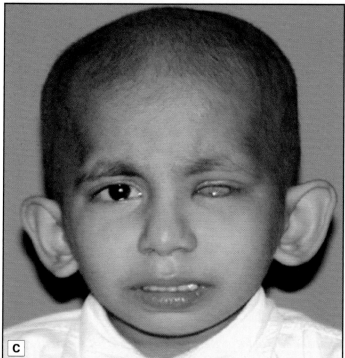
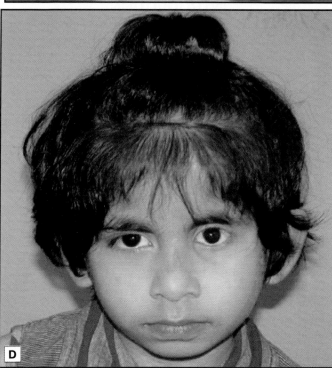

Figure 78-1. Outcome in a case of primary orbital retinoblastoma. A 2-year-old child with primary orbital retinoblastoma in the left eye (A). CT scan showing massive orbital tumor (B). Following three cycles of neoadjuvant chemotherapy, enucleation, orbital external beam radiotherapy, and an additional nine cycles of chemotherapy, the orbital tumor is completely resolved (C). Three years later, the child is free of local and systemic recurrence and has an acceptable cosmetic appearance (D).

Table 78-2. Suggested Protocol for Primary Orbital Retinoblastoma		
Baseline investigations		
CT scan or magnetic resonance imaging		
Bone marrow biopsy		
Cerebrospinal fluid cytology		
Treatment		
Initial chemotherapy		High-dose triple-drug chemotherapy for 3-6 cycles (every 3 weeks)
Surgery	Enucleation	Assessment of orbital tumor by imaging after completion of third cycle
		After completion of third cycle if the orbital tumor is resolved
		Additional 3 cycles of chemotherapy
		After completion of sixth cycle if the orbital tumor is resolved
	Exenteration	After completion of sixth cycle if the orbital tumor is present
External beam radiation		45 to 50 Gy (fractionated) to the orbit
Subsequent chemotherapy		Continuation high-dose chemotherapy for 12 cycles
Follow-up investigations		
Imaging at 12, 18, 24, and 36 months		
Bone marrow biopsy and cerebrospinal fluid cytology at 6, 12, 18, 24, and 36 months		

Our treatment protocol should be considered experimental at present. Further studies are necessary to evaluate whether fewer treatment cycles are equally effective. There are also serious concerns about the long-term carcinogenic effects of high-dose chemotherapy.

Material presented in this chapter was published in Singh AD, Damato BE, Pe'er J, Murphree AL, Perry JD. *Clinical Ophthalmic Oncology*. © Elsevier 2007.

Chapter

79

Metastatic Retinoblastoma

Ira J. Dunkel and Guillermo L. Chantada

INTRODUCTION

Patients with extraocular retinoblastoma have historically had a poor prognosis, but recently significant improvements in survival have been reported. In this chapter, we will review data indicating that the majority of patients with regional extraocular disease can be successfully treated with conventional chemotherapy and external beam radiation therapy and that patients with distant metastatic disease appear to benefit from the addition of high-dose chemotherapy with stem cell rescue.

CLINICAL FEATURES

The presenting signs and symptoms of metastatic retinoblastoma are quite variable and depend on the site or sites of involvement. Reasonably common sites of extraocular disease include the orbit, preauricular lymph nodes, bones, bone marrow, liver, and central nervous system. In patients who have previously undergone enucleation, orbital recurrences often present with the parental observation that the prosthesis is no longer fitting well. More extensive orbital disease may present as a visible mass. Bone disease may present with pain, and bone marrow disease may present with abnormally low blood counts, but often disease at those sites and liver disease may be asymptomatic and discovered only during the extent of disease evaluation. Central nervous system (CNS) disease can occur as optic nerve disease tracking posteriorly into the brain, or as diffuse leptomeningeal involvement.

DIAGNOSTIC EVALUATION

Patients suspected to have extraocular retinoblastoma need extensive evaluation investigating the sites described above (Table 79-1). In anticipation of aggressive chemotherapy, baseline laboratory work should be performed (Table 79-2).

TREATMENT AND PROGNOSIS

Isolated Orbital Retinoblastoma

The management of orbital retinoblastoma is discussed in detail elsewhere (Chapter 78).

Regional Extraocular Retinoblastoma

Recent publications confirm that patients with regional extraocular disease (orbital and/or preauricular disease, optic nerve

margin positivity) may be cured with conventional chemotherapy and external beam radiation therapy. Chemotherapy included vincristine, doxorubicin, and cyclophosphamide (local protocol 87), or vincristine, idarubicin, cyclophosphamide, carboplatin, and etoposide (local protocol 94). The external beam radiation therapy dose was 4500 cGy, administered up to the chiasm for patients with orbital disease and to the involved nodes in patients with preauricular adenopathy.[1-3]

Distant Metastatic Retinoblastoma Without Central Nervous System Involvement

The bulk of the evidence suggested that the prognosis is grim with conventional dose chemotherapy plus radiation therapy.[4,5]

High-dose chemotherapy with ASCR might be beneficial for patients with metastatic retinoblastoma. Overall experience suggests that the addition of high-dose chemotherapy with ASCR is associated with improved survival for patients with metastatic retinoblastoma not involving the CNS. The inclusion of thiotepa in the regimen may be associated with a lower risk of CNS recurrence (the most likely site of failure) owing to the excellent CNS penetration of that agent.[6,7]

Distant Metastatic Retinoblastoma With Central Nervous System Involvement

Fewer data are available regarding the prognosis of patients with metastatic retinoblastoma involving the central nervous system disease treated with high-dose chemotherapy and ASCR.[6,8]

FUTURE RESEARCH

The Children's Oncology Group has proposed a study of multimodality therapy for extraocular retinoblastoma (ARET 0321) (Chapter 81).

REFERENCES

1. Chantada G, Fandino A, Casak S, et al. Treatment of overt extraocular retinoblastoma. *Med Pediatr Oncol.* 2003;40:158-161.
2. Chantada GL, Dunkel IJ, de Dávila MTG, et al. Retinoblastoma patients with high risk ocular pathological features: who needs adjuvant therapy? *Br J Ophthalmol.* 2004;88:1069-1073.
3. Antoneli CBG, Steinhorst F, Ribeiro KCB, et al. Extraocular retinoblastoma: a 13-year experience. *Cancer.* 2003;98:1292-1298.

Table 79-1. Systemic Work-Up for Suspected Metastatic Disease	
Organ/System	Tests
Central nervous system	Brain and orbit MRI with and without contrast
	Lumbar puncture for CSF cytology
	Spine MRI with and without contrast (if CNS disease is present or appropriate focal neurological signs are present)
Visceral organs	Abdominal CT with IV contrast
Bone and bone marrow	Bone scan
	Bone marrow aspirate and biopsy

Table 79-2. Laboratory Work-Up for Suspected Metastatic Disease

Complete blood count with differential

Liver function studies

Estimate of glomerular filtration rate via either timed urine collection for creatinine clearance or nuclear medicine renal function study

Audiogram

LDH determination may also be useful to provide an estimate of the total body tumor burden

4. Kingston JE, Hungerford JL, Plowman PN. Chemotherapy in metastatic retinoblastoma. *Ophthalm Paediatr Genet.* 1987;8:69-72.

5. Schvartzman E, Chantada G, Fandino A, et al. Results of a stage-based protocol for the treatment of retinoblastoma. *J Clin Oncol.* 1996;14:1532-1536.

6. Namouni F, Doz F, Tanguy ML, et al. High-dose chemotherapy with carboplatin, etoposide and cyclophosphamide followed by a haematopoietic stem cell rescue in patients with high-risk retinoblastoma: a SFOP and SFGM study. *Eur J Cancer.* 1997;33:2368-2375.

7. Dunkel IJ, Aledo A, Kernan NA, et al. Successful treatment of metastatic retinoblastoma. *Cancer.* 2000;89:2117-2121.

8. Jubran RF, Erdreich-Epstein A, Buturini A, et al. Approaches to treatment for extraocular retinoblastoma. Children's Hospital Los Angeles experience. *J Pediatr Hematol Oncol.* 2004;26:31-34.

Chapter

80

Retinocytoma or Retinoma

Arun D. Singh, Aubin Balmer, and Francis Munier

INTRODUCTION

There are several lines of evidence that suggest the existence of a benign variant of retinoblastoma.[1,2] The ophthalmoscopic appearance of certain retinal tumors closely resembles that of a successfully treated retinoblastoma. These tumors were called retinoma.[3] Histopathologic studies have demonstrated that these tumors are composed of well-differentiated, benign-appearing mature retinal cells with a characteristic absence of mitoses and necrosis (Figure 80-1).[4] An alternate term, *retinocytoma*, has been used to describe these tumors. Other less frequently used terminology includes spontaneously regressed retinoblastoma, spontaneously arrested retinoblastoma, and retinoblastoma group 0.[5,6] Although retinocytoma has in the past been referred to as spontaneously regressed retinoblastoma, there are no convincing cases in the literature wherein spontaneous regression of retinoblastoma was documented. Overall, retinocytoma or retinoma are the preferred terminology because they imply more specifically a benign tumor arising from a retinal cell.[3,4]

CLINICAL FEATURES

The incidence of retinocytoma in the general population is not known, but is presumably underestimated. The proportion of retinoma among the population with retinoblastoma is estimated between 2% and 10%. The majority (60%) of patients with retinocytoma are asymptomatic, and the diagnosis is made either on routine eye examination or when retinoblastoma is diagnosed in another family member, prompting an eye examination.[2,3] Leukocoria, a common initial feature of retinoblastoma, is not a presenting feature of retinocytoma.[3]

The ophthalmoscopic appearance of retinocytoma resembles the spectrum of retinoblastoma regression patterns observed after irradiation (Box 80-1). A translucent retinal mass (88%), calcification (63%), retinal pigment epithelial alteration (54%), and chorioretinal atrophy (54%) are four diagnostic ophthalmoscopic features of retinocytoma (Figure 80-2).[1-3] Retinoma is characterized by absence of any prior treatment and is non-progressive.

DIFFERENTIAL DIAGNOSIS

The features of retinocytoma outlined above are characteristic and often resemble the type I regression of a treated retinoblastoma. A retinoma may sometimes present like a type II regression (Figure 80-1B), similar to an astrocytic hamartoma.

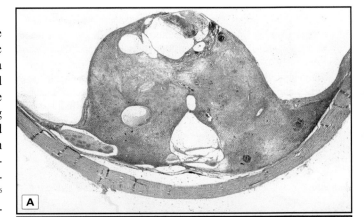

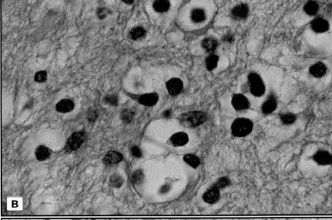

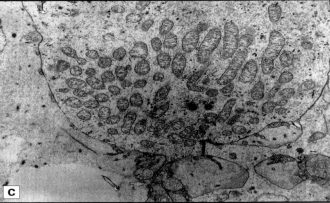

Figure 80-1. Histopathology of retinocytoma. Macroscopic view showing pseudocystic appearance (A). On light microscopy, the tumor is composed of benign cells (B). Note photoreceptor differentiation on electron microphotograph (C).

Box 80-1. Retinocytoma

- Retinocytoma is a benign manifestation of RB1 gene mutation
- The ophthalmoscopic appearance resembles the spectrum of retinoblastoma regression patterns observed after irradiation
- Presence of a translucent grayish retinal mass, calcification, retinal pigment epithelial alteration, and chorioretinal atrophy with or without associated staphyloma are diagnostic features
- Retinocytoma is not associated with retinal exudation or prominent feeder vessels
- Retinocytoma lacks growth over short periods of observation (weeks to months)
- Retinocytoma can undergo malignant transformation into retinoblastoma

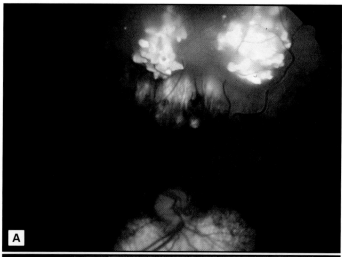

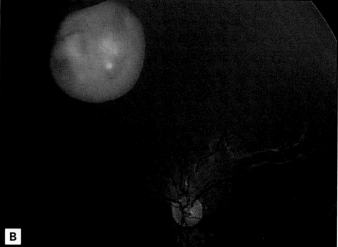

Figure 80-2. Retinocytoma. Note translucent grayish retinal mass, calcification, and retinal pigment epithelial alteration (A). Chorioretinal atrophy may not be present in the early stages (B).

With a flat, pigmented chorioretinal scar (type IV regression), a retinoma may be mistaken for inflammatory chorioretinal lesions as found in toxoplasmosis (Table 80-1).

TREATMENT

By definition, retinoma is non-progressive and does not require treatment; annual ocular examination should be performed for possible risk of malignant transformation. Genetic testing and counseling for RB1 mutations should also be considered.

REFERENCES

1. Balmer A, Munier F, Gailloud C. Retinoma and phthisis bulbi: benign expression of retinoblastoma. *Klin Monatsbl Augenheilkd.* 1992;200:436-439.
2. Singh AD, Santos CM, Shields CL, et al. Observations on 17 patients with retinocytoma. *Arch Ophthalmol.* 2000;118:199-205.
3. Gallie BL, Ellsworth RM, Abramson DH, Phillips RA. Retinoma: spontaneous regression of retinoblastoma or benign manifestation of the mutation? *Br J Cancer.* 1982;45:513-521.
4. Margo C, Hidayat A, Kopelman J, Zimmerman LE. Retinocytoma. A benign variant of retinoblastoma. *Arch Ophthalmol.* 1983;101:1519-1531.
5. Aaby AA, Price RL, Zakov ZN. Spontaneously regressing retinoblastomas, retinoma, or retinoblastoma group 0. *Am J Ophthalmol.* 1983;96:315-320.
6. Abramson DH. Retinoma, retinocytoma, and the retinoblastoma gene. *Arch Ophthalmol.* 1983;101:1517-1518.

Table 80-1. Differential Diagnosis of Retinocytoma

Feature	Retinoblastoma	Retinocytoma	Astrocytic Hamartoma	Myelinated Nerve Fibers
Calcification	White, chunky	White, chunky	Yellow, spherical	Absent
Chorioretinal atrophy	Absent	Present in older patients but absent in early retinocytoma	Absent	Absent
RPE changes	Present	Present	Absent	Absent
Feeder vessels	Present	Absent (except sclerosed and tortuous)	Absent	Vessels obscured
Exudation	Absent	Absent	May be present	Absent
Growth*	Present	Absent	Absent	Absent
Association	13q deletion syndrome	13q deletion syndrome	Tuberous sclerosis	None

*Short-term growth observed over weeks to months.
RPE, retinal pigment epithelium.

Children's Oncology Group Trials for Retinoblastoma

Anna T. Meadows, Murali Chintagumpala, Ira J. Dunkel, Debra Friedman, Julie A. Stoner, and Judith G. Villablanca

INTRODUCTION

The establishment of the Children's Oncology Group (COG) in 2001 from the four existing pediatric cooperative groups brought together the major institutions treating children with cancer in the United States, Canada, and several other countries.

FOUR CHILDREN'S ONCOLOGY GROUP RETINOBLASTOMA PROTOCOLS

During the 4 years of its existence, the committee met to deliberate the methods by which these questions might be practically addressed. Four distinct protocols emerged, each dealing with a subset of retinoblastoma patients with specific aims, methods, statistical analyses, and expectations regarding outcome. The protocols are listed in Table 81-1.

COG ARET 0332: A Study of Unilateral Retinoblastoma With and Without Histopathologic High-Risk Features and the Role of Adjuvant Chemotherapy

Patients with the high-risk features listed in Table 81-2 will receive chemotherapy consisting of six cycles of standard dose carboplatin, vincristine, and etoposide (Chapter 74) given once every 4 weeks. All other patients will be treated with enucleation alone.

COG ARET 0331: Trial of Systemic Neoadjuvant Chemotherapy for Group B Intraocular Retinoblastoma

A total of six cycles of chemotherapy with standard dose vincristine and carboplatin (Chapter 74) is planned. Response to chemotherapy will be determined following the first cycle of vincristine and carboplatin. Local ophthalmic therapy will be delivered before the second to sixth cycles as clinically indicated. Patients whose disease remains stable will continue on therapy; those who develop progressive disease at any time will be treated at the investigator's discretion.

COG ARET 0231: A Single-Arm Trial of Systemic and Subtenon Chemotherapy for Groups C and D Intraocular Retinoblastoma

Children with newly diagnosed bilateral retinoblastoma with at least one Group C or D eye will receive intravenous high-dose carboplatin, etoposide, and vincristine for six courses, with sub-Tenon carboplatin given on the day before or the first day of courses 2–4. Local ophthalmic therapy will be given as clinically indicated, starting with the third course of CEV, and may include cryotherapy, laser, and/or radioactive plaque. Cryotherapy will not be given at the same time as sub-Tenon carboplatin, to avoid toxicity. An event will be defined as the need for any non-protocol chemotherapy external beam radiotherapy, and/or enucleation of a Group C/D eye, or death. New retinal tumors and/or edge recurrences of previous retinal tumors that can be treated successfully by laser, cryotherapy, and/or plaque only will not be considered protocol failures. A central review of Retcam images will be performed by three ophthalmologists at diagnosis to confirm eye group, and after chemotherapy courses 3 and 6 to confirm response.

COG ARET 0321: A Trial of Intensive Multi-Modality Therapy for Extraocular Retinoblastoma

Patients will receive four cycles of induction chemotherapy consisting of vincristine, cisplatin, cyclophosphamide, and etoposide. Autologous hematopoietic stem cells will be harvested after clearance of bone marrow disease. Patients with regional extraocular disease (stratum stages 2 and 3) will then receive external beam radiation therapy (Table 81-3). Those with distant metastatic (stratum stage 4a) or central nervous system (stratum stage 4b) disease will receive consolidative high-dose carboplatin, thiotepa, and etoposide chemotherapy followed by autologous stem cell rescue, and will then be considered for external beam radiation therapy (depending on response to induction chemotherapy).

Table 81-1. The Children's Oncology Group Retinoblastoma Protocols

COG Protocol # ARET-	Protocol		Participants	Investigators
	Short Name	Full Name		
0332	Histopathologic risk factors	A Study of Unilateral Rb with and without Histopathologic High-Risk Features and the Role of Adjuvant Chemotherapy	Group-wide	Chintagumpala, Chevez-Barrios, Eagle, Albert, O'Brien
0331	Group B	Trial of Systemic Neoadjuvant Chemotherapy for Group B Intraocular Retinoblastoma	Limited institution	Friedman, Murphree
0231	Group C/D	A Single-Arm Trial of Systemic and Subtenon Chemotherapy for Groups C and D Intraocular Retinoblastoma	Limited institution	Villablanca, C. Shields
0321	Extraocular disease	A Trial of Intensive Multi-Modality Therapy for Extraocular Retinoblastoma	Group-wide	Dunkel, Abramson

Table 81-2. High-Risk Histopathologic Features in an Enucleated Eye That Qualify for Adjuvant Chemotherapy Under COG ARET-0332

Feature	Details
Massive choroidal invasion	Posterior uveal invasion grades IIC and IID (as defined in pathology guidelines of the protocol)
Any posterior uveal invasion with any optic nerve involvement (optic nerve head, pre- and post-lamina cribrosa)	Both posterior uveal invasion and optic nerve involvement are required
Optic nerve involvement posterior to the lamina cribrosa is an independent finding	

Table 81-3. Three Extraocular Retinoblastoma Stratification Groups for COG ARET-0321

Stage	Inclusion Criteria	Exclusion Criteria
Stage 2 or 3	Orbital disease (including microscopic trans-scleral invasion seen on enucleation pathology), optic nerve margin (+), and/or regional nodal disease	No other sites of metastases
Stage 4a	Overt distant metastatic disease (such as bone, bone marrow, and/or liver)	No detectable CNS involvement
Stage 4b	Overt CNS involvement (brain parenchyma, leptomeninges, CSF cytology). Patients with trilateral retinoblastoma will be included	Extradural/dural disease, but without parenchymal or leptomeningeal disease should not be included and will be considered to be stage 4a

Material presented in this chapter was published in Singh AD, Damato BE, Pe'er J, Murphree AL, Perry JD. *Clinical Ophthalmic Oncology.* © Elsevier 2007.

Retinoblastoma:
At-Risk Pregnancies

Lisa Paquette and David A. Miller

INTRODUCTION

Recent advances in imaging technology have enabled evaluation of the fetus to become more accessible and the information obtained exquisitely more detailed. Specifically, fetal magnetic resonance imaging (MRI) and fetal ultrasound, including three-dimensional ultrasound, are being increasingly used for prenatal diagnosis. The diagnosis of retinoblastoma in utero is expected to become a reality as the techniques available with fetal ultrasound and MRI are applied to the at-risk fetus. The exact role that prenatal detection of retinoblastoma will play in the clinical management of this disease is still to be determined.

ULTRASOUND OF THE FETAL EYE

Figures from our institution help illustrate the fetal ultrasound imaging capabilities of the normal and abnormal eye (Figure 82-1).

MRI OF THE FETAL EYE

Some images from our institution may help illustrate what capabilities exist for the ophthalmic applications of fetal MRI (Figure 82-2).

CARE OF THE FETUS AND NEONATE WITH RETINOBLASTOMA

We have an IRB-approved pilot study to validate the use of three-dimensional ultrasound and MRI to evaluate fetal eyes. The next step may be to pursue early (34 to 35 weeks of gestation) safe delivery so that treatment of prenatally documented intraocular disease can begin as early as possible. Unfortunately, if retinoblastoma is diagnosed in utero, there is currently no action that can be taken until the baby is born.

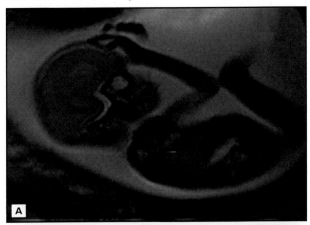

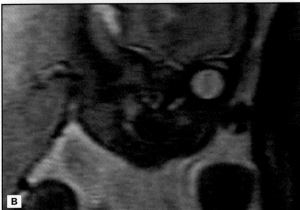

Figure 82-2. Fetal magnetic resonance imaging (A). Easy visualization of the eyeball (B).

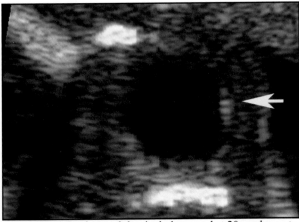

Figure 82-1. Fetal transabdominal ultrasound at 20 weeks gestation. Sagittal view of the eye. Lens is clearly visible (arrow).

Future Directions

A. Linn Murphree

Assessment of future needs resulted in the identification of the following six strategic goals:

Goal 1: Introduce programs to educate the general population and primary care providers about the early signs of intraocular retinoblastoma—Programs targeting the reduction in the number of cases with delayed diagnosis are proving effective in mid-developed countries such as Mexico, Brazil, and Argentina (Chapter 68).

Goal 2: Eliminate maternal diet deficiency and papillomavirus infections—This goal makes the assumption that both maternal diet deficiency and human papillomavirus infection play a role in the etiology of the nonheritable form of retinoblastoma. If these data are confirmed, a program of distribution of prenatal vitamins and an effective vaccine against human papillomavirus infection should have a dramatic impact on the disproportionately high incidence of nonheritable retinoblastoma, especially in Africa and Southeast Asia.

Goal 3: Develop targeted, locally delivered, less toxic, and less expensive therapeutic approaches to intraocular disease—Most eyes are lost to retinoblastoma because of dissemination of the tumor into the vitreous and subretinal space. There is a great need to consistently achieve intraocular therapeutic levels of agents that is not limited by systemic toxicity. The chemotherapeutic agents currently used (carboplatin, etoposide, and vincristine) are small molecules and should enter the eye easily in an appropriate trans-scleral delivery system. Use of a trans-scleral delivery system that consists of a small, impermeable refillable silicone reservoir that is firmly attached to the episclera with minimally invasive conjunctival surgery provides sustained delivery of high levels of agent to the vitreous and the posterior retina, and the potential for an inexpensive route for delivering tumor-targeted biotherapies.[1]

Goal 4: Adoption of a universally used stage and group classification—As discussed in Chapter 69, there has been a broad international movement to adopt the International Stage and Group Classification. Four COG retinoblastoma protocols based on this classification are open and recruiting patients (Chapter 81).

Goal 5: Development of an automated, inexpensive screening examination for RB1 mutations—The universal availability of quick and inexpensive screening for RB1 mutations in the germline would transform the clinical care of retinoblastoma.

Goal 6: Employing metastasis suppressor genes to prevent metastases—The exploitation of the genes and pathways to block growth at distant sites hold promise for precisely targeted therapy, especially among populations unable to support the massive non-specific, resource-intensive therapy currently employed in developed countries.[2,3]

REFERENCES

1. Carvalho R, Krause ML, Murphree AL, et al. Characterization and validation of refillable episcleral drug delivery devices for unidirectional and controlled transscleral drug delivery. *Invest Ophthalmol Vis Sci.* 2005;46:E-Abstract 499.
2. Berger JC, Vander Griend DJ, Robinson VL, et al. Metastasis suppressor genes: from gene identification to protein function and regulation. *Cancer Biol Ther.* 2005;4.
3. Kauffman EC, Robinson VL, Stadler WM, et al. Metastasis suppression: the evolving role of metastasis suppressor genes for regulating cancer cell growth at the secondary site. *J Urol.* 2003;169:1122-1133.

Chapter

84

Examination Techniques

Mehryar Taban and Julian D. Perry

INTRODUCTION

The history aids in establishing a probable diagnosis and in guiding the initial work-up and therapy. Important historical elements will be discussed in Chapter 88.

EXAMINATION

External Examination

The examiner should inspect the patient visually for symmetry of periocular structures, such as the brows, eyelids, canthi, and surrounding soft tissues. Visual inspection should include observation for obvious globe deviation.

Pupils

All patients with suspected orbital disease should undergo the swinging flashlight test to determine the presence or absence of an afferent pupillary defect.

Extraocular Motility

Ductions and versions are tested in each patient. The cover–uncover test is performed in each cardinal position to measure any phoria or tropia. Patients with suspected restrictive disease may undergo forced duction testing.

Eyelid Position and Function

Eyelid position is characterized by the marginal reflex distances (MRD). The MRD1 represents the distance from the center of the upper eyelid margin to the corneal light reflex in millimeters. The MRD2 represents the distance from the center of the lower eyelid margin to the corneal light reflex. Levator function is measured as the extent of upper eyelid excursion from downgaze to upgaze with the brows fixated. If present, scleral show is measured from each limbus to the corresponding eyelid margin with the eye in the primary position.

The upper eyelid should be everted to inspect the palpebral lobe of the lacrimal gland. Lymphoma can result in a salmon-colored conjunctival mass that is only visible in the fornix.

Globe Position

The Hertel exophthalmometer quantifies the anterior protrusion of the eye by measuring the distance in millimeters from the lateral orbital rim to the front surface of the cornea. The Luedde exophthalmometer measures globe protrusion unilaterally from the lateral orbital rim. The Naugle exophthalmometer measures anterior globe position relative to the superior and inferior orbital rims. This method provides accurate assessment for patients with lateral rim fractures or defects. The McCoy Facial Trisquare (Paget Instrument Co, Kansas City, MO) provides quick and accurate measurements when viewed superimposed over the face.

Palpation

The examiner should palpate any abnormal areas for tenderness or a mass, assess the degree of resistance to retropulsion of each globe, and check for local adenopathy.

Resistance to Globe Retropulsion

The examiner places both forefingers over the anterior portion of the globe with the eyelids closed and gently pushes posteriorly on the globe.

Slit-Lamp Examination

The corneal surface is evaluated for signs of exposure, and the posterior pole is evaluated for signs of ocular or optic nerve compression or congestion.

Fundus Examination

Orbital mass lesions may result in choroidal folds, optic disc edema, pallor, or shunt vessels.

Cranial Nerves V and VII

Sensation to light touch in each dermatome of the trigeminal nerve is tested using a tissue, including testing of the corneal blink reflex. Each motor branch of the facial nerve is evaluated. Bell's phenomenon testing is performed in all patients with lagophthalmos.

Lacrimal System

Secretory function is measured with Schirmer's test. Excretory function is determined by irrigation with or without Jones' test.

Material presented in this chapter was published in Singh AD, Damato BE, Pe'er J, Murphree AL, Perry JD. *Clinical Ophthalmic Oncology.* © Elsevier 2007.

Imaging Techniques

Patrick De Potter

INTRODUCTION

Ultrasonography, color Doppler imaging (CDI), computed tomography (CT), and magnetic resonance imaging (MRI) are the most important imaging tools for the clinician in the field of orbital oncology. Catheter diagnostic angiography has a limited role in the diagnostic approach to orbit lesions, except for evaluating vascular abnormalities suggesting the diagnosis of carotid cavernous fistula. The role of positron emission tomography with [2–18F] fluoro-2-deoxy-D-glucose (FDG) in evaluation of orbital tumors is limited because FDG accumulates in extraocular muscles in proportion to their contractile activities and decreases lesion conspicuity in regions with high physiological tracer uptake.

TECHNIQUES OF ORBITAL IMAGING

Ultrasonography is a non-invasive, simple, fast, and economical imaging technique that allows easy detection of an orbital lesion before any decision can be made as to whether further evaluation with CT or MRI is necessary (Figure 85-1).[1,2] However, it is limited by the requirement for skilled operators and because penetration of the deeper regions of the orbit at energy levels acceptable for the retina cannot be achieved.

CDI has proved to be effective in the display of the normal orbital and intraocular vasculature, tumor vascularization, and echographic differentiation of tumors from subretinal hemorrhage.[3] In patients with carotid–cavernous fistula or dural cavernous arteriovenous malformations, CDI clearly demonstrates the dilated, arterialized superior ophthalmic vein with high-velocity blood flow towards the transducer.[4] In addition, CDI may be able to differentiate meningioma from glioma of the optic nerve. It may also be effective in confirming the diagnosis of orbital varices by showing the dynamic changes throughout inspiration and expiration.[5]

Computed Tomography

The basis of CT is the measurement of different tissue absorption values (Hounsfield units) of a given tissue to neighboring structures, following exposure to X-rays.

Conventional CT provides excellent details of the eye, orbital soft tissues, and bony orbit, and has an established role in the evaluation of orbital trauma and orbital diseases (Box 85-1). However, there are several drawbacks, including relatively long exposure times and increased radiation exposure (approximately 75 mGy of radiation). Although reconstructions in the sagittal and coronal planes can be obtained from conventional CT data, these images are of poor quality under practical conditions.

Helical CT, also known as spiral or volume acquisition CT, acquires data in a continuous fashion. With the use of image-reconstruction algorithms, multiple very thin-sectioned and multiplanar computer-reformatted images can be produced that are superior to those obtained from standard incremental axial CT images (Figure 85-2).[6] In addition, acquisition time is reduced, a great advantage with children and unstable patients.

Three-dimensional (3D) CT a computerized post-processing technique, allows a unique topographic overview of selected anatomic or pathologic structures that have been isolated (a process called segmentation) from the image tissue volume.[7]

MRI is based on a physical phenomenon called the nuclear magnetic resonance effect on the atomic nuclei, primarily hydrogen atoms of water molecules in human tissues. MR images of patients are obtained by inducing electromagnetic signals from the magnetic dipole movements of 1H nuclei and then converting those signals into cross-sectional images.

Although CT and MRI studies are complementary, MRI provides superior soft tissue contrast. Its multiplanar capability with outstanding tissue contrast and the absence of ionizing radiation make MRI an especially suitable technique for imaging orbital structures (Box 85-2).[8] Moreover, the superficial location of the eye and eyelids permits the use of surface coils, which improve the display of anatomic details.

INTERPRETATION OF IMAGING STUDIES

Interpretation of imaging studies is facilitated by evaluating radiological characteristics such as anatomic location, appearance, content, post-contrast enhancement features, and bone characteristics.[8]

Location Computed Tomography

Location CT provides similar information to MRI on the location and extent of a lesion in the anterior orbital space, the globe, the intraconal–extraconal space, orbital fat, extraocular muscles, cavernous sinus, and temporal fossa. CT remains the imaging modality of choice in the evaluation of lesions located in the lacrimal gland fossa, the paranasal sinuses, and the adjacent

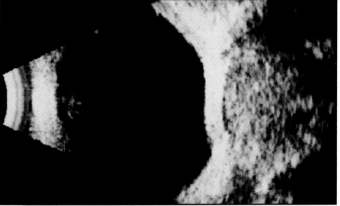

Figure 85-1. B-scan ultrasound of cavernous hemangioma displays a well-defined oval echogenic lesion deforming the globe.

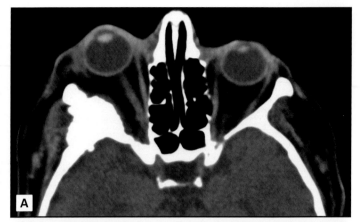

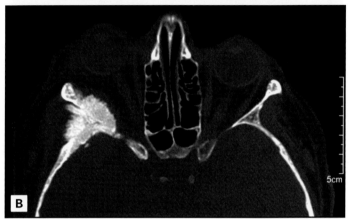

> **Box 85-1. Indications of Orbital CT**
>
> - Evaluation of patient with proptosis with suspicion of osseous, fibro–osseous, fibrous lesions
> - Evaluation of patient with clinical diagnosis of lacrimal gland lesion
> - Evaluation of orbital trauma
> - Detection of calcification
> - Contraindication for MRI (claustrophobia, metallic implants, allergy to contrast agent)

bony orbit. Owing to the superior soft tissue contrast resolution of MRI, it is the study of choice for lesions infiltrating the optic nerve, optic nerve sheath, and orbital apex.

Appearance

An orbital lesion may be described as having a regular (round or oval) or irregular (infiltrative) configuration. Its margin characteristics may be well circumscribed or diffuse.

Content

Information on the content of the lesion (cystic or solid; homogeneous or heterogeneous) can be obtained by both CT and MR imaging techniques. MRI images identify tissue compounds such as melanin, methemoglobin, deoxyhemoglobin, ferritin, and proteinaceous material. Punctate or conglomerate increased densities on CT scans or foci of signal void on MRI may be seen in trauma, vascular tumors, optic nerve sheath tumors (meningioma), epithelial lacrimal gland tumors, and malignant osseous tumors (osteosarcoma). In general, MR images provide more information about the content of the lesion than do CT images. However, CT is best suited for the detection of calcification.

Contrast Enhancement

The pattern of contrast enhancement (present or absent; homogeneous or heterogeneous) of orbital lesions guides in forming a differential diagnosis. The enhancement characteristics of an orbital lesion are best identified on fat-suppressed post-contrast T1-weighted images. No enhancement is documented in hemorrhagic processes, dense scar tissue, fluid collections, or necrotic portions of a tumor. Minimal contrast enhancement sug-

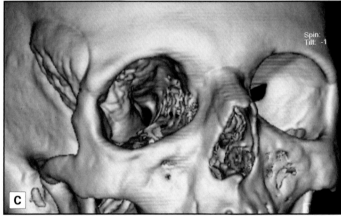

Figure 85-2. Axial CT images of a right sphenoid wing meningioma. Helical CT scan showing a right hyperostotic sphenoid wing (A), bone windows (B), and three-dimensional scan (C).

gests a chronic or sclerosing orbital inflammation, tissue fibrosis, or post-therapeutic scar tissue. Moderate to marked contrast enhancement is usually noticed in solid tumors as well as in acute inflammatory orbital lesions. Linear enhancement surrounding a non-enhancing well-delineated lesion suggests the cystic nature of the lesion. A well-defined linear or void signal within an enhancing lesion may suggest air, high-flow blood vessels (artery or vein), fragments of cortical bone, or foreign body. Gadolinium-enhanced MRI has proved to be the best-suited imaging modality for assessing the progression of fibrovascularization tissue into porous orbital implants (hydroxyapatite and porous polyethylene).

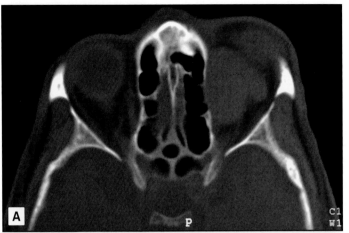

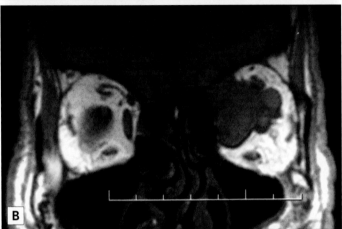

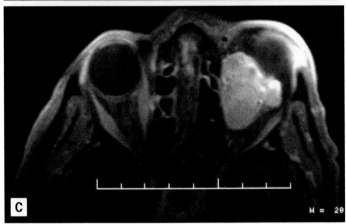

Figure 85-3. Left orbital schwannoma. Axial CT image showing a well-circumscribed orbital mass (A). Coronal pre-contrast T1-weighted image. The lesion shows a slight heterogeneous appearance (B). Axial postcontrast T1-weighted image displaying heterogeneous enhancement (C).

Bone Characteristics

Bone molding by a well-circumscribed orbital mass suggests a congenital lesion (dermoid cyst, lymphangioma) or a slowly growing benign tumor (cavernous hemangioma, neurofibroma, neurilemmoma, or benign lacrimal gland tumor). Bone erosion is usually seen with more aggressive inflammatory lesions, primary tumors, and secondary tumors.

Bone lysis is observed in very aggressive primary tumors, secondary malignant tumors, and inflammatory lesions (idiopathic orbital inflammation, eosinophilic granuloma).

Box 85-2. Indications of Orbital MRI

■ Location and extent of orbital lesion
■ Evaluation of orbital, intracanalicular, and prechiasmal optic pathways
■ Evaluation of patient with proptosis (hemorrhagic, neoplastic, fibrosclerotic, mucinoid/cystic degeneration)
■ Evaluation of patient with progressive bluish lid swelling (capillary hemangioma vs lymphangioma)
■ Evaluation of tumor response after radiotherapy or chemotherapy
■ Evaluation of anophthalmic socket when orbital tumor recurrence is suspected
■ Orbital trauma when ferromagnetic material is excluded
■ Identification of fibrovascular ingrowth within biocompatible implant

---

Bone infiltration by the tumor is best seen on CT with bone algorithm reconstruction and identified on MRI as a discontinuity of cortical signal void and loss of high signal intensity of the fat in the bone marrow.

Hyperostosis is observed with benign osseous tumors (meningioma), malignant bone tumors (osteosarcoma), and metastatic tumors such as from prostate carcinoma. In general, osseous speculation and inhomogeneous density are findings suggestive of a malignant tumor.

RADIOLOGICAL DIFFERENTIAL DIAGNOSIS

Orbital tumors can be classified into one of seven radiological patterns (well-circumscribed solid, ill-defined solid, circumscribed cystic, enlarged optic nerve, enlarged lacrimal gland, enlarged extraocular muscles, and anomalies of the bony orbit) to obtain a reliable differential diagnosis (Box 85-3).

Well-circumscribed solid orbital tumors are cavernous hemangioma, neurilemmoma, neurofibroma, fibrous histiocytoma, and hemangiopericytoma (Figure 85-3). These tumors usually present as a well-defined, oval to round intraconal orbital mass on MRI.

Ill-defined solid orbital tumors in children include capillary hemangioma, lymphangioma, plexiform neurofibroma, idiopathic orbital inflammation, and metastasis. In adults, idiopathic orbital inflammation, metastasis, primary orbital tumor, and lymphoproliferative disorder are more frequent causes.

Well-circumscribed cystic lesions are dermoid cyst, colobomatous cyst, teratoma, meningoencephalocele, lymphangioma, acquired inclusion cyst, chronic hematic cyst (cholesterol granuloma), mucocele, subperiosteal hematoma, and parasitic cyst (Figure 85-4).[8]

Enlarged optic nerve can be due to juvenile pilocytic astrocytoma, malignant glioma, secondary spread from intraocular tumor (retinoblastoma, uveal melanoma, melanocytoma), CNS lymphoma, systemic metastatic disease, and optic neuritis.[9] In all these diseases, the optic nerve may assume a tubular, fusiform, lobular configuration. The differential diagnosis of an enlarged

Box 85-3. Radiological Patterns of Orbital Tumors

- Well-circumscribed solid tumor
- Ill-defined solid tumor
- Circumscribed cystic tumor
- Enlarged optic nerve
- Enlarged lacrimal gland
- Enlarged extraocular muscles
- Anomalies of the bony orbit

optic nerve sheath includes meningioma, meningeal spread of tumor, meningitis, arachnoidal cyst, hemorrhage, and CSF expansion, as seen with idiopathic intracranial hypertension or orbital apex compression (Figure 85-5).

Enlarged lacrimal gland may be due to non-epithelial or epithelial lesions. Non-epithelial lesions include inflammation and lymphoid tumors, whereas epithelial lesions include dacryops, pleomorphic adenoma, and malignant epithelial tumors (adenoid cystic carcinoma).[8]

Calcification within the enlarged lacrimal gland is highly suggestive of adenoid cystic carcinoma.

Enlarged Extraocular Muscles

The extraocular muscles can be enlarged by infectious, inflammatory, neoplastic, and vascular diseases best seen on postcontrast coronal CT and MR images.[10] In thyroid-associated orbitopathy, the belly of the extraocular muscles is expanded, and unlike in idiopathic myositis, the tendinous attachment to the globe is usually spared. Focal or multifocal nodularity of the extraocular muscle(s) is highly suggestive of metastatic disease (Figure 85-6).[10]

Anomalies of bony orbit CT remains the imaging modality of choice for the evaluation of bone abnormalities (scalloping, deformity, hyperostosis, expansion, and bone marrow invasion) as well as osseous, fibro-osseous, and fibrous tumors.[11]

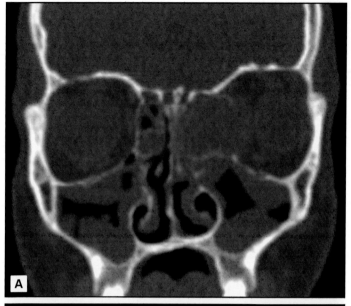

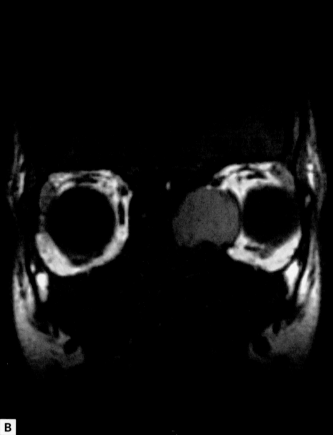

Figure 85-4. Left ethmoidal mucocele with bilateral pansinusitis (A). Coronal CT with bone window suggesting the rupture of the medial orbital wall (B).

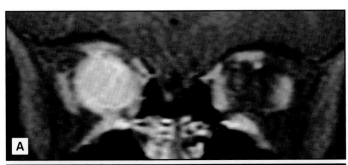

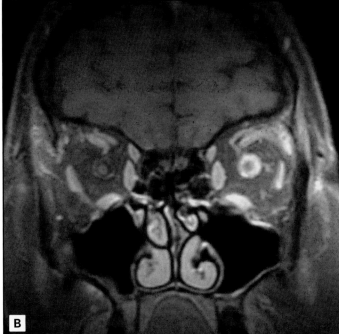

Figure 85-5. Enlarged optic nerve on coronal post-contrast T1-weighted images. Enhancing pattern of juvenile pilocytic astrocytoma within the right optic nerve (A). Rim-like enhancing left optic nerve sheath meningioma (B).

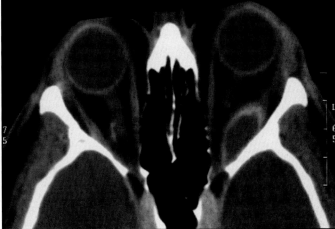

Figure 85-6. Focal enlargement of the left lateral rectus muscle by metastatic carcinoid from the lung. The necrotic tumor does not enhance.

REFERENCES

1. Berges O, Bilaniuk LT. Orbital ultrasonography: ocular and orbital pathology. In: Newton TH, Bilaniuk LT, eds. *Radiology of the Eye and Orbit*. New York, NY: Raven Press; 1990:Chapter 7.

2. Nasr AM, Abou Chacra G. Ultrasonography in orbital differential diagnosis. In: Karcioglu ZA, ed. *Orbital Tumors, Diagnosis and Treatment*. New York, NY: Springer Verlag; 2005:73-83.

3. Lieb WE. Color Doppler imaging of the eye and orbit. *Radiol Clin North Am.* 1998;36:1059-1071.

4. Karam EZ, Destarac L, Hedges TR, Heggerick PA. Abnormal ophthalmic veins: differential diagnosis and management using color Doppler imaging. *Neuro-Ophthalmology.* 1999;22:87-96.

5. Jacquemin C, Bosley T, Mullaney P. Orbital color Doppler imaging of optic nerve tumors. *Int Ophthalmol.* 1999;23:11-15.

6. Rhea JT, Rao PM, Novelline RA. Helical CT and three-dimensional CT of facial and orbital injury. *Radiol Clin North Am.* 1999;37:489-513.

7. Zonneveld FW, Vaandrager JM, van der Meulen JHC, Koornneef L. Three-dimensional imaging of congenital disorders involving the orbit. *Radiol Clin North Am.* 1998;36:1261-1279.

8. De Potter P, Shields JA, Shields CL. *MRI of the Eye and Orbit.* Philadelphia, PA: Lippincott Raven; 1995.

9. Saeed P, Rootman J, Nugent R, et al. Optic nerve sheath meningiomas. *Ophthalmology.* 2003;110:2019-2030.

10. Lacey B, Chang W, Rootman J. Nonthyroid causes of extraocular muscle disease. *Surv Ophthalmol.* 1999;44:187-213.

11. Weinig BM, Mafee MF, Ghosh L. Fibro-osseous, osseous, and cartilaginous lesions of the orbit and paraorbital region. Correlative clinicopathologic and radiographic features, including the diagnostic role of CT and MR imaging. *Radiol Clin North Am.* 1998;36:1241-1259.

Classification of Orbital Tumors

Mehran Taban and Julian D. Perry

INTRODUCTION

Neoplasms of the orbit may be primary, secondary (infiltration from adjacent structure), or metastatic (from distant structures).

DIFFERENTIAL DIAGNOSIS

Many masquerading processes, including infectious and inflammatory diseases, can resemble an orbital tumor. Most can be excluded based on a combination of demographic, clinical, and imaging characteristics (Table 86-1).

CLINICOPATHOLOGICAL CLASSIFICATION

Cystic Lesions

Dermoid cyst is the most common cystic lesion of the orbit.[1] Other cystic lesions include colobomatous cyst, congenital cystic eye, meningocele, and teratoma.

Vascular tumors are divided into no-flow (type 1), low-flow (type 2), and high-flow (type 3) lesions. Cavernous hemangioma and capillary hemangioma are hamartomas (Table 86-2).

Myogenic tumors represents the most common primary orbital malignant neoplasia of childhood. It accounts for 4% of all biopsied orbital masses in children.[1]

Lacrimal Gland Tumors

Approximately half of all lacrimal gland tumors represent epithelial proliferations, and the remainder represent inflammatory or lymphoproliferative lesions (Table 86-3).

Lacrimal Sac Tumors

Epithelial tumors are the most common neoplasms of the lacrimal sac.[2]

Lymphoproliferative Tumors

Lymphoid and leukemic tumors represent a common group of orbital neoplasms (Chapter 95).

Peripheral nerve tumors include neurilemmoma (schwannoma), neurofibroma, alveolar soft-part sarcoma, amputation neuroma, and malignant peripheral nerve sheath tumor.

Optic nerve, meningeal, and other neural tumors consist mainly of optic nerve glioma, malignant optic nerve astrocytoma, and meningioma.

Table 86-1. Orbital Tumors: Simulating Lesions

Category	Subtype
Infectious	Acute bacterial orbital cellulitis
	Invasive fungal infection
	Mycobacterial infection
Inflammatory	Idiopathic orbital inflammation
	Dysthyroid orbitopathy
	Systemic vasculitides
Other	Amyloidosis

Table 86-2. Orbital Vascular Tumors

Category	Subtype	
More common	Capillary hemangioma	Cavernous hemangioma
	Hemangiopericytoma	Lymphangioma (type 1)
	Varix (type 2)	Arteriovenous malformation (type 3)
Less common	Angiosarcoma	Hemangioendothelioma
	Hemangiosarcoma	Kaposi's sarcoma
	Kimura's disease	Vascular leiomyoma/leiomyosarcoma

Table 86-3. Tumors of the Lacrimal Gland

Types	Subtypes
Benign	Pleomorphic adenoma
	Myoepithelioma
Malignant	Adenoid cystic carcinoma
	Malignant mixed tumor (carcinoma arising within pleomorphic adenoma)
	Mucoepidermoid carcinoma
	Adenocarcinoma
Lymphoproliferative	

REFERENCES

1. Shields JA, Bakewell B, Augsburger JJ, Donoso LA, Bernardino V. Space-occupying orbital masses in children. A review of 250 consecutive biopsies. *Ophthalmology.* 1986;93:379-384.
2. Stefanyszyn MA, Hidayat AA, Pe'er JJ, Flanagan JC. Lacrimal sac tumors. *Ophthal Plast Reconstr Surg.* 1994;10:169-184.

Evaluation of a Child With Orbital Tumor

Paul L. Proffer, Jill A. Foster, and Julian D. Perry

HISTORY

As with adults, the history begins with a description of the symptoms, severity, onset, and rate of progression.

Presenting Symptoms

Tumor location and histology determine the presenting symptoms, which can be divided into sensory, motor, and structural or functional (Table 87-1).

EXAMINATION

A systematic evaluation that includes a detailed history, physical examination, and attention to "Krohel's 6 Ps" allows the examiner to narrow the differential diagnosis (Box 87-1).

Globe Displacement

Assess globe position qualitatively with the child in the chin-up position. Although an exophthalmometer may provide an objective measure, patient cooperation may limit its accuracy.

Palpation yields information regarding tumor location, size, and shape.

Pulsation may occur with certain tumors in children, such as absence of the sphenoid wing in the setting of neurofibromatosis.

Periorbital Changes

Neuroblastoma often presents with periorbital ecchymoses. Plexiform neurofibroma often presents with an S-shaped upper eyelid deformity with characteristic skin changes. Lymphangiomas and capillary hemangiomas can be visible through the conjunctiva. Rhabdomyosarcoma often presents with periorbital inflammatory signs.

Head and neck examination of the sinuses, nasopharynx, and adjacent lymphatic drainage areas often helps to limit the differential diagnosis.

LABORATORY EVALUATION

Laboratory evaluation further narrows the differential diagnosis.

Table 87-1. Presenting Features of Orbital Tumors in Children

Category	Entity	Common Symptoms and Signs
Inflammatory	Ruptured dermoid	Acute onset, pain, proptosis
Congenital	Plexiform neurofibroma	Pulsating proptosis (absent sphenoid wing); painless, slow progression
	Dermoid	Proptosis with orbital lesions; painless, slow progression
	Teratoma	Progressive severe proptosis
Vascular	Capillary hemangioma	Slow progression, pain and pulsation rare; blanches with palpation; proptosis if posterior
	Lymphangioma	Painless proptosis but pain with intralesional bleed or upper respiratory infection; conjunctival involvement may aid in diagnosis
Benign	Optic nerve glioma	Axial proptosis, slow progression; Usually painless
Malignant	Rhabdomyosarcoma	Rapid onset painless proptosis; discoloration of overlying skin
Metastasis	Leukemia (chloroma)	Unilateral or bilateral painless proptosis; rapid progression;
	Neuroblastoma	Abrupt progressive proptosis; eyelid ecchymoses

Box 87-1. The 6 Ps of the Orbital Examination

- Proptosis
- Palpation
- Pulsation
- Periorbital changes
- Pain
- Progression

DIAGNOSTIC IMAGING

Imaging is essential to establish the diagnosis, clarify the extent of the disease, and determine the surgical approach (Chapter 85).

BIOPSY

Confirmation of the diagnosis may require surgery. The differential diagnosis determines the possible outcomes of frozen section results and the appropriate extent of surgical excision. An adequate specimen should anticipate the possibility of needing tissue for further testing, including microbiological testing, cell marker studies, or electron microscopy.

Evaluation of an Adult With Orbital Tumor

Benson Chen, Julian D. Perry, and Jill A. Foster

HISTORY

The history begins with a description of the symptoms, severity, onset, and rate of progression. A targeted review of systems reveals additional clues to the etiology.

Presenting Symptoms

Orbital neoplasia presents with a wide spectrum of symptoms, which may be categorized as sensory, motor, structural, or functional in nature (Box 88-1).[1]

Rate of onset and progression help characterize the pathology (Table 88-1).

Past Medical History

Detailed inquiry should also include social history and medications, as this information may elucidate further past medical history not initially provided by the patient.

EXAMINATION

The physical examination of an adult with suspected orbital neoplasia consists of three aspects: complete eye examination, orbital examination, and head and neck evaluation (Table 88-2) (Chapter 84).

LABORATORY EVALUATION

Serologic testing can often support a non-neoplastic etiology in the setting of equivocal physical findings. Thyroid function and antibody testing can provide further evidence for Graves' disease. cANCA titers may reflect underlying Wegner's granulomatosis.

Box 88-1. Common Presenting Symptoms of Orbital Disease

- Sensory: Orbital pain, changes in vision, numbness or tingling
- Motor: Diplopia, ptosis
- Structural: Changes in facial symmetry, globe displacement, visible or palpable mass
- Functional: Dry eyes or tearing

Angiotensin-converting enzyme, serum lysozyme elevation, and chest imaging can help to confirm sarcoidosis.[2]

DIAGNOSTIC IMAGING

Most patients with suspected orbital neoplasia require orbital imaging to further elucidate the etiology of the orbital mass (Chapter 85). The history, physical examination, laboratory tests, and imaging studies will narrow the differential diagnosis to determine the surgical approach and goals (Table 88-3).

BIOPSY

Diagnosis of an orbital tumor ultimately requires confirmatory histology. Although the location of the lesion largely dictates the approach, some tumors require complete excision, whereas others require only biopsy to establish a tissue diagnosis for medical therapy (Table 88-4).

Table 88-1. Onset of Orbital Tumors in Adults				
Congenital	Acute	Subacute	Chronic (Months)	Chronic (Years)
Dermoid	Lymphangioma	Lymphoproliferative	Cavernous hemangioma	Cavernous hemangioma
Epidermoid	Lymphoproliferative	Metastatic lesions	Lymphoproliferative	Lacrimal gland neoplasia
	Metastatic lesions		Metastatic lesions	Lymphoproliferative
	Secondary tumors		Optic nerve meningioma	Metastatic lesions
			Secondary tumors	Optic nerve glioma
				Optic nerve meningioma
				Secondary tumors
				Vascular neoplasia

Table 88-2. Clinical Findings of Common Orbital Neoplasms

Clinical Finding	Etiology
Salmon-colored cul-de-sac mass	Lymphoma
Eyelid ecchymoses	Neuroblastoma, leukemia, capillary hemangioma
Prominent temple with pulsations	Sphenoid wing meningioma
Optociliary shunt vessels	Meningioma (or glioma)
Frozen globe	Metastases
Gaze-evoked amaurosis	Orbital apex tumors

Table 88-3. Normal Hertel Exophthalmometry Values

	Male Mean	Normal Limit	Female Mean	Normal Limit
Asian	13.9	18.6	13.9	18.6
Caucasian	16.5	21.7	15.4	20.1
African-American	18.5	24.7	17.8	23.0

REFERENCES

1. Krohel GB, Stewart WB, Chavis RM. *Orbital Disease: A Practical Approach*. New York, NY: Grune & Stratton; 1981.
2. Leone CR. Painful orbital swelling. In: van Heuven WAJ, Zwaan J, eds. *Decision Making in Ophthalmology*. St Louis, MO: Mosby; 2000:88-89.

Table 88-4. Benign Versus Malignant Orbital Tumors

	Benign Tumors	Malignant Tumors
Duration of symptoms	Long (years)	Short (months)
Pain	None	Present
Vision impairment	Little	Present
Motility impairment	Little	Present
Degree of exophthalmos	Minor	Marked
Imaging findings	Circumscribed mass	Infiltrative mass
	Bone intact	Bone eroded

Non-Specific Orbital Inflammation

Roberta E. Gausas, Kimberly Cockerham, and Madhura Tamhankar

INTRODUCTION

Non-specific orbital inflammation (NSOI) is defined as a benign inflammatory process of the orbit characterized by a polymorphous lymphoid infiltrate with varying degrees of fibrosis, without a known local or systemic cause.[1] The diagnosis is arrived at after all specific causes of inflammation have been eliminated.

PATHOGENESIS

The pathogenesis of NSOI remains controversial, although it is generally believed to be an immune-mediated process.

CLINICAL FEATURES

The symptoms and clinical findings in NSOI may vary widely, but are dictated by the degree and anatomic location of the inflammation. The five most common orbital locations or patterns, in order of occurrence, are the extraocular muscles, lacrimal glands, anterior, apical, or diffuse orbital inflammation.[2]

Symptoms

Nonspecific orbital inflammation may be acute (within hours or days), subacute (days to weeks), or chronic (weeks to months) in onset. The most typical presentation is of acute-onset pain, redness, eyelid swelling, chemosis, and proptosis. In atypical cases, pain may be absent.[3] Chronic NSOI presents with a mass effect, inflammation, and/or infiltration, resulting in variable deficits in function or vision.[4]

Signs

The clinical findings vary based on the anatomic pattern of the inflammation. In addition to pain and lid swelling, diffuse inflammation of the globe can manifest as uveitis, papillitis, and exudative retinal detachment (Figure 89-1).[5]

Variants

Four clinical and pathological variants of NSOI deserve special mention: orbital myositis, orbital apex syndrome, sclerosing inflammation, and granulomatous inflammation. Classically, orbital myositis is distinguished from thyroid-related orbitopathy, the most common cause of muscle enlargement, by tendon involvement. On imaging studies, myositis is characterized by

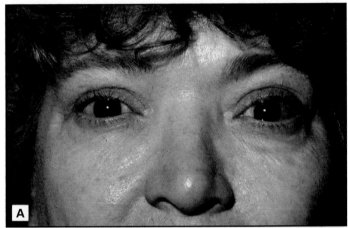
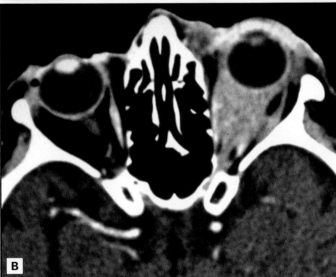

Figure 89-1. Diffuse orbital inflammation. Patient with painful proptosis and limited motility of left eye (A). Orbital CT reveals periocular and retrobulbar involvement of multiple tissues (B).

thickening not only of the extraocular muscle belly, but also of the tendon. In contrast, thickening of the muscle tendon is not seen in thyroid-associated orbitopathy.

Box 89-1. Orbital Inflammation: Diagnostic Steps

- Contrast-enhanced magnetic resonance imaging with fat suppression
- Hematologic work-up
  - Complete blood count
  - Serum electrolytes
  - Sedimentation rate
  - Antinuclear antibody
  - Anti-ds DNA
  - Antineutrophil cytoplasmic antibody
  - Angiotensin-converting enzyme level
  - Rapid plasma reagin
- Biopsy (if indicated)

Orbital Apex Syndrome

Inflammation in the posterior orbit may present with findings of an orbital apex syndrome, which includes ophthalmoplegia, optic neuropathy, and proptosis (Figure 89-2).

Sclerosing Inflammation

A distinct sclerosing form of orbital inflammation has been identified, which is characterized by dense fibrous replacement.[6]

Granulomatous Inflammation

Another distinct form displays granulomatous inflammation similar to sarcoidosis but is not associated with systemic sarcoidosis.[7]

DIAGNOSTIC EVALUATION

Imaging

Although high-resolution orbital computerized tomography (CT) may demonstrate variable enhancement after administration of iodinated contrast material, contrast-enhanced magnetic resonance imaging (MRI) with fat suppression is the imaging study with the highest yield and should be performed when available.

Hematology

The diagnostic evaluation of a patient with suspected orbital inflammation should include a full hematologic work-up (Box 89-1).

Biopsy

Although some authors have advocated empiric steroid treatment while reserving orbital biopsy for atypical, non-steroid-responsive or recalcitrant cases, many others feel that almost all infiltrative lesions should be biopsied, except for possibly two clinical scenarios: orbital myositis and orbital apex syndrome. Given the low morbidity of the procedure and the high incidence of systemic disease involving the lacrimal gland, biopsy is recommended for isolated inflammation of the lacrimal gland.[5]

DIFFERENTIAL DIAGNOSIS

NSOI is a diagnosis of exclusion, to be made only after all other specific causes of orbital inflammation have been eliminated (Table 89-1).

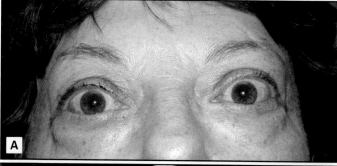
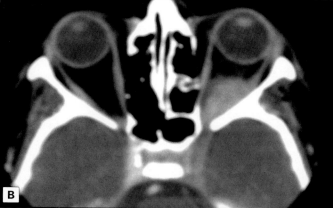
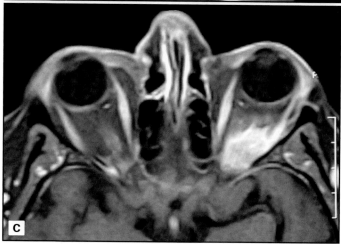

Figure 89-2. Apical orbital inflammation. Patient with painful proptosis and optic neuropathy. Although the periorbital area and anterior segment are quiet (A), neuroimaging reveals an infiltrating lesion involving the orbital apex on a CT scan (B) and MRI (C).

TREATMENT

As the pathogenesis of NSOI remains unknown, management is directed toward the common consequence of the inflammatory cascade: tissue inflammation and destruction.

Steroids

High-dose oral corticosteroids are commonly employed as the initial anti-inflammatory agent. The recommended starting dose for prednisone is 1 mg/kg/day, with a maximum adult dose of 60 to 80 mg/day. The recommended taper is 10 mg/day every 1 to 2 weeks. Typically, the response is quick, with resolution of pain and proptosis within 24 to 48 hours after onset of the treatment.

Steroid-Sparing Agents

Avoiding steroid-associated complications via alternative therapies is often desirable. Options include methotrexate (15 to 25 mg/week), azathioprine, cyclosporin, and tacrolimus. A multidisciplinary approach that utilizes the expertise of rheumatologists and/or oncologists is beneficial in organizing such treatment plans.[7]

Radiation

External beam radiation has been used in the treatment of orbital inflammation with an efficacy of 50% to 80% (Chapter 8).

Surgery

Although incisional biopsy may play an important role in establishing a correct diagnosis, the treatment of NSOI is generally medical.

PROGNOSIS

Although rapid resolution of pain and recovery of vision with steroid treatment is the common clinical course, the risk of recurrence ranges from 37% to 55%.[8] NSOI is not a precursor of lymphoma.

REFERENCES

1. Kennerdell JS, Dresner SC. The non-specific orbital inflammatory syndromes. *Surv Ophthalmol.* 1984;29:93-103.
2. Rootman J. Inflammatory diseases of the orbit. Highlights. *J Fr Ophthalmol.* 2001;24:155-161.
3. Mahr MA, Salomao DR, Garrity JA. Inflammatory orbital pseudotumor with extension beyond the orbit. *Am J Ophthalmol.* 2004;138:396-400.
4. Mombaerts I, Goldschmeding R, Schlingemann RO, Koornneef L. What is orbital pseudotumor? *Surv Ophthalmol.* 1996;41:66-78.
5. Rootman J, Nugent R. The classification and management of acute orbital pseudotumors. *Ophthalmology.* 1982;89:1040-1048.
6. Weissler MC, Miller E, Fortune MA. Sclerosing orbital pseudotumor: a unique clinicopathologic entity. *Ann Otol Rhinol Laryngol.* 1989;98:496-501.
7. Raskin EM, McCormick SA, Maher EA, Della Rocca RC. Granulomatous idiopathic orbital inflammation. *Ophthalm Plast Reconstr Surg.* 1995;11:131-135.
8. Yuen SJ, Rubin PA. Idiopathic orbital inflammation: distribution, clinical features, and treatment outcome. *Arch Ophthalmol.* 2003;121:491-499.

Table 89-1. Differential Diagnosis of Orbital Inflammation

Categories	Subtypes	
Thyroid-associated orbitopathy		
Infections	Bacterial	Spread from sinusitis
		Tuberculosis
		Syphilis
	Fungal	Mucormycosis
		Aspergillosis
	Parasitic	Echinococcosis
		Cysticercosis
Vasculitis	Wegener's granulomatosis	
	Polyarteritis nodosa	
	Hypersensitivity angiitis	
	Systemic lupus erythematosus	
	Giant cell arteritis	
Granulomatous inflammation	Sarcoidosis	
	Xanthogranulomatous	
	Foreign body granuloma	
	Erdheim-Chester disease	
	Sjögren's syndrome	
Non-inflammatory disorders	Lymphoid disorder	
	Dural-cavernous sinus arteriovenous fistula	
	Retained orbital foreign body	
Non-specific orbital inflammation (by exclusion)		

Chapter

90

Vascular Orbital Tumors

Benson Chen and Julian D. Perry

INTRODUCTION

The Orbital Society created a new classification of vascular lesions based on hemodynamic behavior. This new system guides management and prevents high-risk and unnecessary surgical intervention.[1]

VASCULAR MALFORMATIONS

The Orbital Society's hemodynamic classification divides vascular malformations into three categories by flow characteristics: no-flow (type 1), venous-flow (type 2), and arterial flow (type 3) (Table 90-1).

No-Flow (Type 1) Vascular Malformations

These vascular malformations consist of hemodynamically isolated lymphatic or combined lymphatic and venous channels. Historically classified as hamartomas or lymphangiomas, lymphatic malformations typify this class of hemodynamic behavior.

Clinical Features

More than half of these lesions are diagnosed at birth (59%), with the rest typically presenting within the first few years of life. Unilateral proptosis, or swelling, exacerbates with respiratory infections and with prolonged recumbent positioning.[2] The spontaneous hemorrhage that typifies this malformation creates blood-filled "chocolate" cysts.

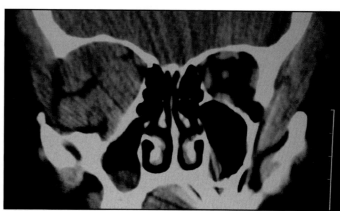

Figure 90-1. Coronal CT imaging study shows lobulated appearance of lymphangioma (type 1 vascular lesion). Note surgical absence of the lateral wall.

Diagnostic Evaluation

Imaging studies show no evidence of venous or arterial flow (Figure 90-1). Gadolinium-enhanced MRI optimally delineates the cystic compartments of these lesions, which can be intraconal, extraconal, or both. Old and new hemorrhages appear as fluid levels.

Treatment

Treatment remains risky, controversial, and only marginally effective, but common techniques include surgical debulking and sclerotherapy.[3] Acute hemorrhage causing compressive optic neuropathy requires emergency surgical decompression or cyst evacuation.

Table 90-1. Diagnostic Features of Orbital Vascular Lesions				
Type	Flow	Imaging		Treatment
		Doppler US Angiography	CT MRI	
Lymphangioma (type I)	No flow	No flow	No enhancement Fluid levels	Debulking
Varix (type II)	Venous flow	Venous flow	Contrast enhancement Flow voids	Sclerotherapy, ligation and excision
AV malformation (type III)	Arterial flow	Arterial flow	Contrast enhancement Flow voids	Embolization then debulking

AV, arteriovenous; US, ultrasound; CT, computed tomography; MRI, magnetic resonance imaging.

Venous-Flow (Type 2) Vascular Malformations

Type 2 vascular malformations consist of venous and mixed venous/lymphatic channels that communicate with the venous system. Increased venous pressure may or may not cause distention, depending on the extent of the communication.

Clinical Features

Non-distensible venous malformations behave clinically similar to type 1 lymphatic malformations, with frequent episodes of spontaneous thrombosis and hemorrhage. Doppler and contrast imaging show evidence of venous flow. Distensible venous malformations have a larger direct communication with the venous system and typically exhibit higher flow. These lesions less frequently exhibit spontaneous thrombosis and hemorrhage. Distensible combined venous and lymphatic malformations possess both type 1 and 2 flow characteristics.

Diagnostic Evaluation

Color Doppler and directional ultrasound detect venous flow. CT and MRI reveal diffuse contrast-enhancing lesions (Figure 90-2). MR imaging best delineates these lesions and may reveal fluid levels. MR angiography detects the venous flow through distensible lesions.

Treatment

Surgical management for venous malformations in the orbit is notoriously difficult. Intralesional Nd:YAG laser, delivered by optical fiber, has been recommended as a less invasive technique.[4] Other treatment modalities, including irradiation, electrocoagulation, cryotherapy, and compression, may be used alone or preoperatively to reduce bleeding complications. Resistant lesions may ultimately require surgical treatment, which carries a high risk of severe complications.

Arterial-Flow (Type 3) Vascular Malformations

These malformations display arterial-flow hemodynamics characterized by antegrade shunting of blood into the venous system.

Clinical Features

AVMs typically present in children with progressive swelling, proptosis, redness, and pain. A bruit may be audible, and proptosis is characteristically pulsatile (Figure 90-3).

Diagnostic Evaluation

Angiography remains the standard for diagnosis and evaluates the internal and external carotid arterial systems, as well as the orbital venous system.

Treatment

Surgery alone risks bleeding and ex-sanguination. Preoperative endovascular embolization and gluing of the nidus significantly reduces the risks of ligation and debulking surgery. Owing to the rapid development of a collateral circulation and inflammation, excision is generally performed within 24 to 48 hours after embolization.[5,6]

INFANTILE CAPILLARY HEMANGIOMA

Infantile capillary hemangioma represents the most common vascular tumor in children. An increased incidence in females, a

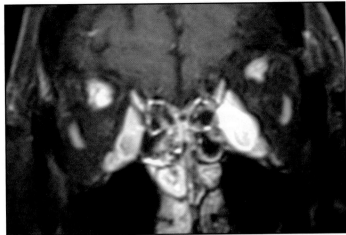

Figure 90-2. Coronal contrast-enhanced MRI shows bilateral contrast-enhancing lesions consistent with type 2 vascular lesions.

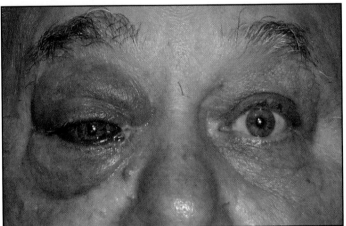

Figure 90-3. External photograph demonstrates severe arterialization and proptosis of the right eye in a patient with a type 3 orbital vascular lesion.

hormonal responsive growth pattern, and immunohistochemical markers suggest a placental origin of this benign tumor.[7]

Clinical Features

Typical presentation is within the first few months of life, with progressive unilateral swelling and proptosis, frequently with a visible dark blue anterior orbital component. Superficial extensions of lesions typically blanch on compression. Parents may report expansion of the lesions with crying.

Diagnostic Evaluation

These lesions are characterized hemodynamically by dilated inflow and outflow channels on imaging.

Treatment

These lesions exhibit a rapid growth phase over the first few months, followed by a gradual involutional phase and regression over 4 to 7 years. Most infantile capillary hemangiomas benefit from conservative observation because of a high rate of spontaneous involution. Life-threatening, visually impairing, and disfiguring lesions require treatment. Although superficial lesions respond well to a variety of treatments, including argon, YAG, and pulsed dye laser, and immunomodulating topical creams, deeper lesions often require steroids or surgical management (Chapter 99).[8]

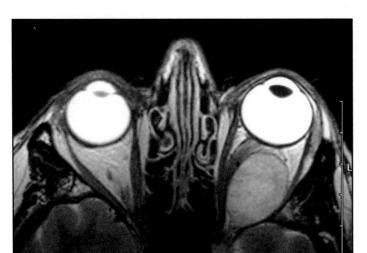

Figure 90-4. MRI of cavernous hemangioma. The lesion is circumscribed and appears hyperintense on T2-weighted images.

CAVERNOUS HEMANGIOMA

Cavernous hemangioma, the most common benign orbital tumor in adults, is characterized as a hamartoma, but these lesions may behave as low-flow arterial side vascular malformations.[9]

Clinical Features

Cavernous hemangioma typically presents in a middle-aged adult with slowly progressive, painless proptosis. It is not infrequent for cavernous hemangioma to be detected incidentally when imaging studies of the brain are performed for unrelated symptoms.

Diagnostic Evaluation

CT scanning typically reveals a well-circumscribed, multiloculated, intraconal mass. Lesions appear hypo- or isointense on T1-weighted images and hyperintense on T2-weighted images (Figure 90-4).

Treatment

Patients without significant symptoms can be followed to detect evidence of progression. For symptomatic patients, lateral orbitotomy remains the standard approach to most intraconal cavernous hemangiomas, which typically lie lateral to the optic nerve.[9]

HEMANGIOPERICYTOMA

Hemangiopericytomas are characterized by a spectrum of pericyte proliferation, and varying levels of cellular atypia implies malignant transformation or metastasis.[10]

Clinical Features

Hemangiopericytoma typically presents in middle-aged adults as slowly progressing unilateral proptosis, often with pain and vision loss.

Treatment

Although the majority of these lesions are benign, the high rate of malignant transformation and recurrent disease mandates aggressive en bloc excision with wide margins. Adjunctive radiation therapy may be of benefit.[11]

REFERENCES

1. Harris GJ. Orbital vascular malformations: a consensus statement on terminology and its clinical implications. Orbital Society. *Am J Ophthalmol.* 1999;127:453-455.
2. Greene AK, Burrows PE, Smith L, Mulliken JB. Periorbital lymphatic malformation: clinical course and management in 42 patients. *Plast Reconstruct Surg.* 2005;115:22-30.
3. Hall N, Ade-Ajai N, Pierro A, et al. Is intralesional injection of OK-432 effective in the treatment of lymphangioma in children? *Surgery.* 2003;133:238-242.
4. Werner JA, Dunne AA, Folz BJ, et al. Current concepts in the classification, diagnosis and treatment of hemangiomas and vascular malformations of the head and neck. *Eur Arch Otorhinolaryngol.* 2001;258:141-149.
5. Goldberg RA, Garcia GH, Duckwiler GR. Combined embolization and surgical treatment of arteriovenous malformation of the orbit. *Am J Ophthalmol.* 1993;116:17-25.
6. Hayes BH, Shore JW, Westfall CT, Harris GJ. Management of orbital and periorbital arteriovenous malformations. *Ophthalmic Surg.* 1995;26:145-152.
7. Mulliken JB, Glowacki J. Hemangiomas and vascular malformations in infants and children: a classification based on endothelial characteristics. *Plast Reconstruct Surg.* 1982;69:412-422.
8. Egbert JE, Paul S, Engel WK, Summers CG. High injection pressure during intralesional injection of corticosteroids into capillary hemangiomas. *Arch Ophthalmol.* 2001;119:677-683.
9. McNab AA, Wright JE. Cavernous haemangiomas of the orbit. *Aust NZ J Ophthalmol.* 1989;17:337-345.
10. Karcioglu ZA, Nasr AM, Haik BG. Orbital hemangiopericytoma: clinical and morphologic features. *Am J Ophthalmol.* 1997;124:661-672.
11. Croxatto JO, Font RL. Hemangiopericytoma of the orbit: a clinicopathoaligic study of 30 cases. *Hum Pathol.* 1982;13:210-218.

Benign Tumors of the Orbit

Bhupendra Patel

INTRODUCTION

Benign orbital tumors may be congenital or, more frequently, acquired. Benign tumors are more commonly of vascular (Chapter 90), neural (Chapter 92), meningeal, fibroytic, and osseous origin. Benign tumors may also arise from the lacrimal gland (Chapter 93) and lacrimal sac (Chapter 94).

DERMOID AND EPIDERMOID CYSTS

Dermoids cysts are the most common orbital cysts, representing up to 5% of all orbital tumors.[1] Epidermoid cysts have a single layer of keratinized or non-keratinized epithelium without evidence of adnexal structures. Most epidermoid cysts are traumatic in origin.[2] Dermoids, on the other hand, are choristomas with adnexal structures such as hair, sebaceous glands, and lipid. They arise from ectodermal nests pinched off at suture lines. Clinically, dermoid and epidermoid cysts may present very similarly and so are now usually differentiated by location: superficial or deep.

Histopathology of dermoids may show hair, keratin, sebaceous glands, macrophages, lipid globules, multinucleated giant cells, and calcium.

Diagnostic Evaluation

On CT scans, the majority of orbital dermoids have some adjacent bony changes, which are rounded and well defined (Figure 91-1). A well-defined wall is seen with a center of fat density. Some will show calcification and fluid levels.

Treatment

The surgical aim is to remove the dermoid completely. Dermoids presenting in childhood are removed soon after presentation to avoid traumatic rupture. Most can be safely removed via an anterior or anterolateral orbitotomy.

MUCOCELE

Mucoceles occur mostly in adults; 60% affect the frontal sinus, 30% occur in the ethmoid sinus, and 10% occur in the maxillary sinus. They develop secondary to an obstruction of the ostium of the affected sinus. Mucoceles may result from facial fractures, nasal or sinus surgery, paranasal osteomas, chronic polyposis, or congenital abnormalities.[3]

NEUROFIBROMA AND NEURILEMMOMA (SCHWANNOMA)

Neurofibromas are twice as common as schwannomas in the orbit, and together constitute 4% of all orbital tumors. Isolated, solitary neurofibroma are unassociated with neurofibromatosis.[4,5] Plexiform neurofibromas may involve any of the cranial, sympathetic, and parasympathetic nerves in the orbit. Schwannomas are well-defined, encapsulated, slowly growing tumors that develop as eccentric growths from peripheral nerves. They are usually solitary and may also be associated with neurofibromatosis.

Treatment

Although solitary orbital neurofibroma and neurilemmoma may be easily excised, the involved nerve is necessarily sacrificed. Therefore, care should be taken to identify the involved nerve as a sensory rather than a motor nerve.

MENINGIOMA

Meningiomas constitute 20% of adult and 2% of childhood intracranial tumors. Primary meningioma affects a younger age group, arises within the orbit, and may arise from the optic nerve sheath or the orbital surface of the sphenoid bone. The secondary type extends into the orbit from an intracranial source. These secondary tumors arise from the sphenoid ridge, the basofrontal region, the suprasellar area, the olfactory groove, and the paranasal sinuses.[6] Most adult meningiomas are seen in the fifth decade, with females being affected 75% of the time. Previous ionizing radiation and neurofibromatosis type 2 are predisposing factors.

Clinical Features

Patients may present with proptosis, decreased visual acuity, disc pallor, eyelid edema, disturbance of ocular motility, headaches or orbital pain, and seizures (Figure 91-2). The more medial sphenoidal ridge tumors cause cranial nerve palsies, visual deficits, and venous obstructive signs. A mass may be palpable in the temporal fossa when meningiomas of the greater wing of the sphenoid bone expand laterally.

Diagnostic Evaluation

CT and MRI show hyperostosis, and calcification is seen in 25% of cases (see Figure 91-2). MRI shows a hyperintense lesion

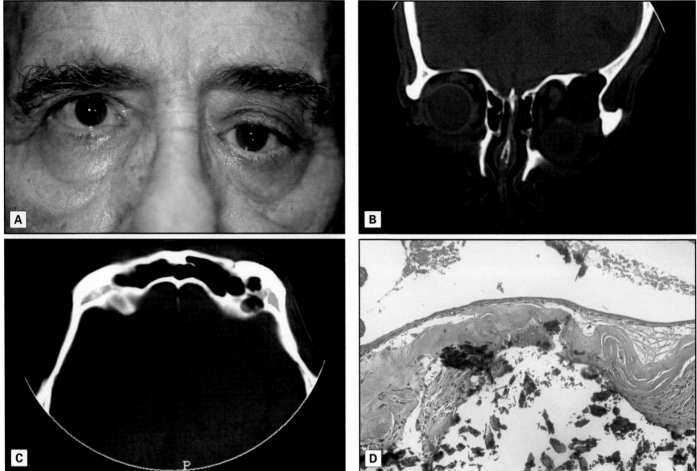

Figure 91-1. Dermoid cyst. A 75-year-old man presented with left proptosis and hypoglobus with double vision of several months duration (A). CT scan demonstrated thinning of the superotemporal orbital wall (B) (coronal view) and a cystic lesion (C) (axial view). The cyst wall is lined with stratified epithelium, and there is keratin within the lumen (D).

against the isointense brain on T1-weighted sequences, allowing delineation of intracranial meningiomas, especially when gadolinium enhancement is used.

Treatment

It is believed that meningioma in patients younger than 20 years are more aggressive and require earlier surgical intervention. Observation is warranted in older patients and where vision is not at risk. Major indications for surgery are disfiguring or severe proptosis, temporal fullness, orbital congestion, and impaired vision. Aggressive excision or debulking of sphenoid wing tumors may allow improved cosmesis, alleviate compressive symptoms, and postpone visual loss. Most patients undergoing surgical resection of sphenoidal ridge meningioma develop recurrences over several years, requiring further surgery or radiation.[7]

FIBROUS HISTIOCYTOMA

Fibrous histiocytoma is the most common mesenchymal orbital tumor in adults, seen most commonly in the middle-aged. They may be benign, locally aggressive, or malignant (Chapter 28). Fibrous histiocytoma is defined as a proliferating, complex admixture of fibroblasts and histiocyte-like cells of biphasic nature in a fibrous or collagenous matrix of varying proportions of capillaries, lipid, and reticulin.[8]

OSTEOMA

Primary osteomas, although rare, are the most common bony tumor of the orbit. They are well-defined benign tumors of bone. Most are seen in the superonasal orbit and arise secondarily from the frontal sinus, ethmoidal sinus, and junctions.[9]

FIBROUS DYSPLASIA

Fibrous dysplasia is a benign developmental disorder characterized by proliferation of fibrous tissue. It is a hamartomatous malformation thought to be an arrest of bone maturation at the woven bone stage. The fibrous tissue replaces and distorts medullary bones. Three forms have been described: monostotic, polyostotic, and McCune–Albright syndrome.[10]

ANEURYSMAL BONE CYST

Aneurysmal bone cyst is a reactive lesion of bone. Aneurysmal bone cyst may arise in the orbit secondary to trauma or as a result of local vascular disturbance.

REFERENCES

1. Shields JA, Shields CL, Scartozzi R. Survey of 1264 patients with orbital tumors and simulating lesions: the 2002 Montgomery Lecture, part 1. *Ophthalmology.* 2004;111:997-1008.

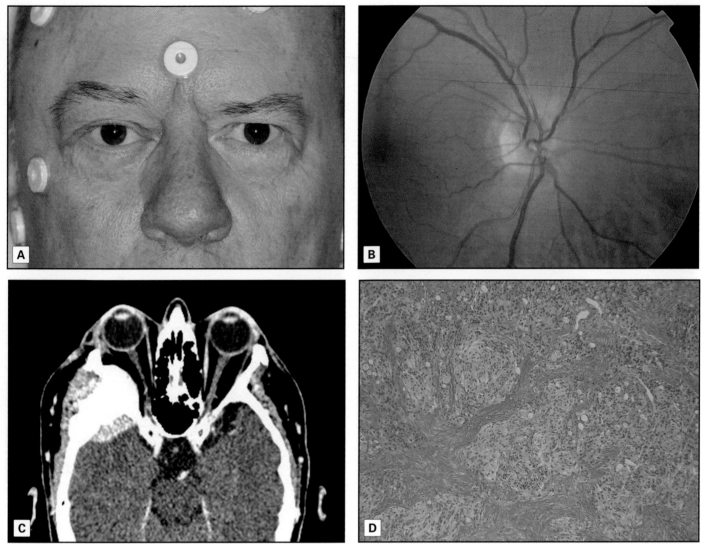

Figure 91-2. Sphenoidal wing meningioma invading orbit. A 58-year-old man presented with a bump on the temple, decreased vision, and right-sided headaches (A). Right optic disc was edematous (B). CT scan demonstrated a right sphenoidal wing hyperostosis with a well-defined and homogenous soft tissue mass extending into the orbit (C). Histopathology shows parallel interlacing bundles of elongated cells. Whorled meningothelial cells are also present (D).

2. Shields JA, Kaden IH, Eagle RC Jr, Shields CL. Orbital dermoid cysts: clinicopathologic correlations, classification and management. *Ophthalm Plast Reconstr Surg.* 1997;13:265-276.
3. Illiff CE. Mucoceles in the orbit. *Arch Ophthalmol.* 1973;89:392-395.
4. Rose GE, Wright JE. Isolated peripheral nerve sheath tumours of the orbit. *Eye.* 1991;5:668-673.
5. Rootman J, Goldberg C, Robertson W. Primary orbital schwannomas. *Br J Ophthalmol.* 1982;66:194-204.
6. Honeybul S, Neil-Dwyer G, Lang DA, Evans BT, Ellison DW. Sphenoid wing meningioma en plaque: a clinical review. *Acta Neurochir (Wien).* 2001;143:749-757.
7. Shrivastava RK, Sen C, Costantino PD, Della Rocca R. Sphenoorbital meningiomas: surgical limitations and lessons learned in their long-term management. *J Neurosurg.* 2005;103:491-497.
8. Jacobiec FA, Howard GM, Jones IS, Tannenbaum M. Fibrous histiocytomas of the orbit. *Am J Ophthalmol.* 1974;77:333-345.
9. Grove AS Jr. Osteoma of the orbit. *Ophthalmic Surg.* 1978;9:23-39.
10. Bibby K, McFadzean R. Fibrous dysplasia of the orbit. *Br J Ophthalmol.* 1994;78:266-270.

Tumors of the Optic Nerve

Jonathan Dutton

INTRODUCTION

Primary tumors of the optic nerve include optic gliomas and optic sheath meningiomas. Both are relatively rare lesions that result in significant visual morbidity.

ANTERIOR VISUAL PATHWAY GLIOMA

Optic pathway gliomas (OPG) are uncommon benign lesions classified as pilocytic astrocytomas.[1,2]

Clinical Features

Ninety percent of cases occur within the first two decades of life. The overall mean age at presentation is 8.5 years for all optic gliomas. About 25% of optic gliomas are confined to the optic nerve alone, but in three quarters of cases, the chiasm is involved.[3,4] Of the tumors that involve the chiasm, 40% extend into the adjacent hypothalamus or third ventricle. The overall incidence of neurofibromatosis type 1 (NF1) among patients with optic gliomas is 39%.[1] Proptosis is a presenting sign in 95% of all patients with optic nerve gliomas (Figure 92-1). Rare symptoms seen with central nervous system (CNS) invasion include nystagmus, seizures, hypothalamic signs, and hydrocephalus (Box 92-1).

Diagnostic Evaluation

CT imaging typically demonstrates a well-outlined fusiform swelling of the optic nerve (Figure 92-2). MRI has proved superior to CT for evaluation of chiasmal, hypothalamic, and optic tract lesions.

Treatment Options

Anterior visual pathway gliomas are neoplasms with the potential to spread into contiguous areas of the optic nerve, chiasm, and adjacent brain. They appear at an early age, grow slowly for a few years, and vision generally stabilizes in most cases.[5] However, indolent growth can be seen in up to 40% of cases. As with most medical decisions, treatment must be individualized based on patient symptoms, findings, and clinical course (Figure 92-3).

Glioma Confined to the Optic Nerve

For gliomas initially confined to the optic nerve and treated conservatively or incompletely excised, recurrence or progression is seen in 17%. The mortality rate is 12%, typically from intracranial extension.

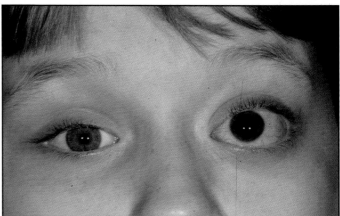

Figure 92-1. External photograph of a child with a left orbital optic nerve glioma showing axial proptosis.

Box 92-1. Benign Optic Glioma

- Proptosis, orbital tumors 94%; chiasmal tumors 22%
- Early visual loss 88%
- Optic disc atrophy 59%
- Optic disc swelling 35%
- Increased intracranial pressure 27%
- Hypothalamic signs 26%
- Nystagmus 24%

Gliomas With Extension to the Chiasm

Gliomas that do not invade the adjacent hypothalamus or third ventricle show results similar to those for untreated optic nerve tumors.

Gliomas With Extension to the Chiasm and Hypothalamus

The prognosis for life is markedly reduced. The mortality rate is 50% or more over 15 years.

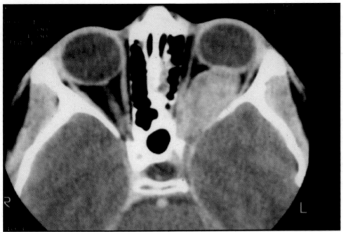

Figure 92-2. External photograph of a child with a left orbital optic nerve.

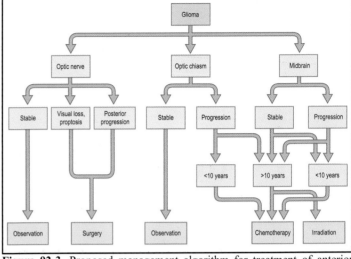

Figure 92-3. Proposed management algorithm for treatment of anterior visual pathway glioma.

Box 92-2. Malignant Optic Glioma

■ Very rapid loss of vision to blindness over weeks to months
■ Optic disc swelling 43%
■ Optic disc atrophy 31%
■ Proptosis 23%
■ Ophthalmoplegia 19%
■ Other neurologic signs 35%

MALIGNANT OPTIC NERVE GLIOMA

Malignant optic nerve glioma has aggressive behavior and a uniformly fatal outcome (Box 92-2).[6]

OPTIC NERVE SHEATH MENINGIOMA

Meningiomas are the second most common brain neoplasms after gliomas. Although most orbital meningiomas are extensions from intracranial sites, primary orbital meningiomas account for 1.3% of all meningiomas.[7]

Clinical Features

Orbital meningioma is a disease primarily of middle age with a slight female preponderance of approximately 60%.[7] Ninety-four percent are unilateral and 6% bilateral. In about 8% of cases, the meningioma is confined to the optic canal. The most frequent presenting symptom is loss of vision, seen in 97% of cases. Proptosis is found on initial examination in 65% of patients (Figure 92-4 and Box 92-3).

Diagnostic Evaluation

Tram-tracking, a radiographic sign in which the denser and thickened optic nerve sheath outlines a central lucency representing the residual optic nerve, is a characteristic of sheath meningioma (Figure 92-5). Calcification, an important finding, is seen in 20% to 50% of patients.

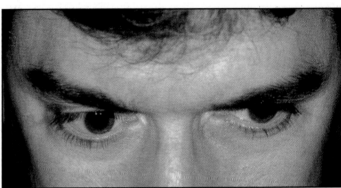

Figure 92-4. External photograph of a patient with a right orbital optic nerve sheath meningioma demonstrating proptosis.

Box 92-3. Optic Nerve Sheath Meningioma

■ Slowly progressive visual loss 96%
■ Proptosis 59%
■ Optic disc atrophy 49%
■ Optic disc swelling 48%
■ Decreased ocular motility 47%
■ Optociliary shunt vessels 30%
■ Increased intracranial pressure 27%

Treatment

The most appropriate therapy for optic sheath meningiomas has been a matter of some controversy.[7-10] The major rationale for treatment is the perceived risk of spread to the contralateral optic nerve. In most cases, radiotherapy may slow or halt tumor progression. However, in cases of treatment failure, surgical excision should be considered (Figure 92-6).

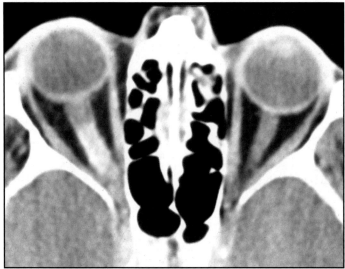

Figure 92-5. Axial CT scan shows a tubular optic nerve sheath meningioma with tram-tracking. The involved sheath enhances brightly, with the uninvolved optic nerve centrally.

Prognosis

Patients with optic sheath meningiomas have an excellent prognosis for life. The prognosis for vision, however, is poor.

REFERENCES

1. Dutton JJ, Byrne SF, Proia AD. *Diagnostic Atlas of Orbital Diseases*. Philadelphia, PA: WB Saunders; 2000.
2. Shields JA, Shields CL, Scartozzi R. Survey of 1264 patients with orbital tumors and simulating lesions: the 2002 Montgomery Lecture, part I. *Ophthalmology.* 2004;111:997-1008.
3. Gayre GS, Scott IU, Feuer W, Saunders TG, Siatkowski RM. Long-term visual outcome in patients with anterior visual pathway gliomas. *J Neuro-Ophthalmol.* 2001;2:1-7.
4. Czyzyk E, Jozwiak S, Roszkowski M, Schwartz RA. Optic pathway gliomas in children with and without neurofibromatosis 1. *J Child Neurol.* 2003;18:471-478.
5. Hoyt WF, Bagdassarian SA. Optic gliomas of childhood: natural history and rationale for conservative management. *Br J Ophthalmol.* 1969;53:793-798.
6. Hoyt WF, Meshel LG, Lessell S, et al. Malignant optic glioma of adulthood. *Brain.* 1973;96:121-132.

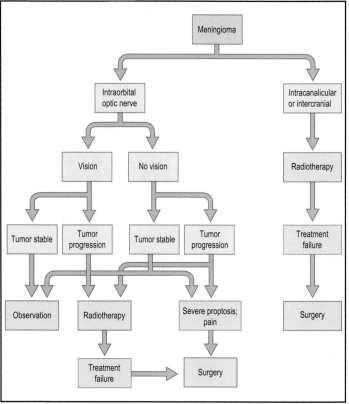

Figure 92-6. Proposed management algorithm for treatment of optic nerve sheath meningioma.

7. Dutton JJ. Optic nerve sheath meningiomas. *Surv Ophthalmol.* 1992;37:167-183.
8. Radhakrishnan S, Lee MS. Optic nerve sheath meningiomas. *Curr Treat Options Neurol.* 2005;7:51-55.
9. Richards JC, Roden D, Harper CS. Management of sight-threatening optic nerve sheath meningioma with fractionated stereotactic radiotherapy. *Clin Exp Ophthalmol.* 2005;33:137-141.
10. Eagan RA, Lessell S. A contribution to the natural history of optic nerve sheath meningiomas. *Arch Ophthalmol.* 2002;120:1505-1508.

Chapter

93

Tumors of the Lacrimal Gland

Omar M. Durrani and Geoffrey E. Rose

INTRODUCTION

Diseases such as dacryoadenitis, sarcoidosis, Wegener's granulomatosis, and other inflammatory or infiltrative conditions account for more than 60% of lacrimal gland masses and may present with signs and symptoms similar to neoplastic lesions (Figure 93-1).[1,2] Most primary tumors of the lacrimal gland are epithelial in origin, with about half being benign (Table 93-1).[3]

CLINICAL FEATURES

Pleomorphic adenomas have a peak incidence in middle age, and patients typically present with upper lid swelling or a mass (Figure 93-2). Pain occurs rarely with pleomorphic adenoma or lacrimal lymphoma, but primary malignant tumors of the lacrimal gland are characterized by a short history and persistent pain (Figure 93-3).[4] Orbital lobe tumors are characterized by progressive inferomedial globe displacement and relatively little proptosis.

DIAGNOSTIC EVALUATION

High-resolution computed tomography (CT), the primary imaging technique for orbital diseases, is valuable in the differentiation of lacrimal gland masses. Because bone changes are poorly shown on MR images, this modality is not as useful as CT in establishing the diagnosis of lacrimal gland lesions.[5]

TREATMENT

Pleomorphic adenoma should be excised intact with a cuff of normal tissue.[6] Palpebral lobe tumors are readily resected through an upper lid skin crease incision. Orbital lobe tumors can be approached through a skin crease incision, which can be extended into the lateral canthal rhytides to allow a lateral osteotomy.[6] If a pleomorphic adenoma has been inadvertently biopsied, the biopsy tract and the tumor should be meticulously excised as recurrence of pleomorphic adenoma is typically infiltrative and may otherwise necessitate extensive tissue resection or exenteration.

Adenoid Cystic Carcinoma

Tumors that are clinically and radiologically localized to the orbit should be debulked and given 55 Gy external beam irradiation or implant brachytherapy.[7]

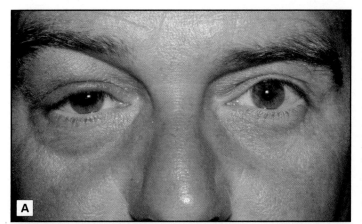
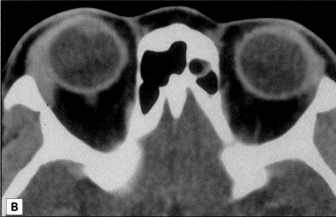

Figure 93-1. S-shaped deformity of the right upper lid caused by subacute dacryoadenitis (A). CT scan showing left lacrimal gland enlargement with molding around the globe (B).

Table 93-1. Primary Lacrimal Gland Neoplasia	
Types	Nomenclature
Benign tumors	Pleomorphic adenoma
	Myoepithelioma*
Malignant tumors	Adenoid cystic carcinoma
	Malignant mixed tumor (carcinoma arising within pleomorphic adenoma)
	Mucoepidermoid carcinoma
	Adenocarcinoma*

*Rare.

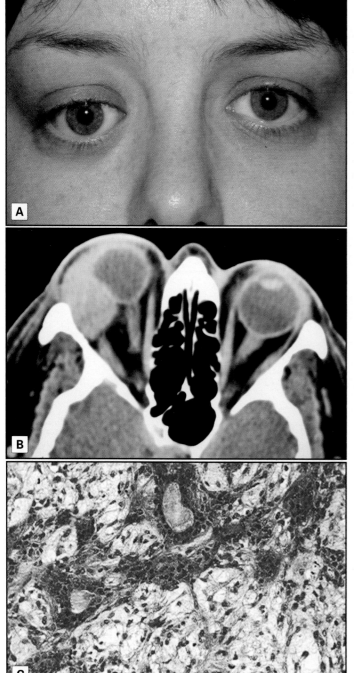

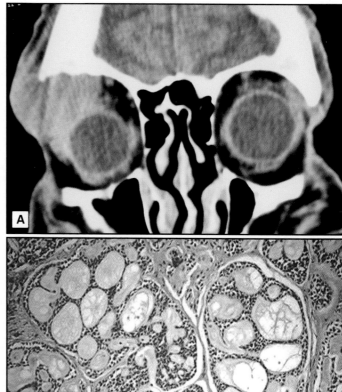

Figure 93-3. Adenoid cystic carcinoma of the right lacrimal gland with destruction of the lateral orbital wall bone and soft tissue invasion of the right temporalis fossa through lateral wall defect (A). Typical cribriform appearance (B). (Hematoxylin and eosin.)

Figure 93-2. Facial asymmetry due to pleomorphic adenoma of the right lacrimal gland (A). CT scan showing marked enlargement of the right lacrimal gland with molding around the globe (B). Epithelial cells centrally with eosinophilic cytoplasm and myoepithelial cells surrounding ducts showing clear lumen (C). (Hematoxylin and eosin.)

Malignant Mixed Tumor

Malignant mixed tumor (malignant transformation within pleomorphic adenoma) is treated with local excision followed by irradiation.[8]

Metastatic tumor of the lacrimal gland carries a poor prognosis and treatment, which is generally palliative and reflects that of the primary tumor.

REFERENCES

1. Shields JA, Shields CL, Scartozzi R. Survey of 1264 patients with orbital tumors and simulating lesions: the 2002 Montgomery Lecture, part 1. *Ophthalmology.* 2004;111:997-1008.
2. Shields CL, Shields JA, Eagle RC, Rathmell JP. Clinicopathologic review of 142 cases of lacrimal gland lesions. *Ophthalmology.* 1989; 6:431-435.
3. Wright JE, Rose GE, Garner A. Primary malignant neoplasms of the lacrimal gland. *Br J Ophthalmol.* 1992;76:401-407.
4. Gamel JW, Font RL. Adenoid cystic carcinoma of the lacrimal gland: the clinical significance of a basaloid histologic pattern. *Hum Pathol.* 1982;13:219-225.
5. Aviv RI, Miszkiel K. Orbital imaging: part 2. Intraorbital pathology. *Clin Radiol.* 2005;60:288-307.
6. Rose GE, Wright JE. Pleomorphic adenoma of the lacrimal gland. *Br J Ophthalmol.* 1992;76:395-400.
7. Brada M, Henk JM. Radiotherapy for lacrimal gland tumors. *Radiother Oncol.* 1987;175-183.
8. Heaps RS, Miller NR, Albert DM, et al. Primary adenocarcinoma of the lacrimal gland. A retrospective study. *Ophthalmology.* 1993;100:1856-1860.

Tumors of the Lacrimal Sac

Jacob Pe'er

INTRODUCTION

Tumors of the lacrimal sac are rare. Lacrimal sac tumors are divided into two major groups: the epithelial tumors, which account for about 75% of reported cases, and the non-epithelial tumors, which account for the remaining 25% (Tables 94-1 and 94-2).[1,2]

CLINICAL FEATURES

Lacrimal sac tumors are usually diagnosed in adults with an average age in the 50s. Benign tumors are diagnosed about a decade earlier than malignant ones.[1,2] Dacryostenosis and/or dacryocystitis due to complete or partial obstruction of the drainage system are common. Lacrimal sac tumors are often found inadvertently at the time of dacryocystorhinostomy (DCR) for presumed dacryostenosis. This is the reason that DCR specimens should always be submitted for pathologic evaluation.[3] The main sign of lacrimal sac tumor is a mass in the area of the lacrimal sac (Figure 94-1); the appearance of a mass above the medial canthal tendon level is most characteristic. Bleeding from the puncta, either spontaneously or on applying pressure to the lacrimal sac, or bleeding from the nose (epistaxis) or a dark bloody nasal discharge are found in some patients, mainly those with epithelial tumors.[2]

DIAGNOSTIC EVALUATION

CT shows a solid mass over the lacrimal sac area, may display dilatation of the lacrimal fossa and/or bony erosion or destruction of the lacrimal fossa, and, in advanced cases, may show invasion into neighboring structures (Figure 94-2). Dacryocystography (DCG) may reveal a filling defect of the sac lumen or a distended sac with uneven or mottled contrast media, or a delay in draining of the contrast material (Figure 94-3). Where the tumor is benign or in the early stages, the lacrimal drainage system may be patent, so that negative results do not rule out a tumor.

Epithelial Tumors

Papilloma may exhibit an exophytic growth pattern, growing toward the sac lumen, or an inverted pattern, growing toward the stroma.

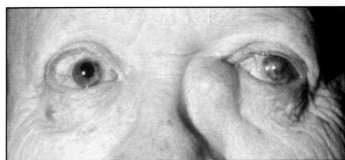

Figure 94-1. A man with a transitional cell carcinoma of the lacrimal sac of the left eye presenting with a mass that reaches a level above the medial canthal tendon. (Courtesy of Mary A. Stefanyszyn, MD.)

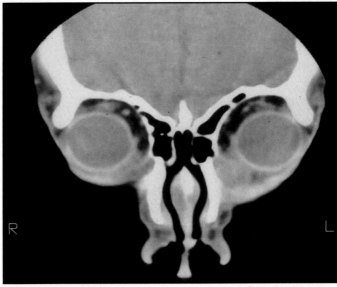

Figure 94-2. A CT scan shows a mass over the left lacrimal sac area. (Courtesy of Mary A. Stefanyszyn, MD.)

Squamous and Transitional Cell Carcinoma

Squamous and transitional cell carcinoma range from a well-differentiated tumor with keratin pearls and intercellular bridges to a poorly differentiated one. Transitional cell carcinoma may show a papillary pattern and be composed of cylindrical epithelial cells.

Table 94-1. Histopathological Classification of Epithelial Tumors of the Lacrimal Sac

Category		Subtype	
Benign	Papilloma	Squamous papilloma	Transitional cell papilloma
		Mixed cell papilloma	Papilloma unspecified
	Oncocytoma		
	Mucocele	Pleomorphic adenoma (mixed tumor)	
	Cyst		Cylindroma
Malignant	Papilloma with carcinoma		
	Carcinoma	Squamous cell carcinoma	Transitional cell carcinoma
		Mixed squamous/transitional carcinoma	Oncocytic adenocarcinoma
		Mucoepidermoid carcinoma	Adenoid cystic carcinoma
		Adenocarcinoma	Adenocarcinoma ex-pleomorphic adenoma
		Eccrine adenocarcinoma	Undifferentiated carcinoma
Secondary tumors			

Table 94-2. Histopathological Classification of Non-Epithelial Tumors of the Lacrimal Sac

Category		Subtype	
Mesenchymal-fibrous tissue	Benign	Fibrous histiocytoma	Lipoma
		Juvenile xanthogranuloma	
	Malignant	Malignant fibrous histiocytoma	
Mesenchymal-vascular	Benign	Capillary hemangioma	Cavernous hemangioma
		Hemangiopericytoma	Angiofibroma
		Hemangioendothelioma	Glomus tumor
	Malignant	Kaposi's sarcoma	
Melanocytic	Benign	Nevi	
	Malignant	Melanoma	
Lymphoproliferative	Benign reactive lymphoid hyperplasia	Malignant lymphoma	
	Leukemic infiltrate (granulocytic sarcoma)	Plasmacytoma	
Neural	Neurofibroma	Neurilemmoma (schwannoma)	
Inflammatory pseudotumors			
Secondary tumors			

Non-epithelial tumors constitute about 25% of lacrimal sac tumors; of these, about half are mesenchymal, one quarter lymphoproliferative, and one quarter melanoma.

TREATMENT

The treatment of choice is complete surgical removal.[4-6] En-bloc excision of the tumor with the periosteum of the fossa and supplemental external irradiation can be added if the tumor is malignant.

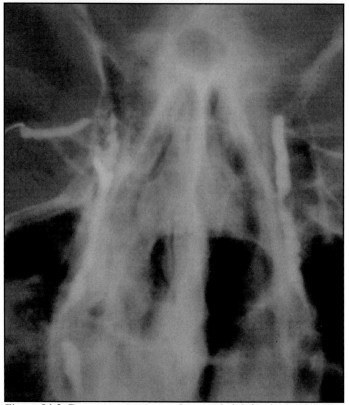

Figure 94-3. Dacryocystogram reveals a mottled defect in the right lacrimal sac compared to the smooth outline of the left lacrimal sac. (Courtesy of Mary A. Stefanyszyn, MD.)

REFERENCES

1. Ni C, D'Amico DJ, Fan CQ, Kuo PK. Tumors of the lacrimal sac: a clinicopathological analysis of 82 cases. *Int Ophthalmol Clin.* 1982;22:121-140.

2. Stefanyszyn MA, Hidayat AA, Pe'er JJ, Flanagan JC. Lacrimal sac tumors. *Ophthalm Plast Reconstr Surg.* 1994;10:169-184.

3. Anderson NG, Wojno TH, Grossniklaus HE. Clinicopathologic findings from lacrimal sac biopsy specimens obtained during dacryocystorhinostomy. *Ophthalmol Plast Reconstr Surg.* 2003;19:173-176.

4. Parmar D, Rose GE. Management of lacrimal sac tumours. *Eye.* 2003;17:599-606.

5. Pe'er J, Hidayat AA, Ilsar M, Landau L, Stefanyszyn MA. Glandular tumors of the lacrimal sac. Their histologic patterns and possible origins. *Ophthalmology.* 1996;103:1601-1605.

6. Pe'er JJ, Stefanyszyn M, Hidayat AA. Nonepithelial tumors of the lacrimal sac. *Am J Ophthalmol.* 1994;118:650-658.

Orbital and Adnexal Lymphoma

David S. Bardenstein

INTRODUCTION

Ocular adnexal lymphoma (OAL) represents the malignant end of the spectrum of ocular adnexal lymphoproliferative disease and has reactive lymphoid hyperplasia (RLH) and RLH with atypia as its benign and intermediate forms, respectively (Box 95-1). OAL can affect the conjunctiva, eyelid, and orbit/lacrimal gland as well as the nasolacrimal drainage system.[1,2] Bilaterality is reported in 10% to 20% of cases.

CLASSIFICATION

OAL is termed solitary if it is the only site involved, secondary when contiguous sites are involved, and systemic if remote sites are involved. General principles of systemic lymphoma staging apply to OAL. The vast majority of OAL are of the non-Hodgkin's B-cell type. Despite the extensive numbers of systemic lymphoma subtypes, most OAL belong to one of five subtypes[3-5]: extranodal marginal zone (EMZL or MALT lymphoma), follicular lymphoma (FL), diffuse large B-cell lymphoma (DLBCL), mantle cell lymphoma (MCL), and lymphoplasmacytic lymphoma (LPL). In all series, most OAL are the EMZL type.

CLINICAL FEATURES

Subjective complaints in OAL include lacrimal gland, orbital, conjunctival mass or apparent eyelid mass, exophthalmos, pain, or diplopia, but many lesions are asymptomatic. In the conjunctiva, the lesions typically have a salmon or flesh-pink color (Figure 95-1). Involvement of the nasolacrimal drainage system can occur (Figure 95-2).

DIAGNOSTIC EVALUATION

Evaluation of OAL involves characterization of the lesion and staging.

Imaging Studies

Contrast-enhanced CT and MRI scans of the orbits will show enhancing lesions, which can be discrete or diffuse (Figures 95-3 and 95-4).

Staging Procedures

Because OAL can co-exist with lymphoma in other sites, staging is performed. This includes a thorough physical examination, CT of the chest, abdomen and pelvis, and MRI of the head.

Box 95-1. Ocular Adnexal Lymphoma

- OAL consists primarily of five types of lymphoma, the most common of which is extranodal marginal zone type (EMZT)
- The diagnosis depends on pathology, immunophenotypic analysis, and molecular genetics studies
- Updated lymphoma classifications allow excellent diagnostic accuracy
- Treatment of local disease consists of radiation and other local modalities with good local control but a variable long-term prognosis
- Low-grade tumors with systemic involvement are treated by observation or local methods
- Chemotherapy is used for high-grade disease with systemic involvement
- Infection and chronic inflammation may play a role in lymphomagenesis, and new treatment modalities may be directed at them

---

Laboratory evaluation includes a full blood count, hepatic enzymes, serum lactate dehydrogenase (LDH), and bone marrow aspiration and biopsy (Table 95-1).

PATHOLOGIC FEATURES

Lesions should be obtained by open biopsy to allow sufficient material for multiple special studies that are employed: pathology, lymphocyte immunophenotypical analysis, and molecular genetic studies to identify gene rearrangements indicative of clonality and/or translocations. Pathologic analysis can identify obvious lymphomas but cannot reliably differentiate lymphoma types (Figure 95-5). The immunophenotypic expressions of the various types can be carried out qualitatively on tissue sections or quantitatively on dispersed cells (flow cytometry). Molecular genetic analysis of OAL is important in two ways. Identification of over-expressed heavy chain gene rearrangements is indicative of clonality and typically represents malignancy.[6] Tumor cells can be analyzed for translocations that may be indicative of a specific lymphoma type.

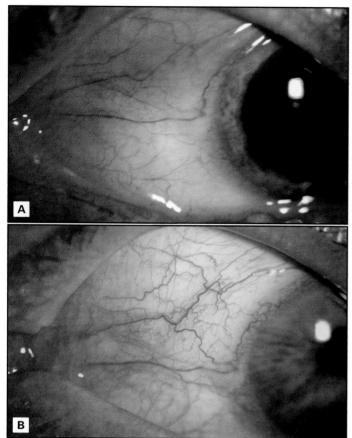

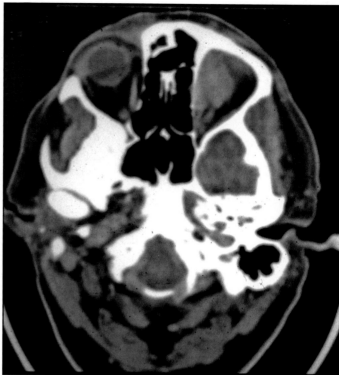

Figure 95-3. Axial CT scan of patient in Figure 95-2, showing a superior orbital mass with irregular margins that molds to the orbital wall.

Figure 95-1. Conjunctival lymphoma with typical salmon color and diffuse margins (A). After radiation treatment, there is complete resolution of the mass (B).

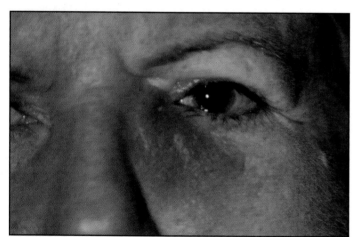

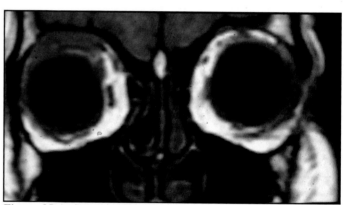

Figure 95-4. Coronal MRI scan (T1-weighted image) demonstrating bilateral orbital involvement.

Figure 95-2. Clinical view of lymphoma involving the nasolacrimal sac region.

TREATMENT

The treatment of OAL is an area of controversy, progress, and change. With the recognition that the vast majority of OAL are of the EMZL/MALT type and that there may be an infectious basis for this subgroup, a possibility of deferring cytotoxic modalities has been raised.

Surgery

Complete excision should generally be reserved for localized and isolated lesions of the conjunctiva.[7]

Cryotherapy may have an application in patients with conjunctival OAL unable to receive other treatment modalities.[7]

Radiation has been the most frequently used modality for the treatment of OAL to avoid surgical complications. Analysis of the radiation dose–response relationship of EMZL revealed that 5-year local tumor control rates were 81% with doses below 30 Gy but 100% with doses higher than that.[4]

Table 95-1. Staging of Non-Hodgkin's Lymphoma	
Indolent lymphomas: EMZL, FL, LPL	
Stage I	Localized disease (Ann Arbor [AA] I, IE & II, IIE)
Stage II	Disseminated disease (Ann Arbor [AA] III & IV)
Aggressive lymphomas: DLBCL, MCL	
Stage I	Localized or extranodal disease (Ann Arbor [AA] I or IE)
Stage II	Two or more nodal sites; three or more extranodal sites
Stage III	Stage II with additional poor prognostic features

E, extranodal disease.

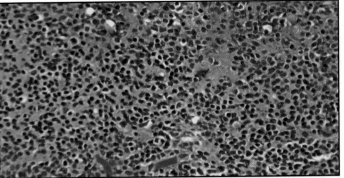

Figure 95-5. Photomicrograph of monomorphic lymphocytes typical of EMZL-type ocular adnexal lymphoma. (Hematoxylin and eosin, original magnification x100.)

Chemotherapy

Because OAL frequently presents as localized disease (stage IE), chemotherapy is rarely used unless it is DLBCL.

Antimicrobial Treatment

There is increasing evidence of a role for chronic infection in OAL. Both *C. psittaci* and *H. pylori* have been identified to date.[8,9] Follow-up data from the *C. psittaci* detection study suggest a therapeutic effect in half of patients using a 3-week course of doxycycline, presumably to eradicate the infection that underlies lymphomagenesis. Larger studies are needed to clarify the role of this therapy.

PROGNOSIS

Among OAL, EMZL has a quantitatively better prognosis than other tumor types with regard to spread and lymphoma-related death.[5]

REFERENCES

1. Char DH. Orbital lymphoid lesions. In: Char DH, ed. *Clinical Ocular Oncology*. Philadelphia, PA: Lippincott-Raven; 1997:349-364.
2. Knowles DM, Jakobiec FA, McNally L, et al. Lymphoid hyperplasia and malignant lymphoma occurring in the ocular adnexa (orbit, conjunctiva, and eyelids): a prospective multiparametric analysis of 108 cases during 1977 to 1987. *Hum Pathol.* 1990;21:959-973.
3. Harris NL, Jaffe ES, Stein H, et al. A revised European-American classification of lymphoid neoplasms: a proposal from the International Lymphoma Study Group. *Blood.* 1994;84:1361-1392.
4. Fung CY, Tarbell NJ, Lucarelli MJ, et al. Ocular adnexal lymphoma: clinical behavior of distinct World Health Organization classification subtypes. *Int J Radiat Oncol Biol Phys.* 2003;57:1382-1391.
5. Jenkins C, Rose GE, Bunce C, et al. Histological features of ocular adnexal lymphoma (REAL classification) and their association with patient morbidity and survival. *Br J Ophthalmol.* 2000;84:907-913.
6. White VA, Gascoyne RD, McNeil BK, et al. Histopathologic findings and frequency of clonality detected by the polymerase chain reaction in ocular adnexal lymphoproliferative lesions. *Mod Pathol.* 1996;9:1052-1061.
7. Shields CL Shields JA, Carvahlo C, et al. Conjunctival lymphoid tumors: clinical analysis of 117 cases and relationship to systemic lymphoma. *Ophthalmology.* 2001;108:979-984.
8. Ferreri AJ, Guidoboni M, De Conciliis C, et al. Evidence for an association between Chlamydia psittaci and ocular adnexal lymphomas. *J Natl Cancer Inst.* 2004;96:586-594.
9. Chan CC, Smith JA, Shen DF, et al. Helicobacter pylori (H. pylori) molecular signature in conjunctival mucosa-associated lymphoid tissue (MALT) lymphoma. *Histol Histopathol.* 2004;19:1219-1226.

Malignant Tumors of the Orbit

Bhupendra Patel

INTRODUCTION

Malignant orbital tumors represent a broad spectrum of tumors, which includes primary, secondary (extension from adjacent structures), and metastatic tumors (Chapter 86). In addition, orbital inflammation and infection may clinically simulate an orbital neoplasm (Chapter 89).

Malignant tumors of vascular (Chapter 90), neural (Chapter 92), fibrocytic, and osseous origin are rare in the orbit. Rhabdomyosarcoma is the most frequent primary malignant orbital tumor in children (Chapter 97), and lymphoproliferative disorders including lymphoma are most frequent in older adults (Chapter 95). Malignant orbital tumors may also arise from the lacrimal gland (Chapter 93) and lacrimal sac (Chapter 94). The details of clinical examination (Chapter 84), clinical evaluation (Chapter 87 and Chapter 88), and imaging techniques (Chapter 85) supplement the contents of this chapter. Malignant orbital tumors not covered under other chapters are reviewed herein.

ESTHESIONEUROBLASTOMA

Esthesioneuroblastoma is a tumor of neural crest origin that arises from the sensory olfactory epithelium and can invade the cribriform plate, the ethmoid sinuses, and the orbit. Most esthesioneuroblastomas seen in the orbit have invaded the orbit secondarily.[1]

MALIGNANT PERIPHERAL NERVE SHEATH TUMOR

This rare tumor may develop de novo, following radiotherapy, or secondary to plexiform neurofibroma. About 50% of malignant peripheral nerve sheath tumors are associated with neurofibromatosis.[2]

OSTEOSARCOMA

Osteosarcoma, also called osteogenic sarcoma, is the most common primary malignant neoplasm of bone. Most cases arise de novo but may be secondary to Paget's disease, fibrous dysplasia, radiation therapy, giant cell tumor, osteoblastoma,[3] or seen as a second tumor in patients with familial retinoblastoma, even in the absence of a history of radiotherapy.[4] The maxillary bone is the most frequent orbital site of the tumor.

MALIGNANT FIBROUS HISTIOCYTOMA

Fibrous histiocytoma is the most common mesenchymal orbital tumor in adults, seen most commonly in the middle-aged (Chapter 91).[5] They may be benign, locally aggressive, or malignant (Chapter 28). Patients present with proptosis, a mass effect, reduced vision, double vision, pain, eyelid swelling, and ptosis (Figure 96-1). Malignant fibrous histiocytoma or myxofibrosarcoma may arise de novo or follow orbital radiotherapy, especially in children with the germline mutation of retinoblastoma (Chapter 71). Malignant fibrous histiocytoma requires exenteration. Although metastases are rare, the tumor shows local infiltrative features with a tendency to local recurrence.

LEIOMYOSARCOMA

Leiomyosarcomas are usually seen as radiation-induced tumors following orbital irradiation in children.[6]

LIPOSARCOMA

Liposarcoma is a common soft tissue sarcoma in adults but it rarely arises within the orbit.[7]

SECONDARY ORBITAL TUMORS

Secondary orbital tumors represent contiguous orbital extension of a primary ocular, conjunctival, eyelid, sinus, or intracranial tumor. Basal cell, squamous cell, melanoma, and sebaceous cell carcinoma of the eyelid may secondarily invade the orbit because of late presentation, incomplete excision (sebaceous cell carcinoma), rapid and aggressive growth, or perineural spread (squamous cell carcinoma and melanoma).

Merkel cell carcinoma is an eyelid neoplasm that may arise in the eyelid or periocular region (Chapter 20). It demonstrates rapid growth with a bulging, red appearance and overlying telangiectatic vessels in the elderly (Figure 96-2). The diagnosis is confirmed by the characteristic immunocytochemical and electron microscopic features. The tumor is associated with local recurrence and satellite lesions, regional nodal metastases, and distant metastases in about half of patients. Orbital invasion is associated with tumor recurrence and may lead to intracranial spread.

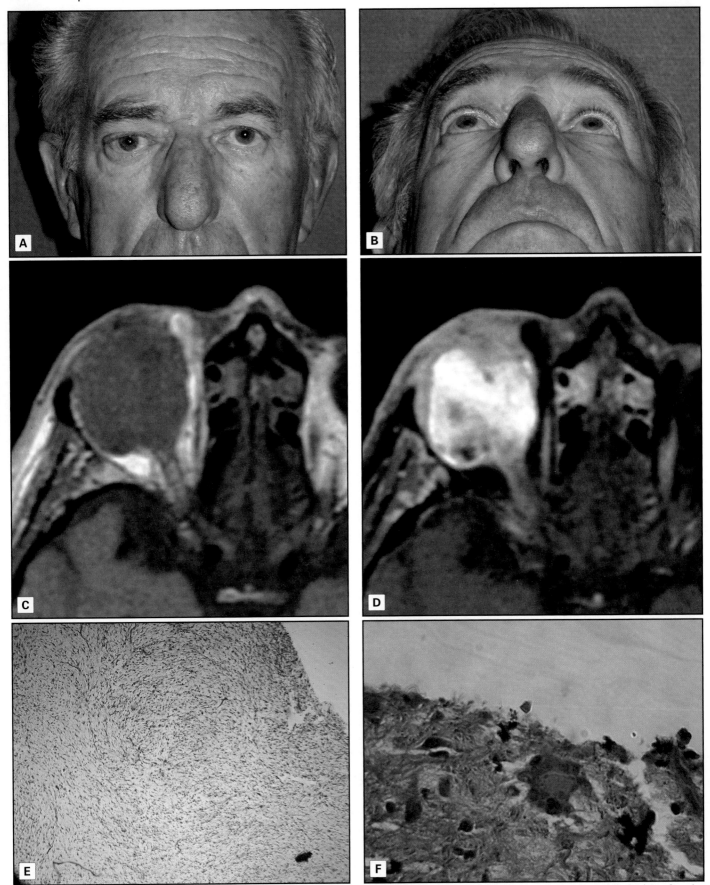

Figure 96-1. Malignant histiocytoma or myxofibrosarcoma. A 75-year-old man with onset of double vision over 2 months and limitation of ocular movements in all fields of gaze. Note hypoglobus (A) and proptosis (B) on the right side. MRI shows a right superior orbital mass (C), which enhances irregularly with gadolinium (D). On histopathology, storiform or cartwheel-like growth pattern is seen (E). Note Touton giant cell (F). Exenteration was performed, and the patient is recurrence free at 4 years.

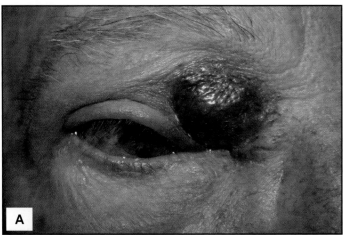

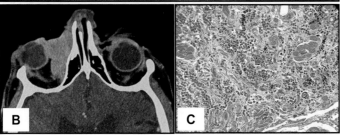

Figure 96-2. Merkel cell carcinoma. A 78-year-old man with a right medial canthal lesion initially biopsied elsewhere and diagnosed as basal cell carcinoma. Note typical budding reddish lesion with overlying vascularity (A). CT scan showed diffuse tumor with orbital invasion but without bone involvement (B). Note relatively large cells with uniformly staining eosinophilic cytoplasm (C).

Category	Feature
Mass effect	Visible or palpable mass
Infiltrative	Diplopia, exophthalmos, enophthalmos
Functional	Neurological deficits
Inflammatory	Pain, chemosis, swelling
Silent	Discovered on imaging or at surgery with no symptoms or signs

Table 96-1. Clinical Features of Orbital Metastases

(Adapted from Goldberg RA, Rootman J. Clinical characteristics of metastatic orbital tumors. *Ophthalmology.* 1990;97:620-624.)

Patients have more rapid onset of symptoms than with other types of orbital neoplasia. Proptosis and motility disturbances with pain are the most common presenting symptoms (Table 96-1).

ORBITAL METASTASES

Approximately 8% of all orbital neoplasia are metastatic in origin. Breast cancer, lung cancer, prostate cancer, and melanoma are the most frequent primary tumors in adults that metastasize to the orbit. In approximately 10% of cases, the primary tumor remains unidentified. In the majority of cases (75%) a diagnosis of pre-existing primary tumor is known, but in about 25% of cases the orbital tumor is the first presentation.[8] Neuroblastoma, Ewing's sarcoma, Wilms' tumor, testicular embryonal sarcoma, and ovarian sarcoma may cause metasases to the orbit in children.[9]

REFERENCES

1. Laforest C, Selva D, Crompton J, Leibovitch I. Orbital invasion by esthesioneuroblastoma. *Ophthalm Plast Reconstr Surg.* 2005;21:435-440.
2. Lyons CJ, McNab AA, Garner A, Wright JE. Orbital malignant peripheral nerve sheath tumors. *Br J Ophthalmol.* 1989;73:731-738.
3. Mark RJ, Sercarz JA, Tran L, et al. Osteogenic sarcoma of the head and neck. The UCLA experience. *Arch Otolaryngol.* 1991;117:761-766.
4. Abramson DH, Ronner HJ, Ellsworth RM. Second tumors in non-irradiated bilateral retinoblastoma. *Am J Ophthalmol.* 1979;87:624-627.
5. Jacobiec FA, Howard GM, Jones IS, Tannenbaum M. Fibrous histiocytomas of the orbit. *Am J Ophthalmol.* 1974;77:333-345.
6. Folberg R, Cleaseby G, Flanagan JA, Spencer WH, Zimmerman LE. Orbital leiomyosarcoma after radiation therapy for bilateral retinoblastoma. *Arch Ophthalmol.* 1983;101:1562-1565.
7. Cai YC, McMenamin ME, Rose G, et al. Primary liposarcoma of the orbit: a clinicopathologic study of seven cases. *Ann Diagn Pathol.* 2001;5:255-266.
8. Goldberg RA, Rootman J. Clinical characteristics of metastatic orbital tumors. *Ophthalmology.* 1990;97:620-624.
9. Levy WJ. Neuroblastoma. *Br J Ophthalmol.* 1957;41:48-53.

Chapter

97

Rhabdomyosarcoma

Benson Chen and Julian D. Perry

INTRODUCTION

Rhabdomyosarcoma (RMS) represents the most common orbital malignancy in children, and patients with this disease often present to the ophthalmologist. Because current therapeutic regimens offer an excellent chance for curing isolated orbital disease, prompt diagnosis and treatment are essential. Much of the success in reducing the morbidity and mortality over the past three decades has been through the collaborative efforts of the Intergroup Rhabdomyosarcoma Studies (IRS) formulated in the 1970s. Treatment of RMS with multiple modalities has transformed the dismal 3-year life expectancy from 25% in the 1960s to about 95% today.[1,2] With such success, clinicians now have the opportunity to focus on minimizing the serious late sequelae of aggressive therapy.

CLINICAL FEATURES

Orbital RMS most commonly presents as a rapidly progressing mass with soft tissue changes suggestive of inflammation, and should be suspected in any pediatric patient developing subacute unilateral proptosis or periorbital swelling.[3] Hertel exophthalmometry typically reveals proptosis and hypoglobus as the lesion occurs most commonly in the supranasal quadrant. Abnormal extraocular motility and ptosis are common findings (Box 97-1).

DIAGNOSTIC EVALUATION

Diagnostic evaluation should proceed urgently. CT imaging typically demonstrates a moderately well-defined homogeneous orbital mass (Figure 97-1). The lesion is isodense to the extraocular muscles and enhances after contrast administration. Signs of adjacent bone destruction are common. MRI studies often show a lesion isointense to the extraocular muscles and hypointense to the orbital fat on T1-weighted studies (Figure 97-2). Gadolinium-DPTA-enhanced MRI studies often show moderate to marked enhancement.

The evaluation proceeds with excisional or incisional biopsy. Initial surgery should debulk as much tumor as possible, with care to preserve vital orbital structures including periosteum, which is a barrier to local spread. Metastases can occur hematogenously to lung and bone. Orbital RMS requires a full metastatic evaluation performed by the pediatric oncologist.[3]

Box 97-1. Signs of Orbital Rhabdomyosarcoma

- Proptosis/hypoglobus
- Palpable mass
- Lid edema or erythema
- Chemosis, exposure keratopathy
- Optic neuropathy or disc edema
- Choroidal folds

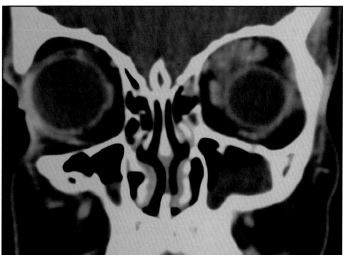

Figure 97-1. Coronal CT of an alveolar rhabdomyosarcoma demonstrates a moderately well-defined superior nasal quadrant lesion that is isodense to the extraocular muscles. Adjacent bony destruction, although common in rhabdomyosarcoma, is not demonstrated in this study.

HISTOLOGY

Light Microscopy

Four major histopathologic variants of RMS exist: embryonal, alveolar, botryoid, and pleomorphic. The majority of orbital RMS are of the embryonal type. The alveolar and botryoid embryonal subtypes are uncommon, and the pleomorphic type is rare in the orbit.[4] The histologic appearance influences the treatment plan and significantly correlates with prognosis (Table 97-1).[5]

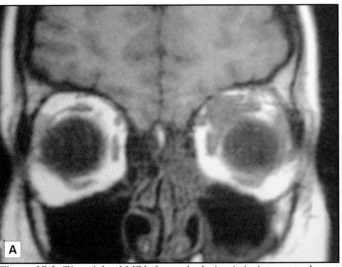 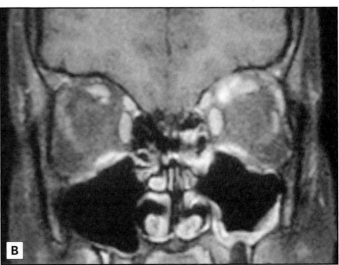

Figure 97-2. T1-weighted MRI shows the lesion is isointense to the extraocular muscles and hypointense to the orbital fat (A). Moderate enhancement with Gadolinium—DPTA (B).

Immunohistochemistry aids in diagnosis and in determining the histologic variant. Numerous immunohistochemical markers such as antibodies against desmin, viment, myogen, and MyoD1 can identify the skeletal muscle-specific expression in an RMS tumor. Caveolin-3 is a new marker that appears highly sensitive and specific for more differentiated RMS tumors and may help to detect residual tumor following chemotherapy.[6]

Electron Microscopy

Electron microscopy may show parallel rays of thick myosin filaments and sarcomeric units with Z-banding.

Molecular Analysis

Translocations of chromosome 13 are specific for alveolar RMS, with t(2;13) associated with a more aggressive form than t(1;13).[7]

TREATMENT

Treatment guidelines have evolved into a sophisticated regimen of multiagent chemotherapy, radiation, and surgery. Successful IRS treatment protocols have allowed current studies to focus on minimizing the long-term side effects of radiation and chemotherapy for patients with a low risk of recurrent disease.[8] In current IRS treatment protocols, group, stage, histology, and patient age contribute to the risk and treatment stratification necessary to optimize outcome (Table 97-2).[8]

PROGNOSIS

Isolated orbital involvement carries the best prognosis of all primary RMS locations, with an overall survival rate of 96% and eye preservation rate of 86%.[2]

FOLLOW-UP

After treatment, patients require serial comprehensive examinations and imaging studies to document their new baseline status and residual tumor size. Follow-up should be every 3 to 4 months for the first year, then every 4 to 6 months for several years thereafter. Secondary biopsy offers low yield with significant risk and should be reserved for patients with clinical indications of recurrence and changes on serial imaging studies.[4]

Table 97-1. International Classification of Rhabdomyosarcoma, Histology, and Prognosis			
Recurrence Risk	Embryonal or Botyroid RMS (ERMS)		Alveolar RMS (ARMS)
Low	Isolated orbital ERMS Orbital ERMS with parameningeal or sinus extension (stage 2, 3)	Group I, II, III Complete surgical resection or gross resection with microscopic residual tumors (group I or II)	
Intermediate		Gross residual tumors (group III)	Orbital ARMS without distant metastasis (stage 1, 2, 3)
	Orbital ERMS with distant metastasis (stage 4)	Group IV Age <10	
High		Group IV Age <10	Orbital ARMS with distant metastasis (stage 4)
RMS, rhabdomyosarcoma.			

SECTION 7 Orbital Tumors

Table 97-2. Current IRS Treatment Protocol by Group, Stage, and Histology

Treatment Category by Recurrence Risk	Treatment Protocol			
	Chemotherapy (by Stage)		Conventional Fractionation Radiation Therapy (by Group)	
Low	Node negative (stage 1, 2)	VA	Group I	No RT
			Group II	40 Gy
	Node positive (stage 3)	VAC		
			Group III	50 Gy
Intermediate	VAC +/-		Group III	50 Gy
	(V, T, C)		Group IV	Local and distant RT
High	CPT-11 then VAC		Group IV	Local and distant RT

V, vincristine; A, actinomycin D; C, cyclophosphamide; T, topotecan; CPT-11, irinotecan; RT, radiotherapy.

REFERENCES

1. Howard GM, Castern VG. Rhabdomyosarcoma of the orbit in brothers. *Arch Ophthalmol.* 1963;70:319-322.
2. Raney RB, Anderson JR, Kollath J, et al. Late effects of therapy in 94 patients with localized rhabdomyosarcoma of the orbit: Report from the Intergroup Rhabdomyosarcoma Study (IRS)-III, 1984-1991. *Med Pediatr Oncol.* 2000;34:413-420.
3. Shields JA, Shields CL. Rhabdomyosarcoma: review for the ophthalmologist. *Surv Ophthalmol.* 2003;48:39-57.
4. Shields CL, Shields JA, Honovar SG, et al. Clinical spectrum of primary ophthalmic rhabdomyosarcoma. *Ophthalmology.* 2001;108:2284-2292.
5. Kodet R, Newton WA, Hamoudi AB, et al. Orbital rhabdomyosarcomas and related tumors in childhood: relationship of morphology to prognosis—an Intergroup Rhabdomyosarcoma Study. *Med Pediatr Oncol.* 1997;29:51-60.
6. Fine SW, Lisanti MP, Argani P, Li M. Caveolin-3 is a sensitive and specific marker for rhabdomyosarcoma. *Appl Immunohistochem Mol Morphol.* 2005;13:231-236.
7. Douglass EC, Rowe ST, Valentine M, et al. Variant translocations of chromosome 13 in alveolar rhabdomyosarcoma. *Genes Chromosomes Cancer.* 1991;3:480-482.
8. Wolden SL, Wexler LH, Kraus DH, et al. Intensity-modulated radiotherapy for head-and-neck rhabdomyosarcoma. *Int J Radiat Oncol Biol Phys.* 2005;61:1432-1438.

Enucleation and Orbital Implants

David R. Jordan and Stephen R. Klapper

INTRODUCTION

The loss of an eye to tumor, trauma, or end-stage ocular disease is devastating. There is a loss of binocular vision, with reduced peripheral visual field, and loss of depth perception. Job limitations may arise, and affected individuals may experience a sense of facial disfigurement. Because eye contact is such an essential part of human interaction, it is extremely important for the patient with an artificial eye to maintain a natural, normal-appearing prosthetic eye. It is now possible to provide the anophthalmic patient with an artificial eye that looks and moves almost as naturally as a normal one.

POROUS ORBITAL IMPLANTS

Hydroxyapatite Implants

In the effort to design a biocompatible, integrated orbital implant, Perry[1] in 1985 introduced coralline (sea coral) hydroxy-apatite (HA) spheres (Bio-Eye, Integrated Orbital Implants, San Diego, CA). The HA implants represented a new generation of buried, integrated spheres with a regular system of interconnecting pores that allowed host fibrovascular ingrowth (Figure 98-1).[1,2] Fibrovascularization potentially reduced the risk of migration, extrusion, and infection of the implant.[3] The HA implant also allowed secure attachment of the extraocular muscles, which in turn leads to improved implant motility.

Synthetic Porous Implants

Polyethylene (MEDPOR, Porex Surgical Inc, Newnan, GA) implants have a smoother surface than HA implants, which permits easier implantation and provides potentially less irritation of the overlying conjunctiva following placement (Figure 98-2).[4] These implants have a high tensile strength and yet are malleable, which allows sculpting of the anterior surface of the implant. They may be used with or without a wrapping material, and the extraocular muscles can be sutured directly onto the implant, although most surgeons may find this difficult without predrilled holes.

Synthetic Hydroxyapatite Implants

Implants developed by FCI (Issy-Les-Moulineaux, France) have a chemical composition identical to that of the Bio-Eye.[5] The synthetic FCI implant has gained in popularity as it is less expensive than the Bio-Eye (approximately $480).

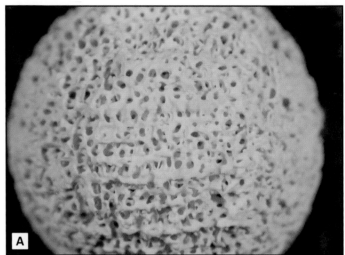

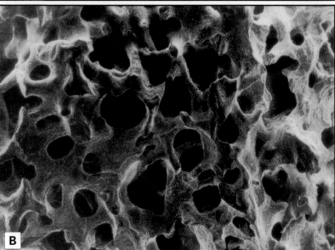

Figure 98-1. The porous architecture of the Bio-Eye hydroxyapatite implant is well visualized (A). Scanning electron microscopy illustrating the porous architecture of a Bio-Eye (B) (222 x 10).

Ceramic Implants

Aluminum oxide (Al_2O_3) is a ceramic implant biomaterial that permits host fibrovascular ingrowth similar to the Bio-Eye.[6] The Bioceramic implant is lightweight and has a uniform pore structure and excellent pore interconnectivity (Figure 98-3).

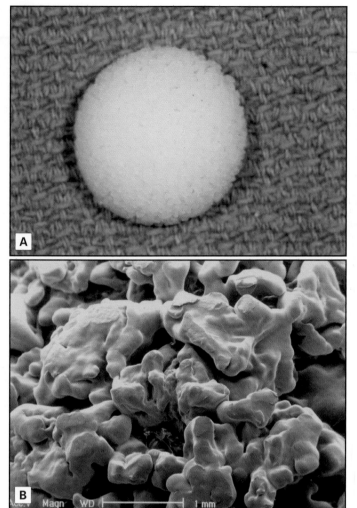

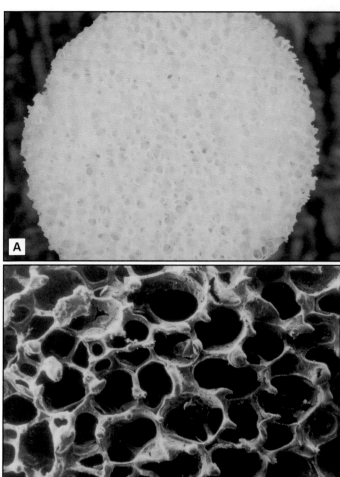

Figure 98-2. On gross examination, the porous polyethylene implant appears to have more of a channel system than pores (A). Scanning electron microscopy of a porous polyethylene implant (222 x 10) illustrating the smooth surface of the architecture as well as the channel system (B).

Figure 98-3. The porous architecture of an aluminum oxide (Bioceramic) implant is well visualized (A). Scanning electron microscopy illustrating the more uniform porous architecture of the aluminum oxide orbital implant (B) (222 x 10).

IMPLANT SELECTION

Surgeons have their own preferences regarding the use of spherical versus shaped, wrapped versus unwrapped, and pegged versus unpegged implants. Costs, hospital budgets, and marketing pressures also play a role in implant selection.

When deciding which implant to use, these authors divide the various products into three categories: porous spheres that may potentially be pegged (HA—coralline or synthetic; porous polyethylene; aluminum oxide); quasi-integrated implants (Universal implant, Quad MEDPOR); and standard non-porous sphere (polymethylmethacrylate, silicone).

If the patient is healthy and between the ages of 15 and 65 years, a porous implant (Bioceramic) that can potentially be pegged is our first choice as it offers the highest degree of movement.[7] If a peg is not being remotely considered, the advantage of using a porous spherical implant are diminished, as the movement associated with a non-pegged porous orbital implant is equal to that of a wrapped nonporous spherical implant.[8] However, the advantage of fibrovascular ingrowth and the potentially diminished risk of implant migration remain reasons to consider using a porous implant.

A standard sphere (PMMA, silicone), wrapped, centered within the muscle cone, and attached to the four rectus muscles, is another alternative if pegging is not a consideration. Although prosthetic movement occurs, it is not as much as that seen with a mounded implant or pegged porous implant. A standard sphere placed into the orbit, without a wrap and without connection to the rectus muscles, is the least desirable choice as it offers little movement, and the implant is prone to migration.

VOLUME CONSIDERATIONS

Approximately 70% to 80% of the volume of an individual's normal globe should be replaced with the orbital implant.[9] This generally allows for a prosthetic volume that is approximately 2 mL.[9] Larger prostheses often result in progressive lower eyelid laxity and malposition owing to the weight of the prostheses on the eyelid. Larger prostheses may also have limited socket excursion.[9]

ORBITAL IMPLANT WRAPPING

Placement of an HA or Bioceramic implant within the soft tissue of the eye socket is facilitated by a smooth wrapping material that diminishes tissue drag.[1] In addition, the wrap facilitates precise fixation of the extraocular muscles to the implant surface.[1] The advantages of placing an unwrapped implant include simplification of the procedure, decreased operating room time, reduced cost, avoidance of a second surgical site for harvesting autogenous wrap, and a decreased risk of disease transmission.[10]

If a wrap is used, human donor sclera has traditionally been the first choice.[1,2] The use of such material has, however, recently fallen out of favor with both surgeons and patients because of the potential risk of transmission of HIV, hepatitis B or C, and prions (Creutzfeldt–Jakob disease).

Specially processed human donor pericardium, fascia lata, and sclera are marketed as safe alternative implant wraps for preserved human donor tissues (Biodynamics International Inc, Tampa, FL). These wraps have the convenience of a long (up to 5 years) shelf life; however, they are currently priced at levels that may exceed the cost of the implant itself.

PEGGING POROUS ORBITAL IMPLANTS

Despite the improved motility, many surgeons and patients still elect to avoid peg placement because of the satisfactory results without pegging and the possibility of pegging-related complications.[11]

REFERENCES

1. Perry AC. Advances in enucleation. *Ophthalmic Plast Reconstr Surg.* 1991;4:173-182.

2. Dutton JJ. Coralline hydroxyapatite as an ocular implant. *Ophthalmology.* 1991;98:370-377.

3. Nunery WR, Heinz GW, Bonnin JM, Martin RT, Cepela MA. Exposure rate of hydroxyapatite spheres in the anophthalmic socket: histopathologic correlation and comparison with silicone sphere implants. *Ophthalmic Plast Reconstr Surg.* 1993;9:96-104.

4. Karesh JW, Dresner SC. High density porous polyethylene (Medpor) as a successful anophthalmic implant. *Ophthalmology.* 1994;101:1688-1696.

5. Jordan DR, Munro SM, Brownstein S, Gilberg SM, Grahovac SZ. A synthetic hydroxyapatite implant: the so-called counterfeit implant. *Ophthalmic Plast Reconstr Surg.* 1998;14:244-249.

6. Jordan DR, Mawn L, Brownstein S, et al. The bioceramic orbital implant: a new generation of porous implants. *Ophthalmic Plast Reconstr Surg.* 2000;16:347-355.

7. Guillinta P, Vasani SN, Granet DB, Kikkawa DO. Prosthetic motility in pegged versus unpegged integrated porous orbital implants. *Ophthalmic Plast Reconstr Surg.* 2000;19:119-122.

8. Custer PL, Kennedy RH, Woog JJ, Kaltreider SA, Meyer DA. Orbital implants in enucleation surgery, a report by the American Academy of Ophthalmology. *Ophthalmology.* 2003;110:2054-2061.

9. Kaltreider SA. The ideal ocular prostheses. Analysis of prosthetic volume. *Ophthalmic Plast Reconstr Surg.* 2000;16:388-392.

10. Long JA, Tann TM, Bearden WH, Callahan MA. Enucleation: is wrapping the implant necessary for optimal motility. *Ophthalmic Plast Reconstr Surg.* 2003;19:94-197.

11. Jordan DR, Chan S, Mawn L, Gilberg SM, Brownstein S, Hill V. Complications associated with pegging hydroxyapatite orbital implants. *Ophthalmology.* 1999;106:505-512.

Principles of Orbital Surgery

José Perez-Moreiras, Javier Coloma, and Consuelo Prada

INTRODUCTION

Recent advances in the diagnostic and therapeutic areas have extended our knowledge of orbital pathology. Computed tomography (CT), magnetic resonance (MR) imaging, and high-resolution ultrasonography have allowed surgeons to localize orbital tumors and to establish the relationships with vital structures of the orbit. These techniques have also permitted the surgeon to infer possible histology based on imaging characteristics to allow for a better surgical plan.

MICROSURGICAL PRINCIPLES

Surgery for orbital tumors should allow for treatment with conservation of function and cosmesis. Although the main goal of surgery is removal of the tumor and preservation of function, optimal treatment must occasionally sacrifice function or cosmesis. With these principles in mind, any surgical approach must offer optimal visualization of the very delicate structures of the orbit.

INSTRUMENTATION

Surgical loupes are employed by many surgeons to provide less cumbersome magnification, but these may be quite heavy, and they often do not provide the required quality and amount of magnification for use in the orbit, especially in the intraconal space and orbital apex. We strongly recommend the use of a microscope for all cases of orbital surgery, especially for intraconal and orbital apex lesions, where it provides the benefits of magnification, coaxial light illumination, and the possibility of at least two assistants, allowing for better surgical assistance.[1]

The use of surgical microscopes,[2] the possibility of having two assistants during surgery, and improved instrumentation permit small incisions and the avoidance of osteotomy. The microsurgical approach also requires expert anesthetists.

ANESTHESIA

Monitored anesthetic care (MAC) provides for patient comfort and safety by relieving anxiety and producing intraoperative amnesia, and also provides relief from pain and other noxious stimuli, without interfering with the patient's ability to communicate verbally or protect the airway. Surgery under MAC offers many advantages, including preservation of protective reflexes, decreased postoperative pain, decreased nausea and vomiting, reduced cardiovascular and respiratory side effects, and faster recovery. MAC is often used for anterior orbital or conjunctival surgery.

General Anesthesia

Retrobulbar, intraconal, and apical lesions are typically approached with the patient under general anesthesia. The anesthesiologist can help with hemostasis by carefully controlling the blood pressure intraoperatively. Typically, the goal is to keep the mean arterial pressure about 25% lower than the preoperative level.

INDICATIONS FOR SURGERY

The basic indications for oncological surgery of the orbit are incisional biopsy, excisional biopsy, and exenteration. Other indications for orbital surgery include abscess drainage, orbital decompression, and orbital reconstruction in trauma.

Biopsy can be performed by taking a small fragment of the lesion (incisional) or by removing all or most of it (excisional) without injury to underlying orbital structures. When biopsy is performed to confirm a suspected diagnosis (new disease or relapse of a previous disease), the specimen can be taken to the pathologist after completion of the procedure; if biopsy is required for diagnosis, the specimen must be sent to the laboratory during the procedure, and surgery can continue or stop depending on the results. The biopsy specimen must be handled delicately to avoid artifacts that can hinder analysis by the pathologist, especially when a lymphoid lesion is suspected. To prevent surgical artifacts, the surgeon should use blunt instruments, minimize the use of electrical or thermal instruments, and employ delicate forceps to avoid crushing the tissue.

PLANNING THE SURGICAL APPROACH

The surgeon must plan the approach based on the examination and diagnostic images to correctly develop the surgery. Many aspects must be considered to correctly plan orbital surgery.

Tumor Location

Tumor location is one of the most important aspects. Tumors located anterior to the equator of the globe (tumors that cause more displacement than exophthalmos) can often be excised under local anesthesia. If the tumor is localized in the extraperiosteal

Table 99-1. Surgical Approaches to Orbital Tumors

	Location	Approach
Extraconal	Superior	Upper eyelid crease incision
	Inferior	Conjunctiva subtarsal incision
Intraconal	Medial-superior (ON displaced inferiorly)	Upper eyelid crease incision (internal)
	Lateral-superior (ON displaced inferiorly)	Upper eyelid crease incision (whole)
	Lateral-inferior (ON displaced superiorly)	Conjunctiva-tarsal incision (lateral)
	Medial-inferior (ON displaced superiorly)	Conjunctiva-tarsal incision (medial)
Apical	Superior	Medial eyelid crease incision
		Lateral eyelid crease incision
	Inferior	Conjunctiva-tarsal incision
	Superior or inferior	Transfrontal approach

ON, optic nerve.

space, the surgeon should preserve the periosteum without disruption of the orbital cavity. On the other hand, intraconal (intraperiosteal) tumors require blunt dissection of the soft tissue of the orbit.

Relationship to Adjacent Structures

The second most important aspect of proper surgical planning is the relationship between the tumor and adjacent structures. For intraconal tumors, the optic nerve determines the approach (Table 99-1); the surgeon should attempt to approach the tumor opposite to the nerve. For example, if the lesion displaces the nerve inferiorly and laterally, the surgical approach should be from the superior and medial aspect of the orbit.

The relationship of the tumor to the extraocular muscles is also important when planning a surgery in order to avoid muscle injury and consequent postoperative diplopia.

Tumor margins must be known precisely to determine the extent of surgery and the potential degree of secondary damage from surgical intervention. Tumor margins also determine whether the tumor can be completely excised. Well-defined lesions can often be resected en bloc, but in some instances, large tumors, ill-defined tumors, or tumors that will require adjuvant medical therapy require only partial excision to avoid collateral injury.

Tumor Composition

Imaging studies (ultrasonography, MRI, and CT) assist in predicting the histopathology of the mass, especially for well-defined tumors (capsulated, round, oval), and these studies play a fundamental role in determining the need for an osteotomy. Tumors with a myxoid component, such as schwannomas with a pseudocapsule, or cystic lesions with true capsules, can often be drained to reduce their size through a keyhole incision prior to excision without osteotomy. Once the mass has been reached and isolated, an opening in the capsule/pseudocapsule can be made to extract the internal component using a blunt spoon, and the capsule/pseudocapsule can then be excised by freeing adherences using blunt dissection from the adjacent tissues. An ultrasonic

fragmentation device, such as the Cavitron ultrasonic aspirator (Valley Labs, Richmond Hill, Ontario, Canada), may be useful, but longer tips are required for posterior tumors, which limit its use. Other well-defined tumors, such as cavernous hemangiomas and lymphangiomas, can be excised in a similar way. These tumors are reached and isolated, and an incision is made in the pseudocapsule to aspirate the contents and reduce the size enough to allow for removal through a small incision. Drainage often reduces cavernous hemangiomas more dramatically in younger patients than in older patients owing to the less solid nature of the tumor in the younger age group. Using these techniques, a great majority of orbital tumors can be excised completely, without the need for an osteotomy. Some tumors, such as pleomorphic adenomas, have the potential to recur or undergo malignant transformation if the capsule is violated, and these lesions must be excised en bloc. For large or ill-defined lesions where a biopsy is mandatory and osteotomy is not needed, internal structure can aid in the diagnosis but is not essential for surgical planning.

MICROSURGICAL APPROACH TO THE ORBIT

Conjunctival Approach

Bulbar conjunctival incisions are typically reserved for tumors anterior or just posterior to the equator of the globe, generally for small biopsies. A periostomy is made, avoiding damage to limbal stem cells, and dissection is performed until the tumor is reached.

Caruncular Approach

A caruncular approach can be used for removal of tumors located adjacent to the medial wall of the orbit.

Perez-Moreiras Approach

Although this approach is preferred by some authors for orbital decompression, we prefer the Perez-Moreiras approach for decompression of the medial wall and floor (beside the infraorbital rim) through a medial superior eyelid crease incision. We have performed more than 500 orbital decompressions through this approach, with good outcomes.

Superior Orbitotomy

Whenever possible, incisions are made following relaxed skin tension lines. The use of a microscope allows for very small incisions to avoid deforming scars (Figure 99-1). Superior orbitomy is performed for tumors located in the superior orbit, or for intraconal masses that displace the optic nerve inferiorly. The incision is made in the upper eyelid crease for tumors located along the orbital roof, the lacrimal fossa or posteriorly, and the superomedial intraconal space (Figure 99-2). For the latter, the incision extends along the whole length of the superior eyelid crease, and a plane between the orbicularis and orbital septum is dissected to the superior orbital rim. The periosteum is incised approximately 2 mm superior to the rim and is dissected from the bone to expose the entire orbital roof. The supraorbital neurovascular bundle must be respected (and can be dissected, but this is seldom necessary) to avoid postoperative frontal hypoesthesia. At this point, the periorbita is incised 2 mm posterior to the arcus marginalis to access the intraconal space and expose the tumor. When a lacrimal gland tumor is removed using this approach, an osteotomy is usually not necessary (Figure 99-3). For lateral osteotomy, once the zygomaticofrontal process has been exposed, dissection must continue within the temporal fossa between the muscular fascia and the temporal skin layer. An incision in the periosteum at the lateral and external border of the zygomaticofrontal process is made to dissect the temporalis muscle, and the periostium is detached. Relaxing incisions in the muscle may allow for better mobilization of the temporalis muscle. Osteotomy is performed using an oscillating saw at the necessary level according to tumor location. Lateral osteotomy has not been needed for resection of any tumor in our center for several years. The superonasal approach for intraconal tumors requires an incision in only the medial aspect (10 to 15 mm) of the superior eyelid crease (Figure 99-4). A small dissection of the orbicularis from

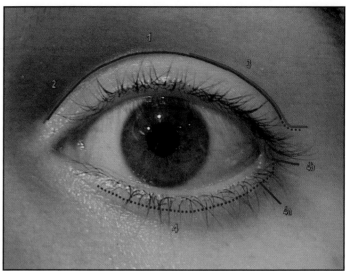

Figure 99-1. Incisions for orbital surgery. Eyelid crease incision (1), medial (2), and external (3). Conjunctival incisions (4, dotted line), subtarsal incision with tarsectomy (4a), and canthothomy–cantholysis (4b).

the septum is recommended in order to facilitate exposure. The septum is then transected, and the medial fat pad is reached. This allows for access medial to the levator muscle, between the aponeurosis and the medial wall. Prolapsing fat can be coagulated using 20 W without causing significant iatrogenic injury; blunt dissection through the orbital fat pads is used until the tumor is reached. It is important to gently displace the superior oblique tendon upward with an orbital retractor in order to avoid any damage to this structure. This approach allows for excellent exposure of the superomedial intraconal space.

Inferior Orbitotomy

We prefer inferior orbitotomy through a transconjunctival approach, as the subciliary approach offers no advantages and risks lid retraction and external scarring. The conjunctiva is

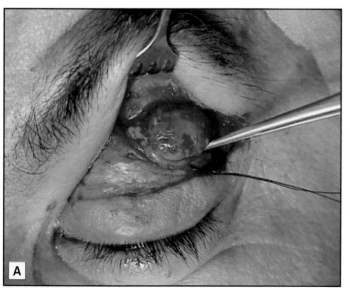

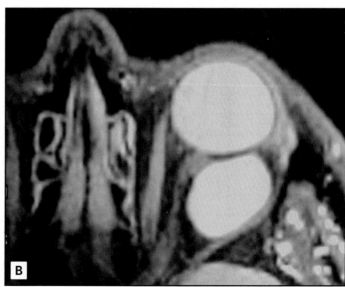

Figure 99-2. Superotemporal approach for intraconal tumor (A). MRI (axial view) shows the intraconal tumor with medial displacement of the optic nerve (B).

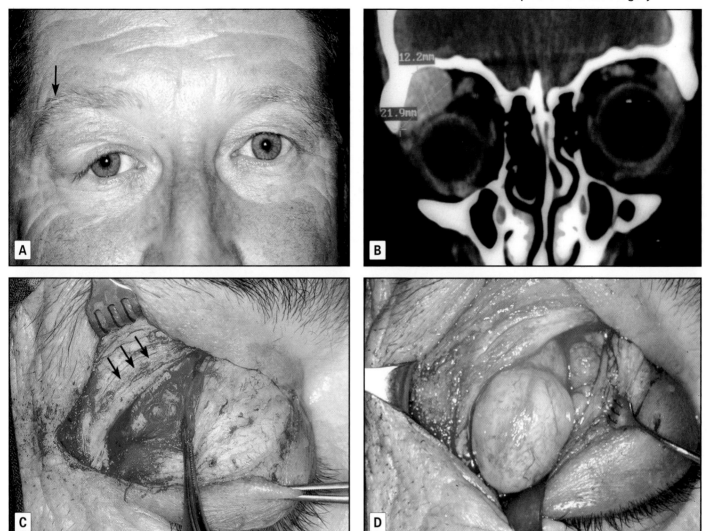

Figure 99-3. Lacrimal gland tumor (pleomorphic adenoma). Clinical appearance (A). CT scan showing a mass expanding the lacrimal fossa (B). Periosteum (arrows) is incised 2 mm from the orbital rim (C), and the tumor is removed en bloc without osteotomy (D).

incised below the tarsal plate in order to detach the retractors from the tarsus. This approach can be performed with or without lateral canthotomy/cantholysis, depending on underlying tissue laxity. If the surgeon prefers to respect lateral canthus anatomy, a tarsectomy can be performed. Once the retractors are detached, blunt dissection between the septum and the orbicularis is performed inferiorly, toward the inferior orbital rim. With the septum widely exposed, we can access the intraconal and extraconal spaces of the inferior and inferolateral orbit, where no important anatomical structures exist (Figure 99-5). Such an approach also permits access to the inferomedial intraconal space; however, this space is very narrow, and careful dissection must be performed to avoid injury to the inferior oblique muscle (Figure 99-6).

Tumors of the orbital apex must be removed by a superior eyelid crease or inferior conjunctival approach. A lateral osteotomy can be performed to allow for greater lateral retraction and access, but a lateral osteotomy alone does not offer significant access to the orbital apex. A transfrontal craniotomy approach may be an alternative for some tumors of the orbital apex.

REFERENCES

1. Nerad J. Oculoplastic surgery. The requisites in ophthalmology. In: *Surgical Approaches to the Orbit*. St Louis, MO: Mosby; 2001:387-418.
2. Alio J, Eiras J, Rabinal F, et al. Microcirugía de los tumores orbitarios. *Arch Soc Esp Oftalmol.* 1982;43(2):226-237.

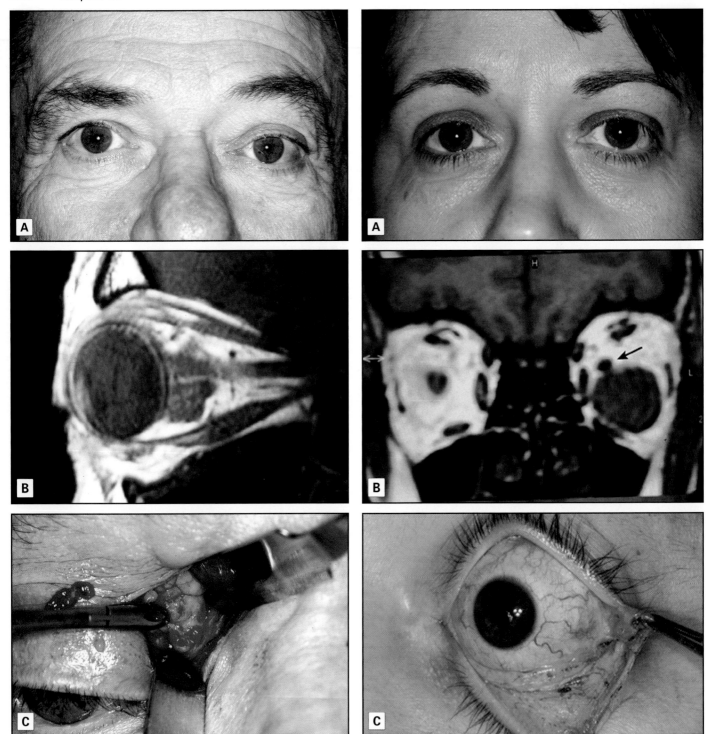

Figure 99-4. Superomedial approach for intraconal tumor. Clinical appearance (A). MRI shows an ill-defined retrobulbar intraconal mass suggestive of lymphoma. Orbital biopsy via superomedial approach (C).

Figure 99-5. Inferolateral conjunctival approach for intraconal tumor. Clinical appearance (A). MRI is suggestive of cavernous hemangioma that has displaced optic nerve superiomedially (arrow) (B). Inferolateral conjunctival approach with tarsectomy (C).

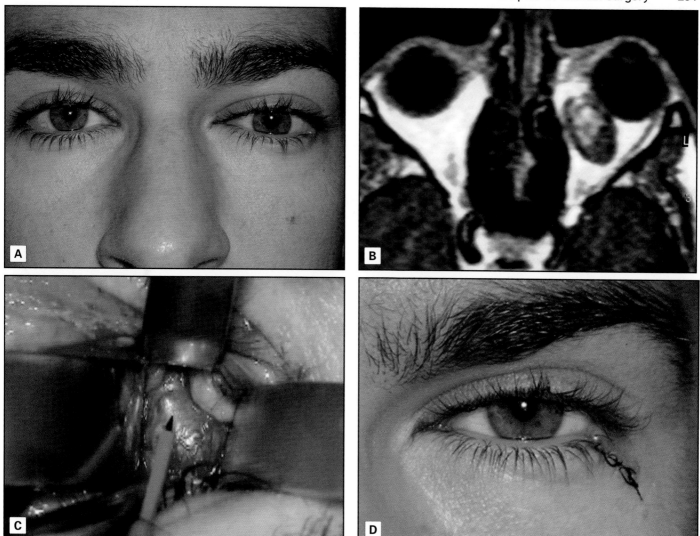

Figure 99-6. Inferomedial conjunctival approach for intraconal tumor. Clinical appearance (A), MRI suggestive of a cavernous hemangioma (B), inferomedial conjunctival approach with tarsectomy (C), and 1 week postoperative appearance (D).

INDEX

acquired immunodeficiency syndrome, 55
acquired tumors of ciliary epithelium, 155
actinic keratosis, 31
adenocarcinoma of retinal pigment epithelium, 152–153
adenoma, 152–153
adjuvant chemotherapy, 26
adnexal lymphoma, 234–236
AIDS. See acquired immunodeficiency syndrome
analysis of cells extracted by fine needle aspiration biopsy, 115
anatomical features, 30
anesthesia, 63, 246
aneurysmal bone cyst, 225
angiogenesis, 6–8
    angiogenic switch, 6
    cooption, 6
    exogenous, 7
    inhibitors of angiogenesis endogenous, 7
    metastatic cascade, 6
    promoters of angiogenesis, 6
    regulation of VEGF, 7
    steps in angiogenesis, 6
    subtypes, 7
    tumor vessels, 6
    vascular endothelial growth factor, 6–7
    VEGF receptors, 7
angiogenic switch, 6
anterior lamellar deficit, lid margin intact, 46–47
anterior visual pathway glioma, 227–228
apoptosis, 11
argon laser, 16
ataxia-telangiectasia, 165

basal cell carcinoma, 33–34
benign conjunctival tumors, 53–54
benign epidermal tumors, 31–32
benign melanocytic tumors, 53–54, 73–76
bilateral diffuse uveal melanocytic proliferation, 160
biopsy, 215–217
brachytherapy, 19, 56, 98–101, 189–192

cancer-associated retinopathy, 159
capillary hemangioma, 43–44
carcinogenic agents, 3
Carney complex, 50
caruncle, tumors of, 54
cavernous hemangioma, 145, 223
cell cycle, 11–12
central nervous system lymphoma, 156–158
CEV toxicity, 187–188

chemotherapy, 3, 25–27
    cell generation cycle, 25
    clinical trials, 26
        phase I, 26
        phase II, 26
        phase III, 26
    combination regimen, 25
    drug development, 25–26
    drug resistance, 25
    mechanism of action, 25
    multimodality therapy, 26–27
        adjuvant chemotherapy, 26
        neo-adjuvant chemotherapy, 27
    side effects, 26
    tumor cell kinetic model, 25
choristoma, 61–62
choroidal melanoma, 81–87
choroidal nevus, 74–75
choroidal osteoma, 127
ciliary body
    hemangioma, 121
    melanoma, 81
    nevus, 74–75
ciliary pigment epithelium tumor, 154–155
ciliochoroidal tumors, 87
circumscribed choroidal hemangioma, 121
clinical trials, 26
Coats' disease, 147–148
cobalt gray equivalents, 18–19
conjunctival melanoma, 59–60
conjunctival nevus, 53–54
conjunctival stromal tumors, 61–62
conjunctival tumors, 14, 51–66
    classification of, 52
conventional radiation therapy, 19
corneal excision, 63
corneal tumors, 51–66
    classification of, 52
counseling, 28, 93, 184–186
    communication, 28
    emotions, 28
    fears, 28
    patients' needs, 28
Cowden syndrome, 50
cross-sectional study, 2
cryotherapy, 13–14, 56
    complications, 14
    conjunctival tumors, 14
    cooling rate, 13

eyelid tumors, 14
freeze-thaw cycle, 13
indications, 14
intraocular tumors, 14
number of repetitions, 14
orbital tumors, 14
tissue injury mechanism, 13
direct effects, 13
indirect effects, 13
cystic lesions, 41

dermolipoma, 62
diode laser, 16
dose, radiation, 18
drawings/photography, 51
drug development, 25–26
drug resistance, 25
dual nature of radiation, 18
dye laser, 16
dysplastic nevus, 39

ellipse sliding flap, 47
endoresection, 108
enucleation, 189–192, 243–245
environmental factors, 80, 172–173
epidemiology, 1–2, 59
bias, 1–2
measures of association, 1
differences in mean score, 1
differences in risk, 1
hazard ratio, 1
odds ratio, 1
relative risk, 1
outcome measures, 1
incidence, 1
mortality, 1
prevalence, 1
quality of life, 1
study designs, 2
case-control study, 2
case series, 2
cohort study, 2
cross-sectional study, 2
randomized controlled trial, 2
systematic review, 2
epidermal inclusion cysts, 41
epidermoid cyst, 224
episcleral radioactive plaque, 98
epithelial cysts, 53
esthesioneuroblastoma, 237
estimation of intraocular tumor basal dimensions, 68
etiology, 3, 33
evaluation, 216
excimer laser, 16
excisional biopsy, 51
exfoliative cytology, 51
exogenous, 7
external beam therapy, 19

eyelid, 14, 29–50
adnexal tumors, 41–42
classification, 30
differential diagnosis, 30
examination, 29
reconstruction, 46
stromal tumors, 43–45

family counseling, 186
fibrohistiocytic tumors, 43
fibrous dysplasia, 225
fibrous histiocytoma, 61, 225
fluorescein angiography, 69
fractionated stereotactic radiotherapy, 105
freeze-thaw cycle, 13
full-thickness eyelid defect, 47–48
fundus drawing, 68

Gardner syndrome, 49
genetic counseling, 184–185
genetic susceptibility, 3
genetic testing, 184–185
genetics, 11–12
apoptosis, 11
cell cycle, 11–12
growth factor signaling pathways, 11
HDM2, 11
Myc, 11
p53, 11
proliferation, 11–12
Rb-p16Ink4a-cyclin D pathway, 11
senescence, 11
telomerase, 11–12
geographic variation in incidence, 172
Gorlin-Goltz syndrome, 50
graft-versus-host disease, 141

hair follicle, tumors of, 42
hamartoma of retina, 153
HDM2, 11
hemangiopericytoma, 223
hereditary benign intraepithelial dyskeratosis, 53
high-frequency ultrasonography, 51
histiocytic tumors, 131–132
holmium laser, 16
human papillomavirus, 55

iatrogenic cancers, 3
chemotherapy, 3
immunosuppression, 3
radiation therapy, 3
imaging techniques, 209–213
immunologic escape, 9
immunology, 9–10
immunologic escape, 9
innate immune responses, 9
specific immune responses, 9
uveal melanoma, 9

anti-uveal melanoma T cells responses, 9
    antibodies against, 9
    HLA expression, 9
    infiltrating immune cells, 9
    tumor antigen expression, 9
immunosuppression, 3
implant selection, 244
incisional biopsy, 51
indirect ophthalmoscopy, 67–68
indocyanine green angiography, 69
infantile capillary hemangioma, 222
inflammation, orbital, non-specific, 218–220
intensity-modulated radiation therapy, 19
interpretation of imaging studies, 209–211
intraepithelial neoplasia, 31
intraocular biopsy, 142–143
intraocular tumors, 14
inverted follicular keratosis, 53
inverted papilloma, 53
iridectomy, 106
iridocyclectomy, 106
iris hemangioma, 121
iris melanoma, 81, 117
iris nevus, 73–74

juvenile xanthogranuloma, 131–132

keratoacanthoma, 31
Knudson's two-hit hypothesis, 170
krypton laser, 16

lacrimal gland choristoma, 62
lacrimal gland tumors, 230–231
lacrimal sac tumors, 232–233
laser therapy, 15–17
    argon laser, 16
    clarity of media, 15
    diode laser, 16
    dye laser, 16
    excimer laser, 16
    holmium laser, 16
    krypton laser, 16
    laser output, 15
    laser properties, 15
    magnification factor, 16
    ruby laser, 16
    spot size, 16
    techniques, 16–17
        indications, 16
        laser photocoagulation, 16
        photodynamic therapy, 16–17
        transpupillary thermotherapy, 16
    tissue absorption, 16
    tissue effects, 15
    treatment variables, 15
    types of lasers, 16
leiomyoma, 131
leiomyosarcoma, 237

lens-sparing radiation therapy, 19
lentigo, 39
leukemias, 140
lipomatous tumors, 43
liposarcoma, 237
lower eyelid defects, 46–48
lymphangiectasia, 61

malignant fibrous histiocytoma, 237
malignant melanoma, 39
malignant optic nerve glioma, 228
malignant peripheral nerve sheath tumor, 237
malignant tumor classification, 4
malignant tumors, 42
measures of association, 1
    differences in mean score, 1
    differences in risk, 1
    hazard ratio, 1
    odds ratio, 1
    relative risk, 1
medulloepithelioma, 154–155
melanocytic epidermal tumors, 31–32
melanocytosis, 75
melanoma-associated retinopathy, 159–160
melanoma of eyelid, 39–40
meningioma, 224
metastasis, 36, 38
metastatic cascade, 6
metastatic process, 4
metastatic retinoblastoma, 200–201
microscopic features of neoplasia, 4
microsurgical approach to orbit, 247–249
microsurgical principles, 246
midline intracranial tumors, 183
Mohs' surgery, 40
mucocele, 224
Muir-Torre syndrome, 50
multimodality therapy, 26–27
    adjuvant chemotherapy, 26
    neo-adjuvant chemotherapy, 27
multiple endocrine neoplasia, 66
multiple hamartoma syndrome, 50
myogenic tumors, 43

neo-adjuvant chemotherapy, 27
neoplasia classification, 4
    benign tumors, 4
    malignant tumors, 4
neurilemmoma, 224
neurocutaneous melanosis, 167
neurofibroma, 49, 61, 224
neurofibromatosis type 1, 162
neurofibromatosis type 2, 162
neurogenic tumors, 45
neuro-oculocutaneous syndromes, 162–167
nevoid basal cell carcinoma syndrome, 50
nevus flammeus, 49
nevus sebaceous syndrome, 165

non-melanocytic epidermal tumors, 31
non-ocular tumors, 181–182
non-specific keratosis, 31
non-specific orbital inflammation, 218–220
nonproliferative radiation retinopathy, 22

ocular adnexal examination, 29
ocular paraneoplastic diseases, 159–161
ocular surface squamous neoplasia, 55–56
oculodermal melanocytosis, 39
ophthalmic outcomes, 102–103
opsoclonus, 160
optic disc melanocytoma, 75
optic nerve, 141
optic nerve sheath meningioma, 228–229
optic nerve tumors, 227–229
optical coherence tomography, 69–71
orbit, malignant tumors of, 237–239
orbital implant wrapping, 244–245
orbital inflammation, non-specific, 218–220
orbital lymphoma, 234–236
orbital metastases, 239
orbital retinoblastoma, 198–199
orbital surgery, 246–251
orbital tumor, 14, 208–251
    classification of, 214
    evaluation of adult with, 216–217
    evaluation of child with, 215
osteoma, 225
osteosarcoma, 237
outcome measures, 1
    incidence, 1
    mortality, 1
    prevalence, 1
    quality of life, 1

paraneoplastic melanocytic proliferation, 160
paraneoplastic optic neuropathies, 160
pathology, 4–5
    diagnostic techniques, 5
    histopathologic sampling, 5
    metastatic process, 4
    microscopic features of neoplasia, 4
    neoplasia classification, 4
        benign tumors, 4
        malignant tumors, 4
    research techniques, 5
    tissue sampling, processing, 4–5
pegging porous orbital implants, 245
perineural spread, 36
phakomatoses, 162–167
photocoagulation, 94
    laser, 16
photodynamic therapy, 16–17
pigmented ocular fundus lesions, 152
polycythemia vera rubra, 141
porous orbital implants, 243–244
precursor lesions, 39

pregnancy, retinoblastoma, 206
primary acquired melanosis, 57–58
primary choroidal lymphoma, 133–135
primary closure, 46–48
primary iridal lymphoma, 135
proliferative hematopoietic disorders, intraocular manifestations, 140–141
proliferative radiation retinopathy, 22
promoters of angiogenesis, 6
proteus syndrome, 66
proton beam radiotherapy, 102–103
pseudoepitheliomatous hyperplasia, 53
pyogenic granuloma, 43, 61

radiation retinopathy, 22–23
    clinical features, 22
    nonproliferative radiation retinopathy, 22
    proliferative radiation retinopathy, 22
    radiation maculopathy, 22
    treatment, 22–23
radiation therapy, 3, 18–20
    brachytherapy, 19
    dual nature of radiation, 18
    radiation parameters, 18–19
        cobalt gray equivalents, 18–19
        radiation dose, 18
        relative biological effectiveness, 18
    radioactive decay, 18
    teletherapy sources, 18
        cobalt-to unit, 18
        cyclotron, 18
        linear accelerator, 18
    teletherapy techniques, 19
        conventional radiation therapy, 19
        external beam therapy, 19
        intensity-modulated radiation therapy, 19
        lens-sparing radiation therapy, 19
        stereotactic radiosurgery, 19
        three-dimensional conformal therapy, 19
    treatment parameters, 19
        fractionation, 19
        target volume, 19
        tissue tolerance, 19
        total dose, 19
radioactive decay, 18
radiotherapy, 102
    ocular complications, 21–24
        conjunctiva, 21
        cornea, 21
        eyelid/periorbital skin, 21
        iris, 22
        lacrimal gland, 22
        lens, 22
        orbit soft tissue, 22
        radiation optic neuropathy, 23–24
        radiation retinopathy, 22–23
        sclera, 22
randomized controlled trial, 2

RB1 gene, 169
Rb-p16Ink4a-cyclin D pathway, 11
reactive epithelial hyperplasia, 53
Reese-Ellsworth classification, 176–177
retention cyst, 41
retina, 140–141
retinal astrocytic hamartoma, 149–150
retinal astrocytic tumors, 149–150
retinal capillary hemangioma, 144–145
retinal cavernous hemangioma, 165
retinal lymphoma, 156–158
retinal pigment epithelium, 144–167
    hamartoma of retina, combined, 153
retinal tumors, 144–167
retinal vascular tumors, 144–146
retinoblastoma, 168–207
    chemotherapy, 187–188
    Children's Oncology Group Trials, 204–205
    fetus with, 206
    neonate with, 206
    pregnancy, 206
    RB1 cancer predisposition syndrome, 179–180
    staging, 176–178
retinoblastoma tumorigenesis, Knudson's two-hit hypothesis, 170
retinocytoma, 202–203
retinoma, 202–203
rhabdomyosarcoma, 240–242
ruby laser, 16

schwannoma, 224
sclerochoroidal calcification, 127
sebaceous cyst, 41
sebaceous gland carcinoma, 37–38
sebaceous gland tumors, 42
seborrheic keratosis, 31
secondary orbital tumors, 237–239
semicircular rotational flap, 47
senescence, 11
sentinel lymph node biopsy, 36, 40
skin graft, 47
slit-lamp examination, 67
solar keratosis, 31
squamous cell carcinoma, 35–36
squamous cell papilloma, 31, 53
stereotactic radiosurgery, 19, 104–105
stereotactic radiotherapy, 104–105
study designs, 2
    case-control study, 2
    case series, 2
    cohort study, 2
    cross-sectional study, 2
    randomized controlled trial, 2
    systematic review, 2
Sturge-Weber syndrome, 165
sunlight exposure, 55
supplemental cryotherapy, 63
sweat gland tumors, 41–42

teletherapy, 18–19, 193–194
    cobalt-to unit, 18
    conventional radiation therapy, 19
    cyclotron, 18
    external beam therapy, 19
    intensity-modulated radiation therapy, 19
    lens-sparing radiation therapy, 19
    linear accelerator, 18
    stereotactic radiosurgery, 19
    three-dimensional conformal therapy, 19
telomerase, 11–12
thermotherapy, 94
three-dimensional conformal therapy, 19
trans-scleral choroidectomy, 106–108
trans-scleral cryotherapy, 189
transillumination, 68
transpupillary thermotherapy, 16
trilateral retinoblastoma, 183
tuberous sclerosis complex, 162
tumor angiogenesis, 6–8
tumor cell kinetic model, 25
tumor vessels, 6
types of lasers, 16

ultrasonography, 69
ultrasound of fetal eye, 206
unilateral retinoblastoma, 184–185
upper eyelid defects, 48
uveal histiocytic tumors, 131–132
uveal lymphoproliferative tumors, 133–135
uveal melanocytoma, 75
uveal melanoma, 9
    anti-uveal melanoma T cells responses, 9
    antibodies against, 9
    brachytherapy, 98–101
    clinical features, 81–84
    COMS results, 109–112
    differential diagnosis, 85–88
    epidemiologic aspects, 78–80
    epidemiology, 78–80
    histopathologic features, 89–91
    HLA expression, 9
    infiltrating immune cells, 9
    management, 92–93
    metastasis, 119–120
    mortality, 116–118
    prognostic factors, 113–115
    proton beam radiotherapy, 102–103
    resection techniques, 106–108
    stereotactic radiotherapy, 104–105
    thermotherapy, 94–97
    tumor antigen expression, 9
uveal metastatic tumors, 136–139
uveal myogenic tumors, 131–132
uveal neural tumors, 125–126
uveal neurofibroma, 125
uveal osseous tumors, 127–130
uveal schwannoma, 125–126

uveal tumor classification, 72
uveal tumors, 67–143
uveal vascular tumors, 121–124

vascular endothelial growth factor, 6–7
vascular malformations, 221–222
vascular orbital tumors, 221–223
vascular tumors, 43–45
vasoproliferative retinal tumor, 145–146

VEGF receptors, 7
vitreous, 140
von Hippel-Lindau disease, 162

Wyburn-Mason syndrome, 145, 165

xanthogranuloma, 131–132
xeroderma pigmentosum, 66

CURBSIDE
Consultation

The exciting and unique *Curbside Consultation Series* is designed to effectively provide ophthalmologists with practical, to-the-point, evidence-based answers to the questions most frequently asked during informal consultations between colleagues.

Each specialized book included in the *Curbside Consultation Series* offers quick access to current medical information with the ease and convenience of a conversation. Expert consultants who are recognized leaders in their fields provide their advice, preferences, and opinions to answer the tricky questions that require ophthalmologists to practice the "art" of medicine.

Written with a similar reader-friendly Q-and-A format and including images, diagrams, and references, each book in the *Curbside Consultation Series* will serve as a solid, go-to reference for practicing ophthalmologists and residents alike.

Series Editor: David F. Chang, MD

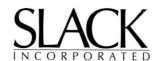